MW00576549

Atlas of Peripheral Nerve Blocks and Anatomy for Orthopaedic Anesthesia

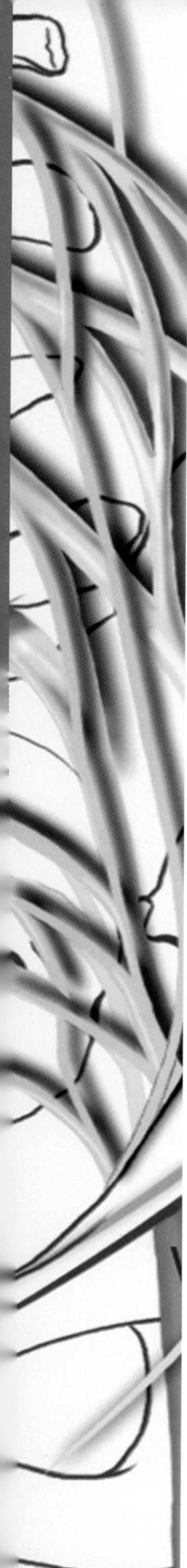

Atlas of Peripheral Nerve Blocks and Anatomy for Orthopaedic Anesthesia

André P. Boezaart
M.B.Ch.B., M.Prax.Med., DA (SA), FFA(CMSA), M.Med. (Anaesth), Ph.D.
Professor of Anesthesia and Orthopaedic Surgery
Director of Acute Pain Medicine and Regional Anesthesia
University of Florida
Gainesville, Florida

Artwork by **Mary K. Bryson,** Bryson BioMedical Illustrations

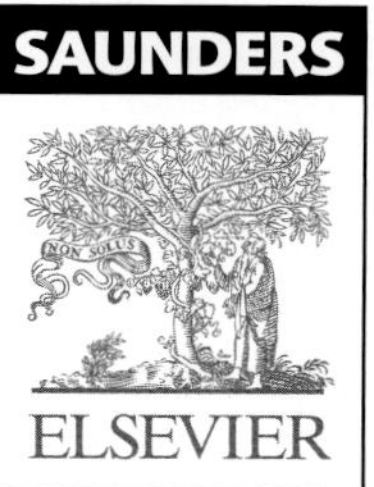

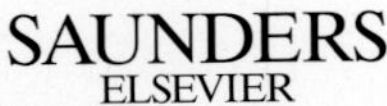

1600 John F. Kennedy Blvd.
Ste 1800
Philadelphia, PA 19103-2899

ATLAS OF PERIPHERAL NERVE BLOCKS AND ANATOMY FOR ORTHOPAEDIC ANESTHESIA

 ISBN 978-1-4160-3941-9

NOTICE

Knowledge and best practice in this field are constantly changing. As new research and experience broaden our knowledge, changes in practice, treatment and drug therapy may become necessary or appropriate. Readers are advised to check the most current information provided (i) on procedures featured or (ii) by the manufacturer of each product to be administered, to verify the recommended dose or formula, the method and duration of administration, and contraindications. It is the responsibility of the practitioner, relying on their own experience and knowledge of the patient, to determine dosages and the best treatment for each individual patient. Neither the publisher nor the author assumes any liability for any injury and/or damage to persons or property arising from this publication.

Library of Congress Cataloging-in-Publication Data

Boezaart, André P.
Atlas of Peripheral Nerve Blocks and Anatomy for Orthopaedic Anesthesia / André P. Boezaart. - 1st ed.
p. ; cm. - (Atlases of anesthesia techniques series)
Includes bibliographical references and index.
ISBN 978-1-4160-3941-9
1. Anesthesia in orthopedics–Atlases. 2. Conduction anesthesia–Atlases. 3. Nerve block–Atlases. I. Title. II. Series.
[DNLM: 1. Anesthesia, Conduction—methods—Atlases. 2. Anesthetics, Local—Atlases. 3. Musculoskeletal System—anatomy & histology—Atlases. 4. Nerve Block—methods—Atlases. WO 517 B673a 2007]
RD751.B64 2007
617.9'6747–dc22

2007007880

Executive Publisher: Natasha Andjelkovic
Multi-Media Producer: David Wisner
Project Manager: Mary Stermel
Design Direction: Karen O'Keefe Owens

Printed in China

Last digit is the print number: 9 8 7 6 5 4 3 2 1

To Karin, my wife, with love and gratitude for her unwavering dedication to the care of our children and for giving meaning to my life.

Contents

Preface, ix

Acknowledgments, xi

Chapter 1. **Proximal Brachial Plexus – Applied Anatomy, 1**
- Phrenic Nerve, 3
- Superior Trunk of the Brachial Plexus, 8
- Suprascapular Nerve, 8
- Dorsal Scapular Nerve, 8
- Nerve to Levator Scapulae, 8
- Accessory Nerve, 13
- Transectional Anatomy (C6), 13

Chapter 2. **Interscalene Block, 21**
- Single-Injection Interscalene Block, 23
- Continuous Interscalene Block, 30

Chapter 3. **Cervical Paravertebral Block, 39**
- Single-Injection and Continuous Cervical Paravertebral Blocks, 41

Chapter 4. **Supraclavicular Block, 55**
- Single-Injection Supraclavicular Block, 57

Chapter 5. **Distal Brachial Plexus: Applied Anatomy, 63**
- Brachial Plexus Cords, 65

Chapter 6. **Infraclavicular Block, 75**
- Single-Injection Infraclavicular Block, 77
- Continuous Infraclavicular Block, 81

Chapter 7. **Nerves in the Axilla: Applied Anatomy, 87**
- Radial Nerve in the Axilla, 89
- Median Nerve in the Axilla, 89
- Ulnar Nerve in the Axilla, 91
- Musculocutaneous Nerve in the Axilla, 93

Chapter 8. **Axillary Blocks, 99**
- Single-Injection Axillary Block, 101
- Continuous Axillary Block, 102

Chapter 9. **Nerves around the Elbow: Applied Anatomy, 107**
- Radial Nerve at the Elbow, 109
- Median Nerve at the Elbow, 109
- Ulnar Nerve at the Elbow, 112

Chapter 10. **Blocks around the Elbow, 119**
- Musculocutaneous Nerve Block at the Elbow, 121
- Radial Nerve Block at the Elbow, 122
- Median Nerve Block at the Elbow, 122
- Ulnar Nerve Block at the Elbow, 123

Chapter 11. **Lumbar Plexus: Applied Anatomy, 125**
Anterior Lumbar Plexus, 127

Chapter 12. **Anterior lumbar Plexus Blocks, 139**
Single-Injection Femoral Nerve Block, 141
Continuous Femoral Nerve Block, 143
Single-Injection Obturator Nerve Block, 153
Single-Injection Lateral Cutaneous Nerve of the Thigh Block, 157

Chapter 13. **Posterior Lumbar Plexus Block, 161**
Applied Anatomy, 163
Continuous Lumbar Plexus Block (Psoas Compartment), 163

Chapter 14. **Sacral Plexus Nerves: Applied Anatomy, 171**
Sciatic Nerve: Subgluteal Area, 173
Sciatic Nerve: Popliteal Area, 176

Chapter 15. **Sciatic Nerve Blocks, 183**
Single-Injection Subgluteal Sciatic Nerve Block, 185
Continuous Subgluteal Sciatic Nerve Block, 186
Single-Injection Popliteal Sciatic Nerve Block, 189
Continuous Popliteal Sciatic Nerve Block, 191

Chapter 16. **The Ankle: Applied Anatomy, 195**

Chapter 17. **Ankle Block, 203**
Ankle Blocks, 205

Chapter 18. **Thoracic Paravertebral Block, 211**
Single-Injection and Continuous Thoracic Paravertebral Blocks, 213

Chapter 19. **PITFALLS IN REGIONAL ANESTHESIA (and how to avoid them), 221**
Introduction, 223
Where Not to Do Blocks, 224
Epinephrine (Adrenaline), 226
Existing Neuropathy, 226
Other Considerations, 230

Preface

The idea for this atlas followed the success of *The Primer of Regional Anesthesia Anatomy*, which was intended as an easily readable visual source of the basic functional anatomy for regional anesthesia. Its companion DVD contained videos of the motor responses following transcutaneous stimulation of individual nerves ("nerve mapping"). To assist with this, medical illustrator Mary Bryson painted the surface anatomy of the nerves on a model, and the concepts of "nerve mapping" and dynamic functional anatomy were illustrated for all the nerves on this model. The goal was to provide as much visual impact of the static and dynamic anatomy as possible with minimum text. Mary received a Certificate of Merit from the Frank Netter Foundation of the Vesalius Trust for the illustrations she created for *The Primer of Regional Anesthesia Anatomy*.

This approach proved successful, and has been continued in this atlas, which is a natural continuation of *The Primer* and contains the relevant peripheral nerve blocks in the appropriate anatomical context. Mary Bryson again provided clear and beautiful illustrations of the applied anatomy. Photographs of dedicated cadaver dissections further illustrate the applied anatomy, and clinical photographs show actual blocks performed on volunteers. All the blocks discussed in this atlas were filmed while being demonstrated on volunteers and, with the functional dynamic anatomy movie clips, arranged on the accompanying DVD.

This atlas consists of chapters dealing first with the details of applied essential anatomy followed by the single-injection and continuous nerve block of the specific areas. The blocks are arranged from the upper extremity to the lower extremity, starting with blocks above the clavicle and ending with ankle blocks and lumbar and thoracic paravertebral blocks. There are of course many more peripheral nerve blocks than those described in this atlas, but the main goal was to focus on the most important, tested and tried blocks rather than present an exhaustive array of blocks. This atlas is thus limited to peripheral nerve blocks that are essential for orthopaedic surgery. Most of the blocks can also be applied to other types of surgery when appropriate. For example, continuous and single-injection thoracic paravertebral block (described in Chapter 18) is more often used in thoracic and breast surgery than in orthopaedic surgery.

The final chapter deals with pitfalls commonly encountered while performing peripheral nerve blocks. Recommendations in this chapter are not strictly based on evidence published in literature; rather, they represent my insight and experience of many years of practicing orthopaedic anesthesia and being an expert witness in medico-legal cases. The points are argued on the basis of anatomical principles, clinical experience, and known facts, which are all referenced in the text. It is my sincere hope that this will help practitioners avoid pitfalls and inspire them to perform only blocks that are clearly indicated and in the best interest of their patients.

André P. Boezaart

Acknowledgments

The idea for producing this atlas came from colleagues who used *The Primer of Regional Anesthesia Anatomy* and its companion DVD. I sincerely thank them and other colleagues for their encouragement, suggestions, and support.

I am incredibly grateful for the support and friendship of my colleagues in the Departments of Orthopaedic Surgery and Anesthesia at the University of Iowa who have greatly enriched my career. A special word of thanks to my good friend and colleague Dr. Rick Rosenquist for his continued support and encouragement and the many constructive debates about regional anesthesia and acute pain management.

I sincerely thank Mary K. Bryson, MAMS, CMI, for the beautiful and clear artwork and Susan McClellen for the excellent photographs. I am indebted to Kathy Fear, MSN, CRNA; Steve Borene, M.D.; Chris Theron, Ph.D.; and Kyle Stahle for their valuable help. Finally, I would like to extend a word of thanks to the editorial and production teams at Elsevier for their guidance and professional support.

Chapter 1

Proximal Brachial Plexus: Applied Anatomy

- Phrenic Nerve
- Superior Trunk of the Brachial Plexus
- Suprascapular Nerve
- Dorsal Scapular Nerve
- Nerve to Levator Scapulae
- Accessory Nerve
- Transectional Anatomy (C6)

PHRENIC NERVE

The phrenic nerve ([1] on Fig. 1-1) originates mainly from C4 and receives a small branch from the C5 root of the brachial plexus. It runs caudad on the belly of the anterior scalene muscle (Figs. 1-4 and 1-6).

The external jugular vein (Fig. 1-5, *top arrow*) is superficial to the brachial plexus. The sternocleidomastoid muscle (*bottom arrow*) partially or completely overlies the phrenic nerve.

If the sternocleidomastoid muscle is removed, as in the dissection shown in Figure 1-6, the phrenic nerve (*arrow*) can clearly be seen on the belly of the anterior scalene muscle.

Phrenic Nerve Surface Anatomy

Superficially, the phrenic nerve lies just behind the posterior border of the sternocleidomastoid muscle, at the level of C6 or the cricoid cartilage (Fig. 1-7, *arrow*). Electrical stimulation of the phrenic nerve causes contractions of the diaphragm, resulting in clear abdominal twitches. If this is encountered during interscalene block, the needle must be redirected approximately 1 cm posteriorly.

(See phrenic nerve transcutaneous stimulation movie on DVD).

Text continued on page 8

1 Phrenic nerve
2 Nerve to Levator Scapulae
3 Spinal accessory nerve
4 Dorsal scapular nerve
5 Suprascapular nerve
6 Superior trunk
7 Middle trunk
8 Inferior trunk
9 Long thoracic nerve
10 Nerves to longus colli and scalene muscles
11 Nerve to subclavius muscle
12 Lateral cord
13 Posterior cord
14 Medial cord
15 Lateral pectoral nerve
16 Medial pectoral nerve
17 Upper subscapular nerve
18 Lower subscapular nerve
19 Medial cutaneous nerve of arm
20 Medial cutaneous nerve of upper arm
21 Axillary nerve
22 Musculocutaneous nerve
23 Radial nerve
24 Median nerve
25 Ulnar nerve

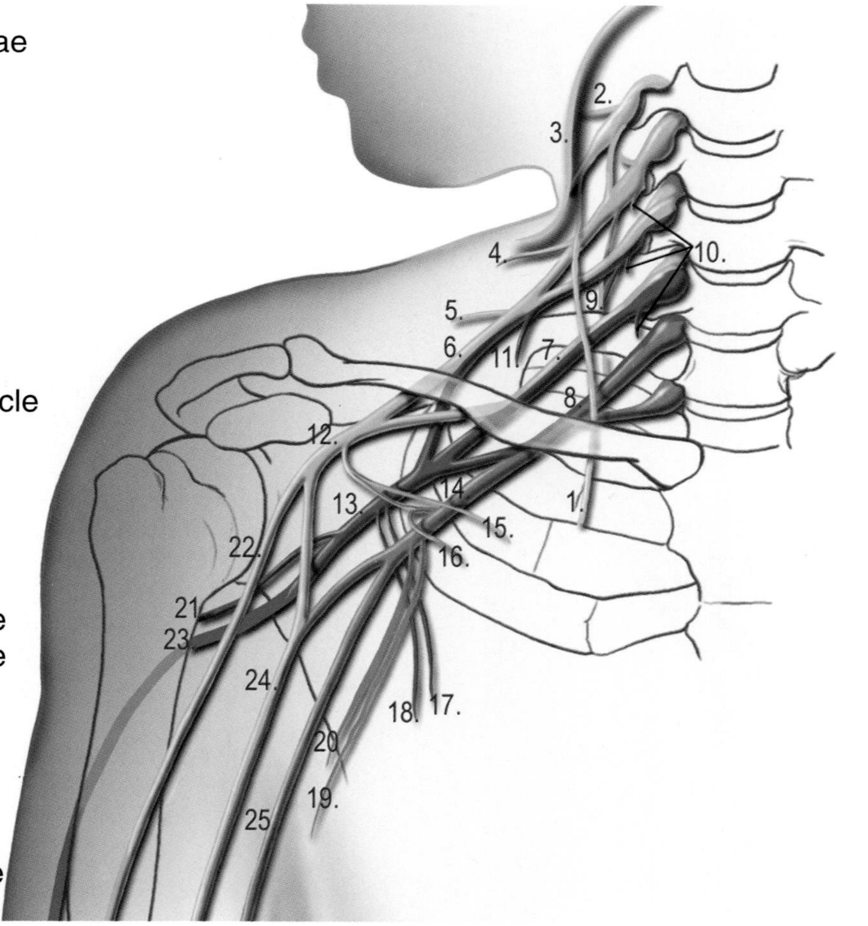

FIGURE 1-1 Schematic representation of the roots, trunks, divisions, cords, and terminal branches of the brachial plexus.

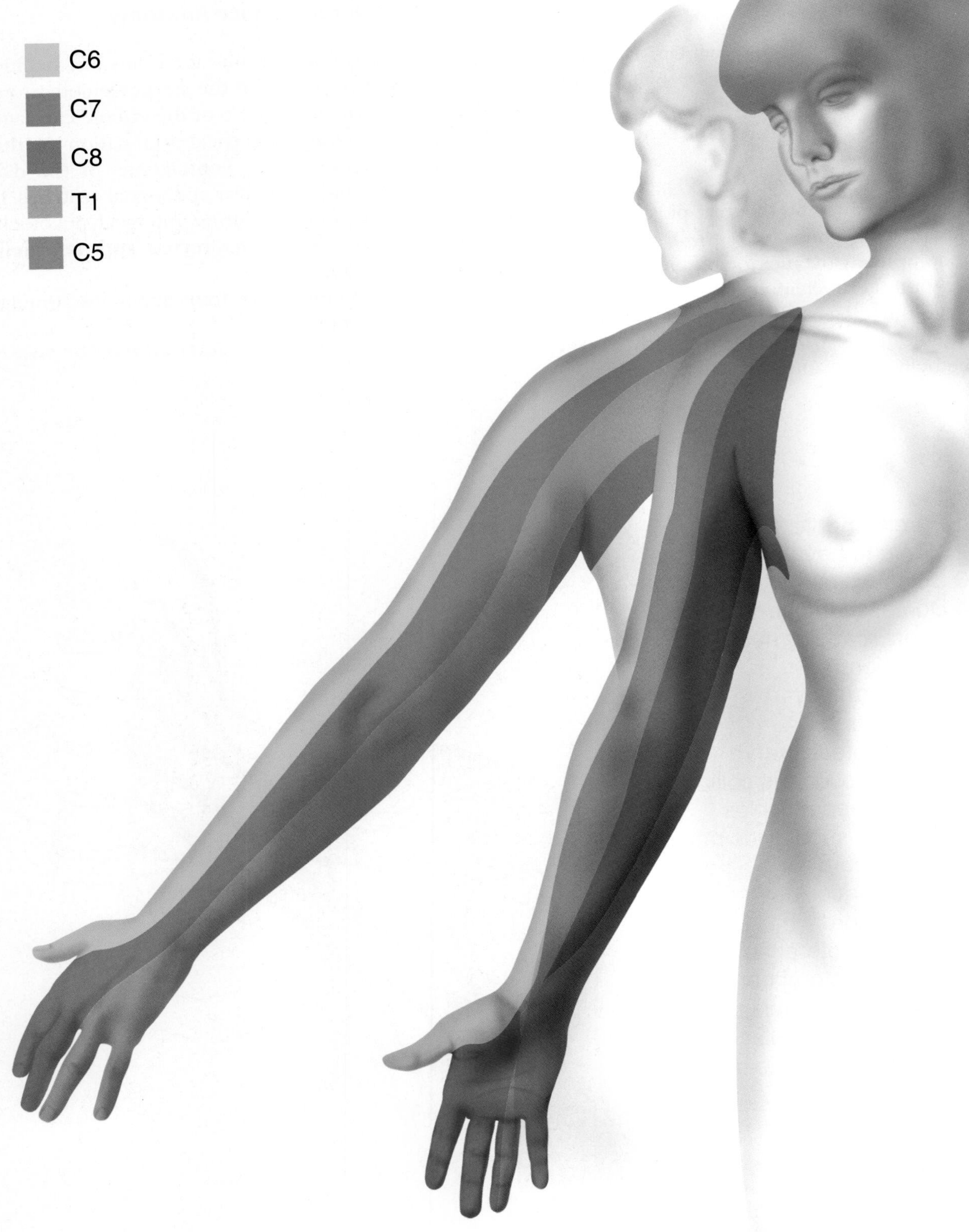

FIGURE 1-2 Dermatomes of the upper limb.

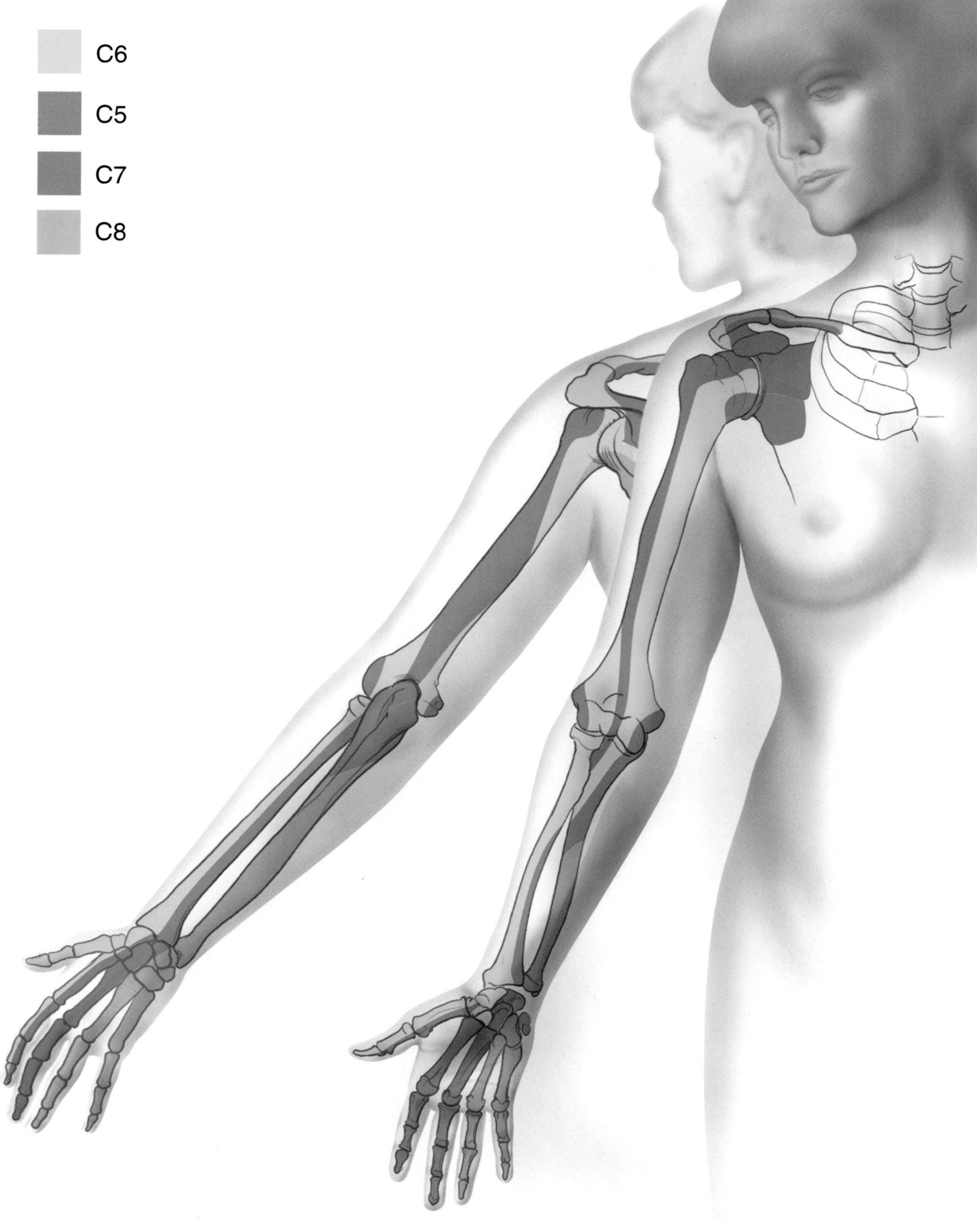

FIGURE 1-3 Osteotomes of the upper limb.

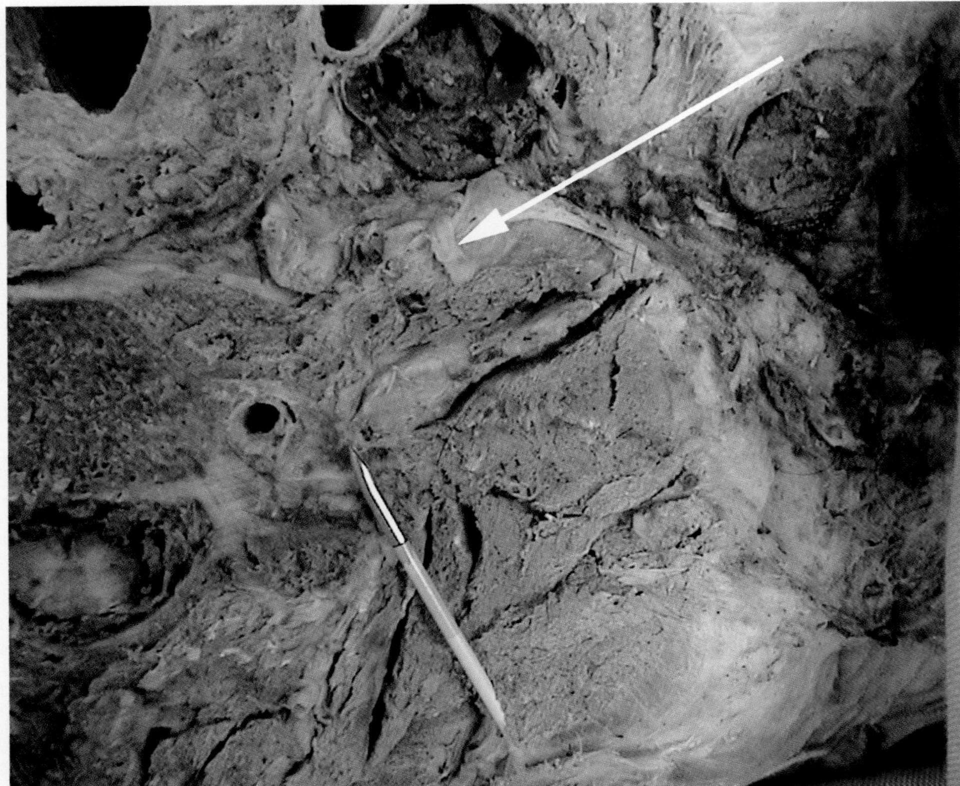

FIGURE 1-4 Transection of the neck at the C6 level. The needle is on the brachial plexus, and the *arrow* indicates the phrenic nerve.

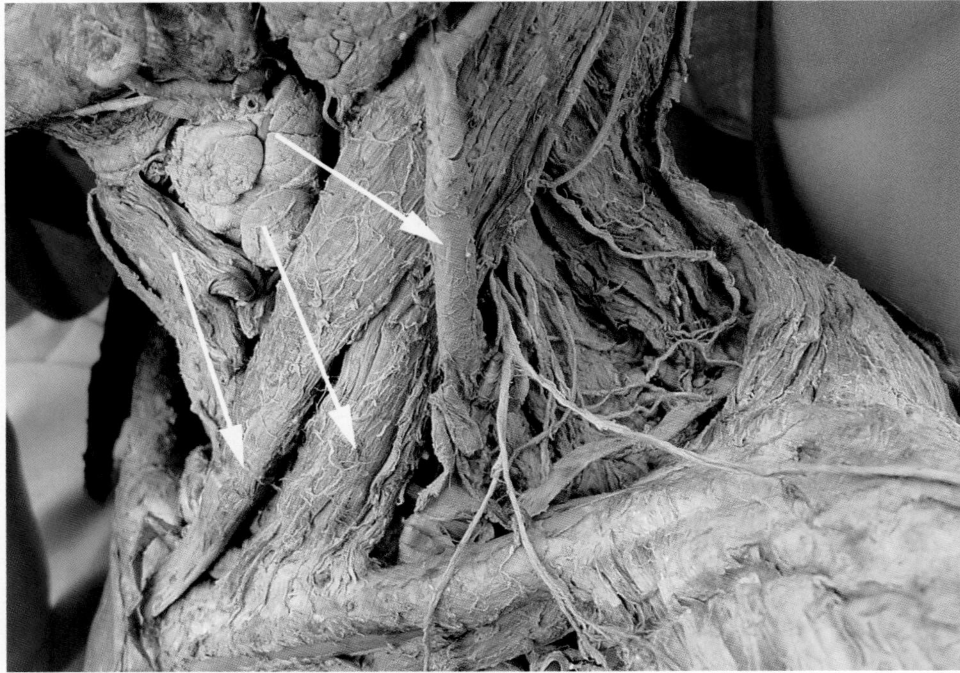

FIGURE 1-5 Lateral view of the posterior triangle of the neck. The *top arrow* indicates the external jugular vein, the *middle arrow* the clavicular head, and the *bottom arrow* the sternal head of the sternocleidomastoid muscle. Note the superficial cervical plexus behind the midpoint of the posterior border of the clavicular head of the sternocleidomastoid muscle.

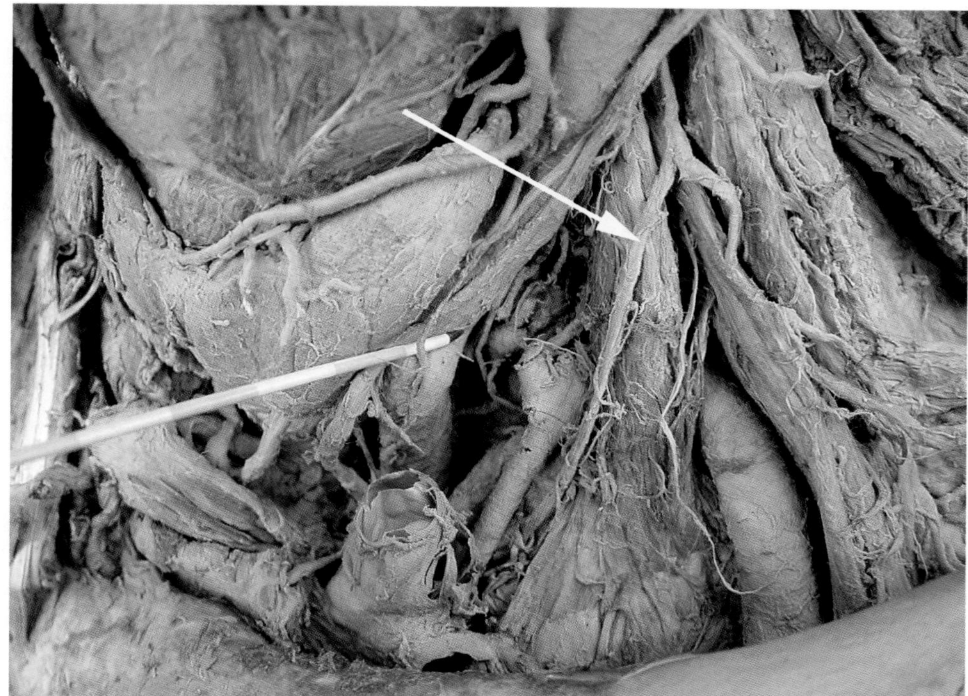

FIGURE 1-6 Lateral view of the neck. The needle retracts the carotid artery, and the stellate ganglion is visible deep to the artery. The *arrow* indicates the phrenic nerve in its position on the belly of the anterior scalene muscle.

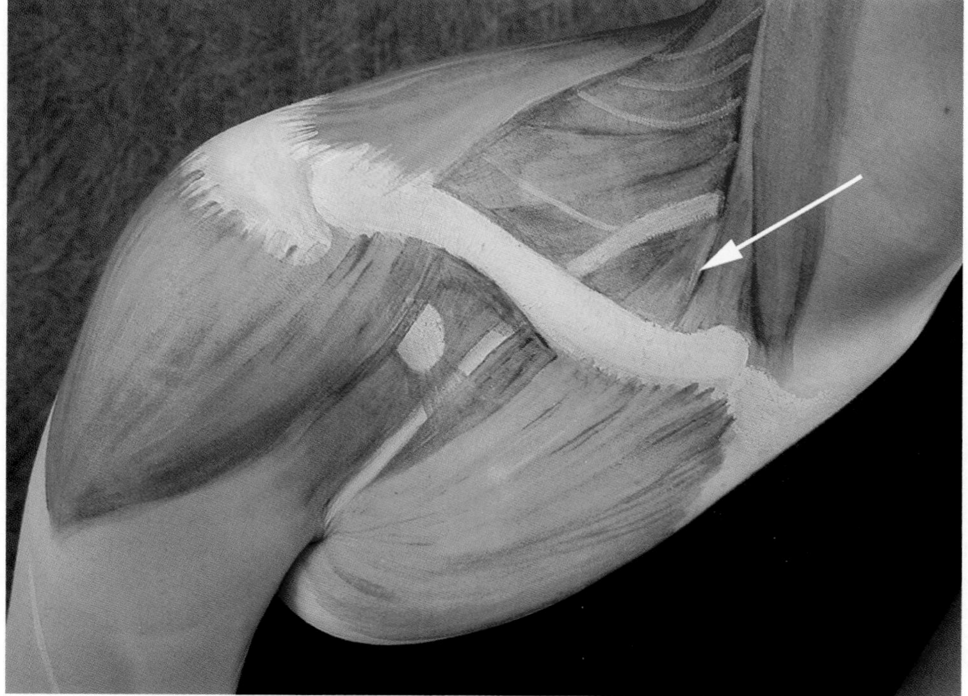

FIGURE 1-7 Anterior view of the posterior triangle of the neck. The *arrow* indicates the surface anatomy of the phrenic nerve behind the clavicular head of the sternocleidomastoid muscle.

SUPERIOR TRUNK OF THE BRACHIAL PLEXUS

The superior trunk of the brachial plexus is a bundle of nerves formed by the fifth and sixth cervical roots (see Fig. 1-1, [6]). Electrical stimulation proximal on the trunk results in a motor response of the triceps muscle, whereas stimulation distally on the same trunk causes biceps muscle twitches.

Figure 1-8 illustrates the area of sensory innervation of the superior trunk of the brachial plexus.

The brachial plexus (Fig. 1-9, *arrow*) lies between the anterior and the middle scalene muscles. Note again the phrenic nerve on the belly of the anterior scalene muscle and the vagus nerve and carotid artery anterior to that.

Superior Trunk Surface Anatomy

The brachial plexus is posterior to the sternocleidomastoid muscle at the level of the cricoid cartilage (Fig. 1-10, *arrow*). This is commonly referred to as *Winnie's point*, and is typically where an interscalene block is performed for shoulder surgery.

Electrical stimulation of the superior trunk of the brachial plexus causes unmistakable twitches of the biceps muscle, as can be seen on the accompanying recording.

(See superior trunk transcutaneous stimulation movie on DVD).

SUPRASCAPULAR NERVE

The suprascapular nerve branches from the superior trunk of the brachial plexus in the lower part of the posterior triangle of the neck (see Fig. 1-1, [5]).

The suprascapular nerve (Fig. 1-11, *arrow*) lies just behind the middle scalene muscle as it passes posterior and disappears under the trapezius muscle. It supplies the supraspinatus and infraspinatus muscles of the rotator cuff.

Suprascapular Nerve Surface Anatomy

The clavicle, when viewed from anterior, sometimes obscures the surface anatomy of the suprascapular nerve (Fig. 1-12, *arrow*). In some individuals it can be stimulated laterally in the posterior triangle of the neck.

Electrical stimulation of the suprascapular nerve results in rotation of the humerus because it innervates the rotator cuff.

(See suprascapular nerve transcutaneous stimulation movie on DVD).

DORSAL SCAPULAR NERVE

The dorsal scapular nerve arises from the posterior aspect of C5 and enters the middle scalene muscle (see Fig. 1-1, [4]).

After entering the middle scalene muscle, the dorsal scapular nerve (Fig. 1-13, *arrow*) appears at its posterior border, between the middle and posterior scalene muscles. It then courses downward beneath the levator scapulae muscle. It supplies both rhomboid muscles on their deep surfaces. It often also gives a branch to the levator scapulae muscle.

Dorsal Scapular Nerve Surface Anatomy

The dorsal scapular nerve (Fig. 1-14, *arrow*) is posterior and superior to the brachial plexus, behind the middle scalene muscle.

Electrical stimulation of the dorsal scapular nerve causes contractions of the rhomboid muscles and medial movement of the scapula. This is often confused with shoulder or arm muscle twitches. Because it is not inside the brachial plexus sheath, blockage of this nerve does not result in successful interscalene block.

(See dorsal scapular nerve transcutaneous stimulation movie on DVD).

NERVE TO LEVATOR SCAPULAE

The nerve to the levator scapulae arises from the C4 cervical root and is not part of the brachial plexus (see Fig. 1-1, [2]).

The nerve to levator scapulae (Fig. 1-15, *arrow*) is posterior and superior to the dorsal scapular nerve.

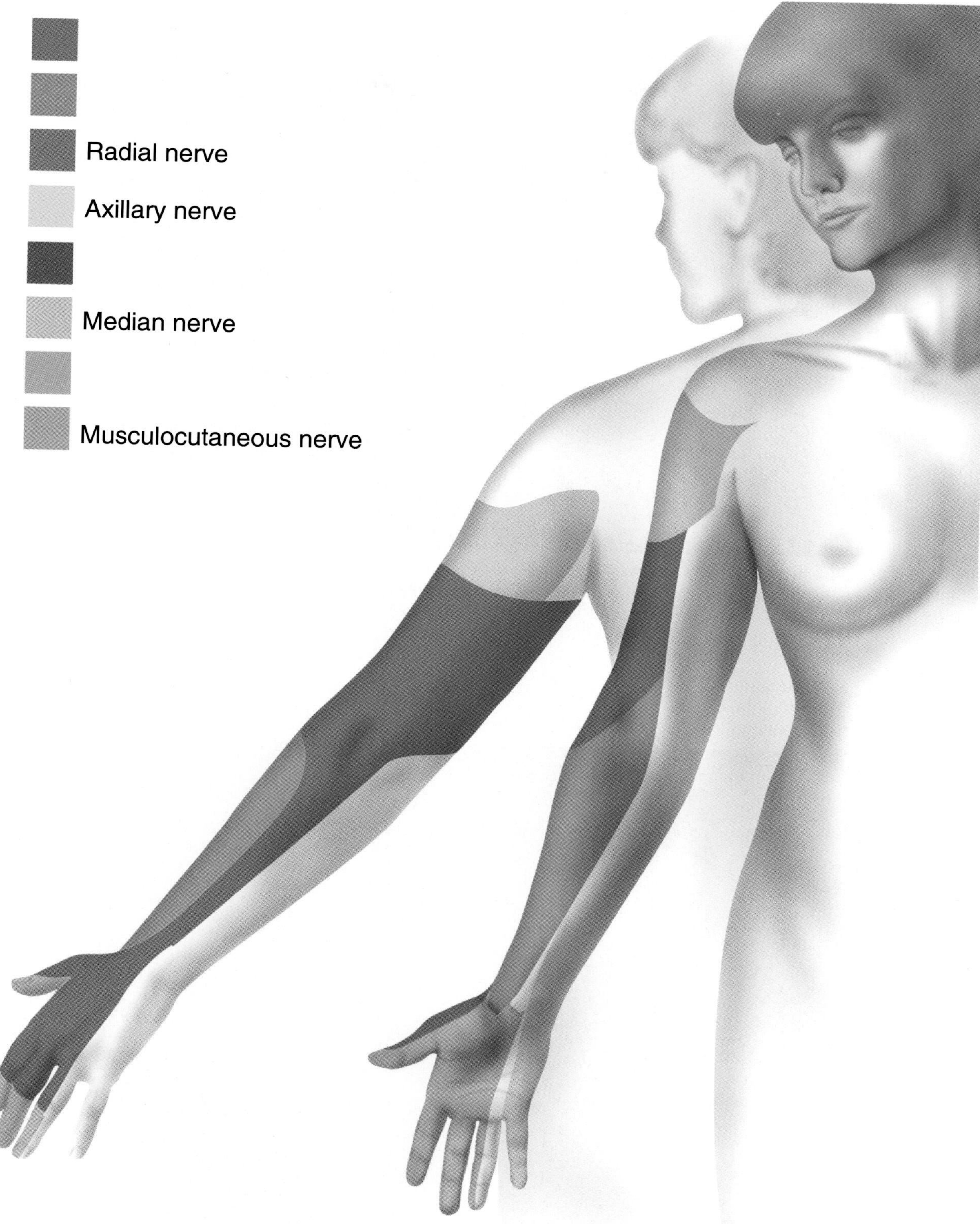

FIGURE 1-8 Neurotomes typically blocked by the interscalene block.

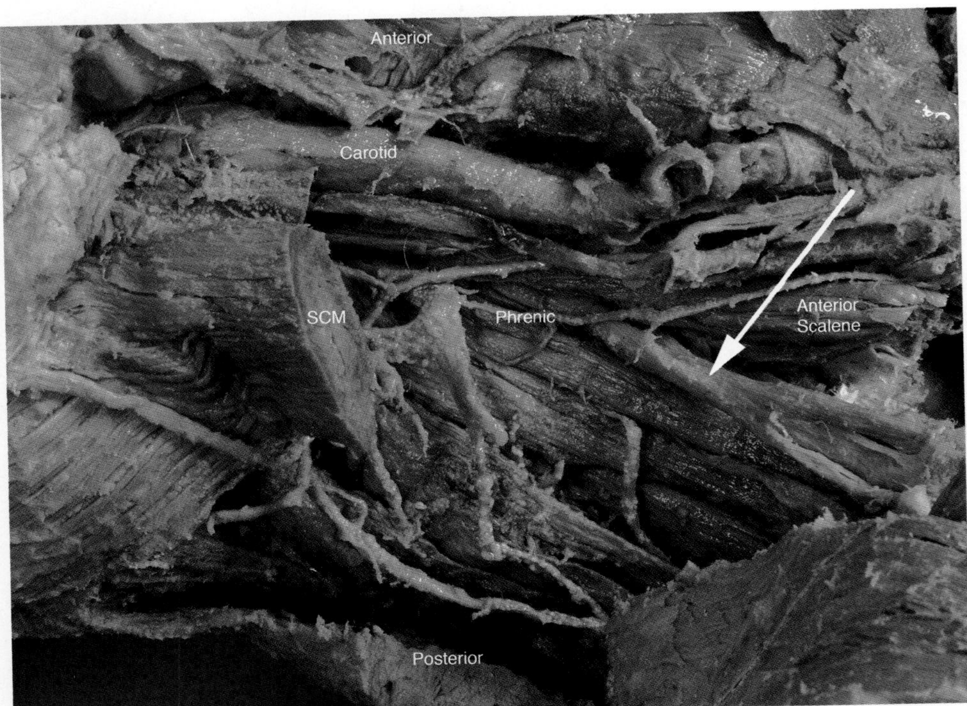

FIGURE 1-9 Dissection of the lateral part of the neck. The *arrow* indicates the brachial plexus between the anterior and middle scalene muscle. The sternocleidomastoid muscle (SCM) is cut away in this dissection.

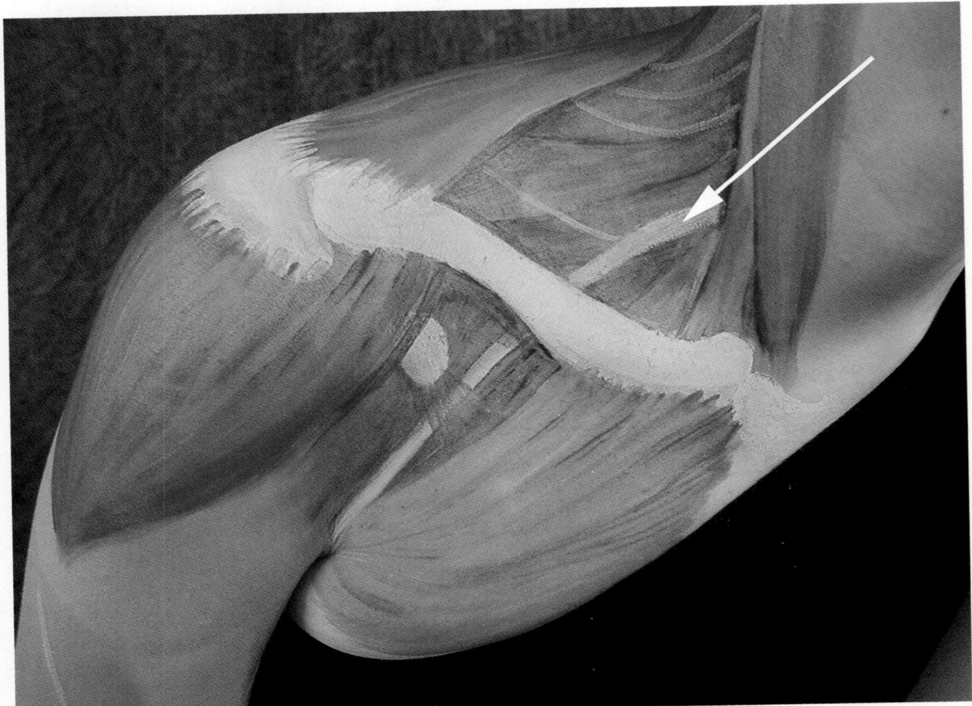

FIGURE 1-10 Anterior view of the posterior triangle of the neck. The *arrow* indicates the surface anatomy of the brachial plexus.

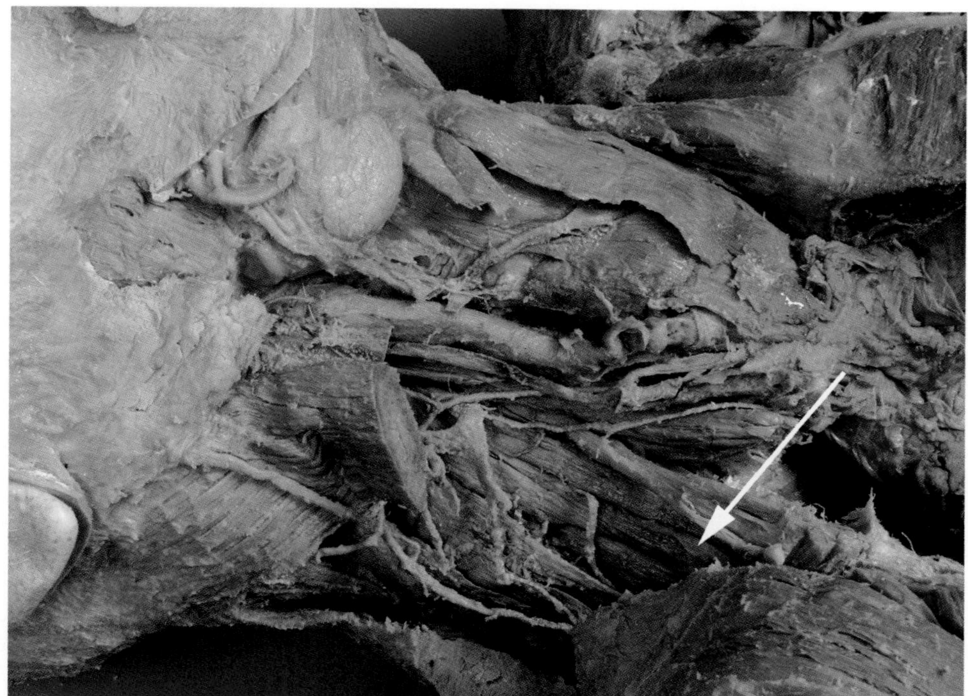

FIGURE 1-11 Lateral view of the neck. The *arrow* indicates the suprascapular nerve between the middle and posterior scalene muscles.

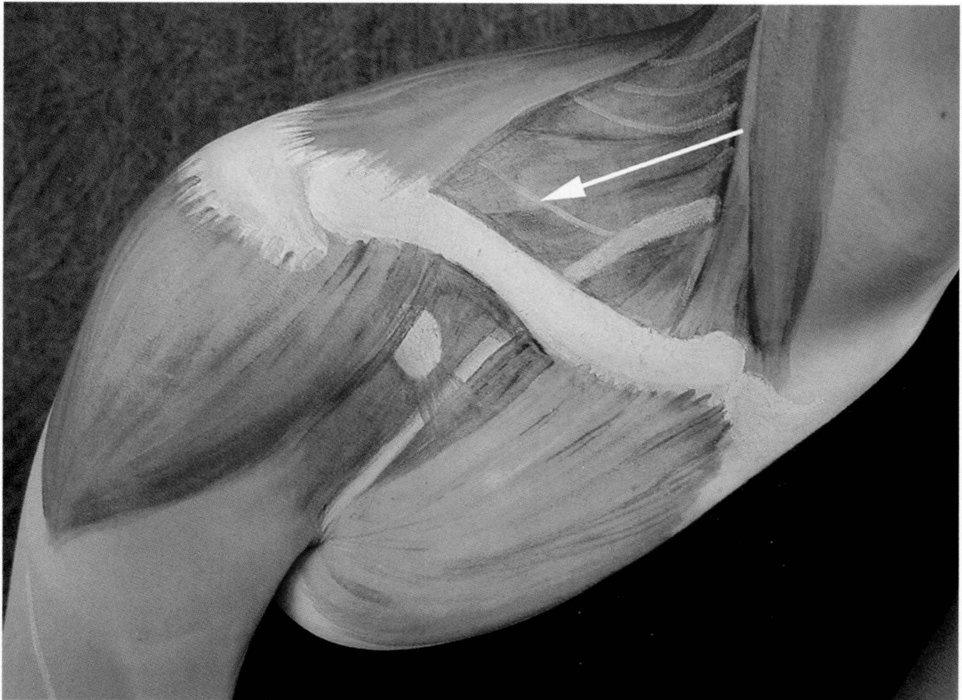

FIGURE 1-12 Anterior view of the posterior triangle of the neck. The *arrow* indicates the surface anatomy of the suprascapular nerve.

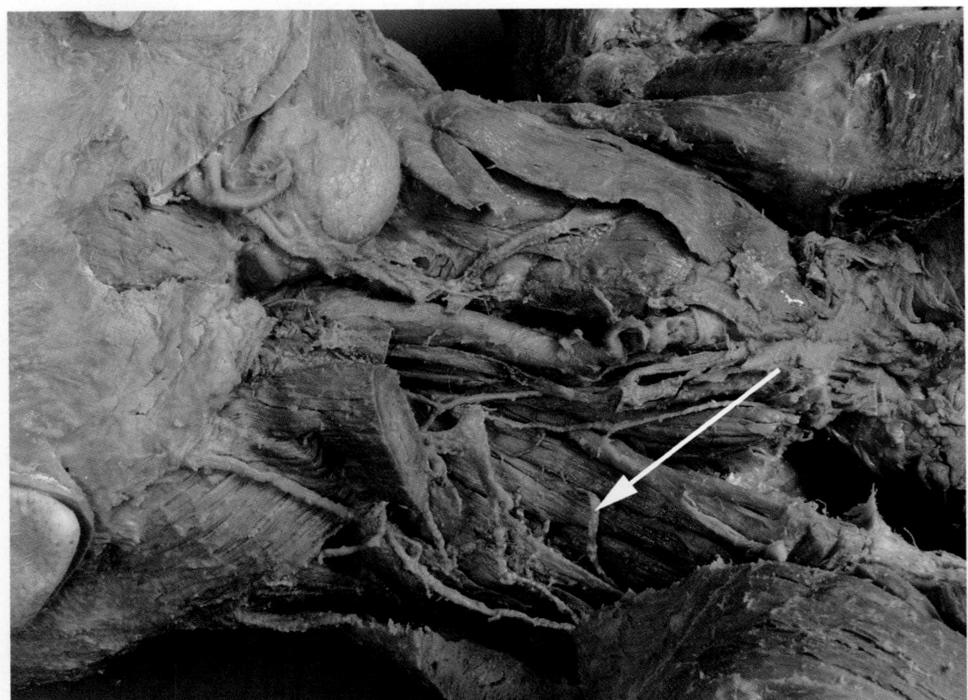

FIGURE 1-13 Lateral view of the neck. The *arrow* indicates the dorsal scapular nerve as it exits between the middle and posterior scalene muscles.

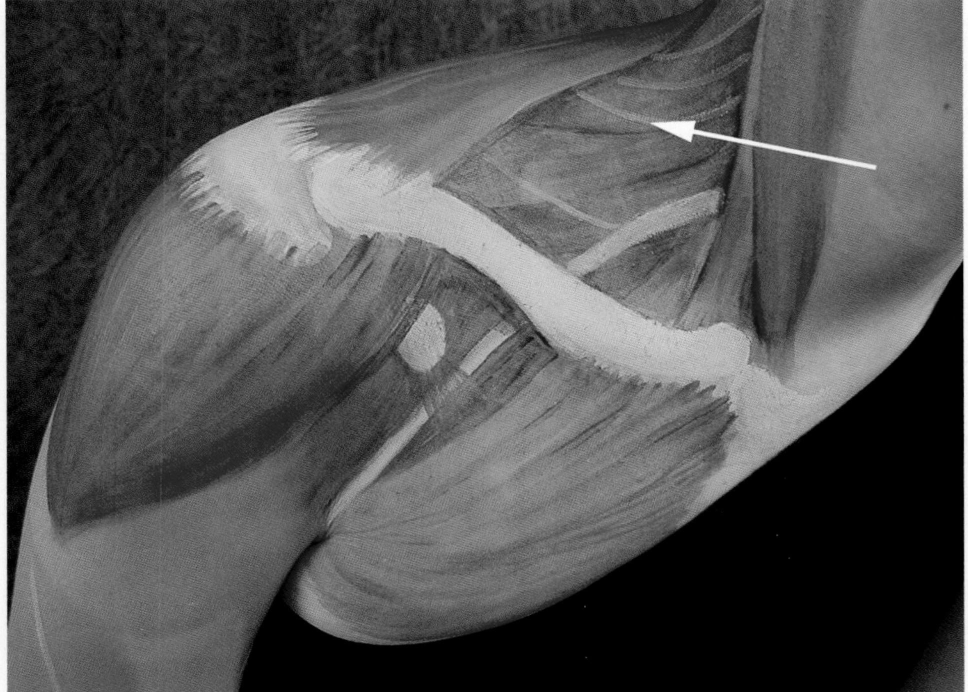

FIGURE 1-14 Anterior view of the posterior triangle of the neck. The *arrow* indicates the surface anatomy of the dorsal scapular nerve.

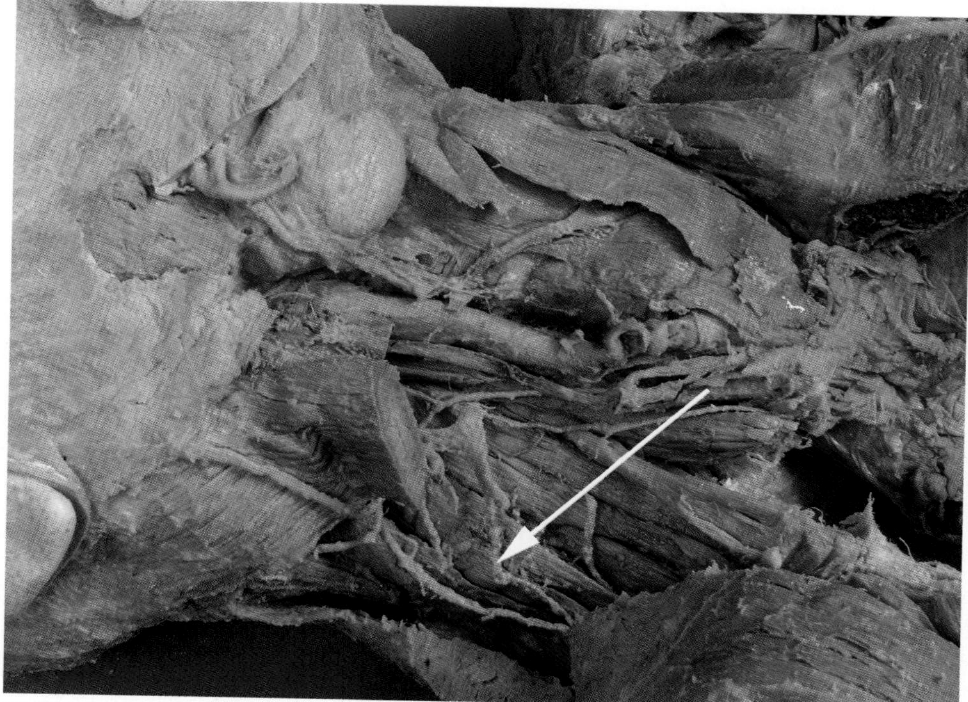

FIGURE 1-15 Lateral view of the neck. The *arrow* indicates the nerve to the levator scapulae muscle.

Nerve to Levator Scapulae Surface Anatomy

The surface anatomy of the nerve to levator scapulae (Fig. 1-16, *arrow*) is superior and posterior to Winnie's point. The only importance of this nerve for the anesthesiologist is to recognize its function, which is innervation of the muscle that elevates the scapula. Like the dorsal scapular nerve, this nerve is not inside the brachial plexus sheath.

Electrical stimulation of the nerve to the levator scapulae causes movement of the scapula. This movement can easily be mistaken for twitches caused by brachial plexus or trapezius muscle stimulation. It is also difficult to distinguish levator scapulae twitches from trapezius muscle twitches. The accompanying recording shows contraction of both these muscles. Both are sometimes confused with brachial plexus stimulation.

(See nerve to levator scapulae transcutaneous stimulation movie on DVD).

ACCESSORY NERVE

The accessory nerve is a cranial nerve and not part of the brachial or cervical plexuses (see Fig. 1-1, [3]). It crosses the posterior triangle of the neck superficially and is easy to stimulate transcutaneously.

The dissection depicted in Figure 1-17 shows the posterior and superior location of the accessory nerve (*arrow*) in the posterior triangle of the neck.

Accessory Nerve Surface Anatomy

The accessory nerve (Fig. 1-18, *arrow*) emerges beneath the posterior border of the sternocleidomastoid muscle, at the junction of its middle and lower thirds. It passes almost vertically downward on the levator scapulae to disappear beneath the anterior border of the trapezius muscle, at the junction of its middle and lower thirds.

Electrical stimulation of the accessory nerve gives the unmistakable motor response of shrugging of the shoulder owing to trapezius muscle contraction.

(See accessory nerve stimulation movie on DVD).

TRANSECTIONAL ANATOMY (C6)

The roots of the brachial plexus emerge from the neuroforamina of the vertebrae. The roots of

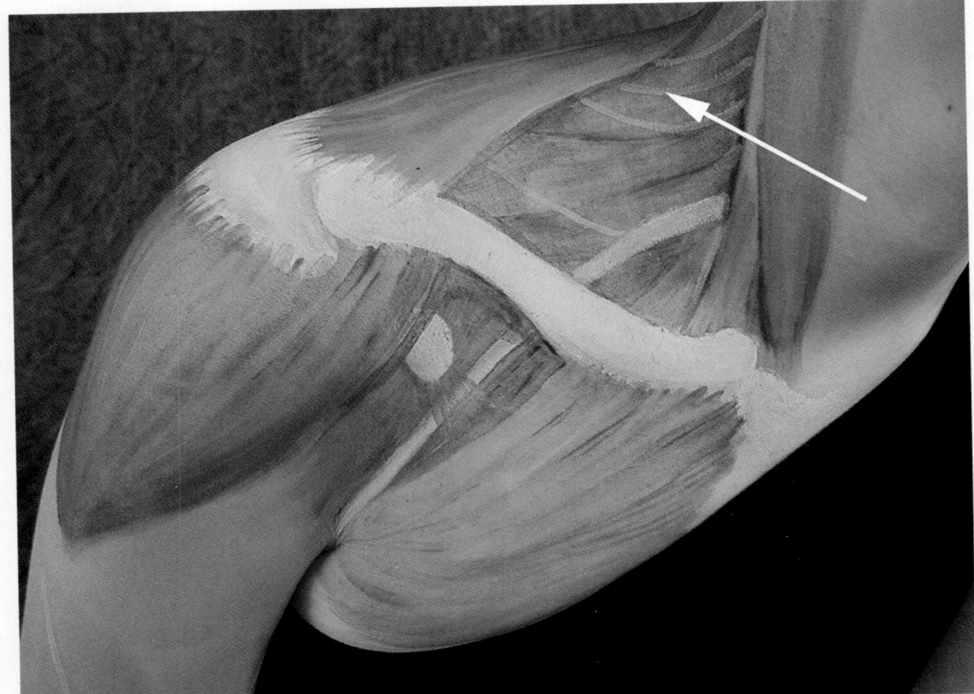

FIGURE 1-16 Anterior view of the posterior triangle of the neck. The *arrow* indicates the surface anatomy of the nerve to the levator scapulae muscle.

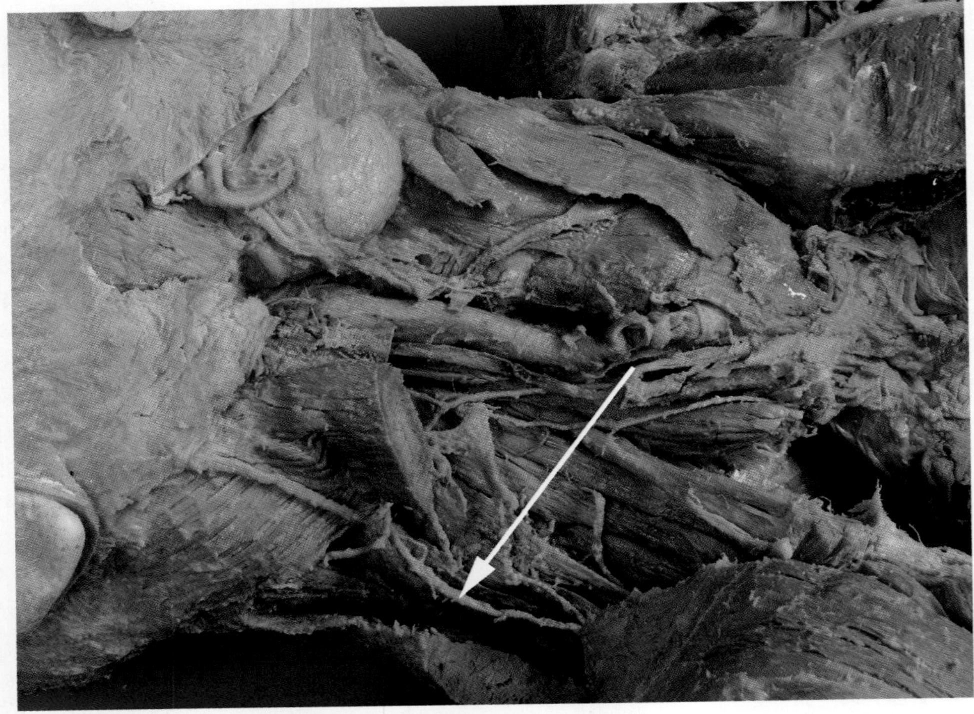

FIGURE 1-17 Lateral view of the neck. The *arrow* indicates the accessory nerve.

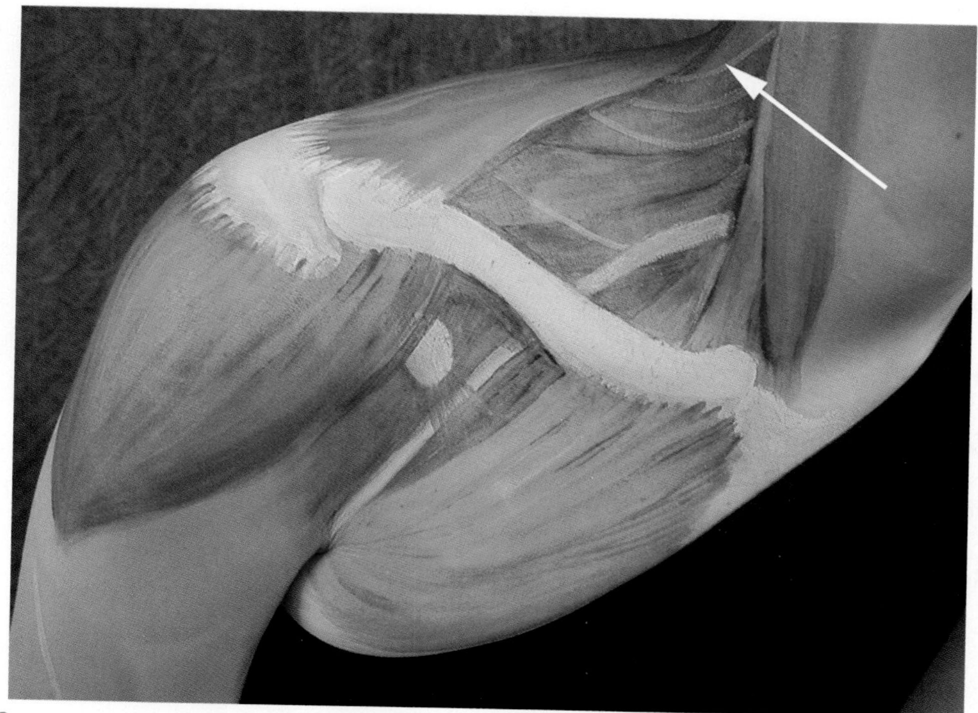

FIGURE 1-18 Anterior view of the posterior triangle of the neck. The *arrow* indicates the surface anatomy of the accessory nerve.

C5 and C6 converge to form the superior trunk, the C7 root continues to form the middle trunk, and the roots of C8 and T1 form the inferior trunk (see Fig. 1-1). The posterior aspects of the roots contain sensory fibers that travel to the dorsal spinal horn of the cord, whereas the anterior aspects of the roots consist mainly of motor fibers from the anterior horn of the spinal cord.

Figure 1-19 demonstrates the neurotomes of the brachial plexus. These neurotomes are typically all blocked during posterior root-level block. The intercostobrachial nerve distribution on the medial aspect of the upper arm is not included in the illustration because the intercostobrachial nerve is not a component of the brachial plexus. Also, there is occasional sparing of the superficial cervical plexus with a posterior approach. Although this is rare, it is easily remedied by the addition of a superficial cervical plexus block, just lateral to the midpoint of the sternocleidomastoid muscle (Fig. 1-5).

Figure 1-20 shows an oblique transection through the neck, from the dorsal spine of C6 to the cricoid cartilage. The arrow (see Fig. 1-20, [1]) indicates the body of C6.

The posterior extensor muscles of the neck (see Fig. 1-20, [2]) are usually tender and should be avoided when approaching the brachial plexus roots from posterior.

There is a "window" through which the brachial plexus can be reached from posterior without penetrating the extensor muscles of the neck. This window is between the trapezius muscle (see Fig. 1-20, [3]) and the levator scapulae muscle (see Fig. 1-20, [4]).

The phrenic nerve (see Fig. 1-20, [5]) lies on the belly of the anterior scalene muscle, with the brachial plexus (see Fig. 1-20, [6]) situated between the anterior scalene muscle (see Fig. 1-20, [7]) and the middle scalene muscle (see Fig. 1-20, [8]).

When approaching the roots of the brachial plexus from posterior, the needle is "walked off" the articular column of C6 or short transverse process of the vertebra (see Fig. 1-20, [9]).

The vertebral artery and vein (see Fig. 1-20, [10]) are situated anterior to the brachial plexus, which makes this approach to the brachial plexus attractive because penetration of these vessels from posterior is unlikely. The bony pars intervertebralis and facet joints, which make up the articular column (see Fig. 1-20, [9]), form a

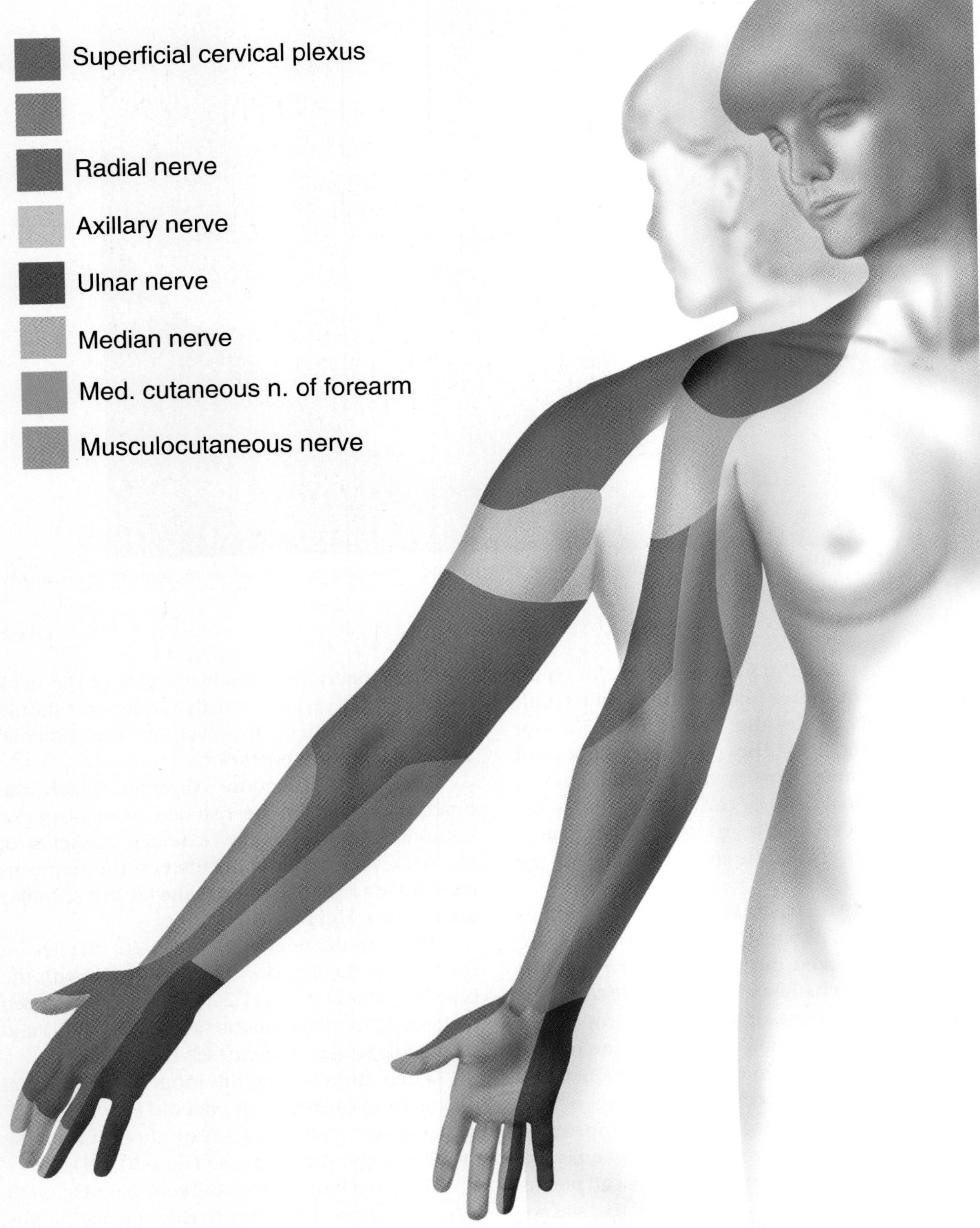

FIGURE 1-19 Neurotomes that can be expected to be blocked by a brachial plexus root block or cervical paravertebral block.

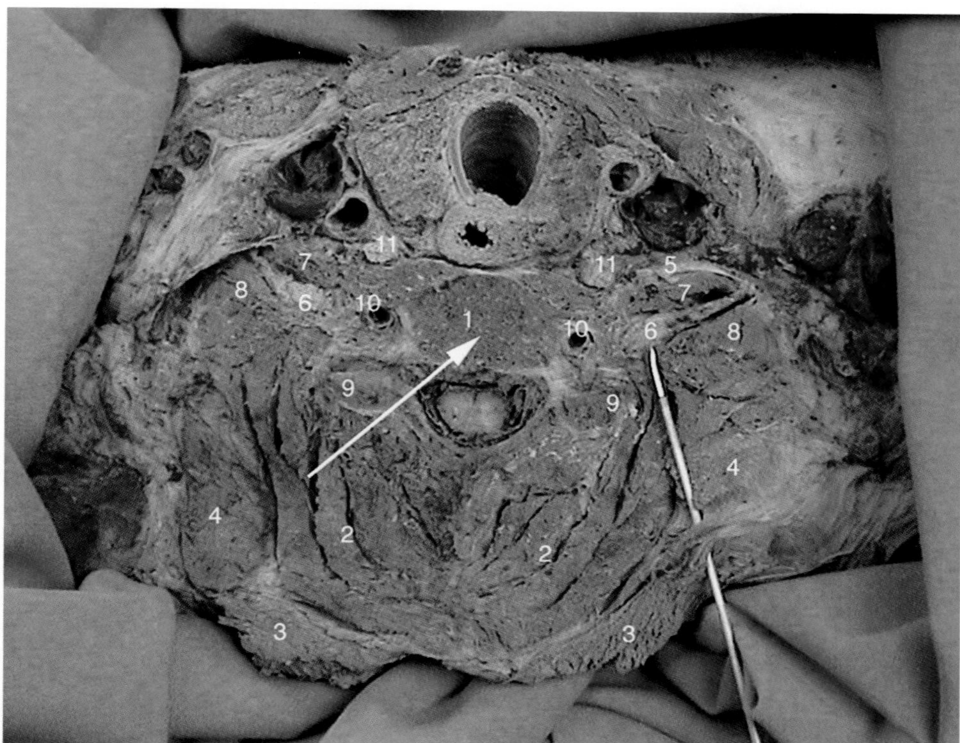

FIGURE 1-20 Transection of the neck. The *arrow* indicates the body of C6. 1, Body of C6; 2, extensor muscles of the neck; 3, trapezius muscle; 4, levator scapulae muscle; 5, phrenic nerve; 6, brachial plexus; 7, anterior scalene muscle; 8, middle scalene muscle; 9, pars intervertebralis [articular column]; 10, vertebral artery and vein; 11, superior cervical (stellate) ganglion.

"wall of bone" that protect the vertebral artery and vein during a posterior approach.

The location of the cervicothoracic sympathetic chain (stellate ganglion) explains why Horner's syndrome is a common companion of nerve blocks in this area (see Fig. 1-20, [11]).

In a magnified transectional view, the phrenic nerve (Fig. 1-21, *arrow*) can be seen on the belly of the anterior scalene muscle. Note that the nerve is outside of the fascia that covers the anterior scalene muscle and brachial plexus. This fascia extends from the paravertebral fascia, which forms the brachial plexus sheath more distally.

Surface Anatomy for Posterior Approach to Brachial Plexus

The surface anatomy for the posterior approach to the brachial plexus (the cervical paravertebral block) starts with a line that is drawn from the dorsal spine of C6 to the suprasternal notch (Fig. 1-22). This line passes through a point in the apex of the "V" formed by the anterior border of the trapezius muscle and the posterior border of the levator scapulae muscle.

The arrows in Figure 1-23 indicate the anterior border of the trapezius muscle.

The arrows in Figure 1-24 indicate the posterior border of the levator scapulae muscle.

The needle is aimed mesiad, anterior, and approximately 30 degrees caudad, toward the suprasternal notch (Fig. 1-25).

The needle, attached to a loss-of-resistance-to-air syringe and a nerve stimulator set at 1.2 to 3 mA, is walked off the bony articular column of the vertebra in a lateral direction. Muscle twitches and loss of resistance to air appear approximately simultaneously.

If surgery is to the shoulder, anterior muscle twitches are sought. These are the major pectoral muscle, biceps, or deltoid muscles, representing the C5/C6 roots. If surgery is to the wrist or elbow, triceps muscle motor response is sought, representing the C7/C8 roots. It is important to place the catheter on the correct root.

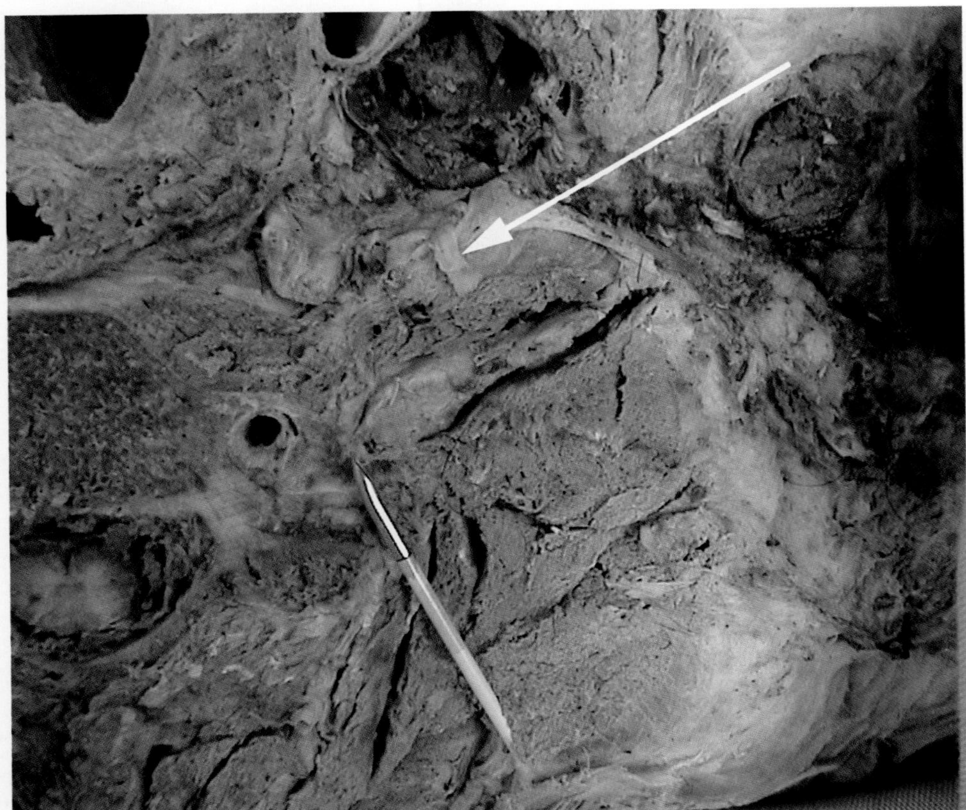

FIGURE 1-21 Magnified view of transection of the neck. The *arrow* indicates the phrenic nerve.

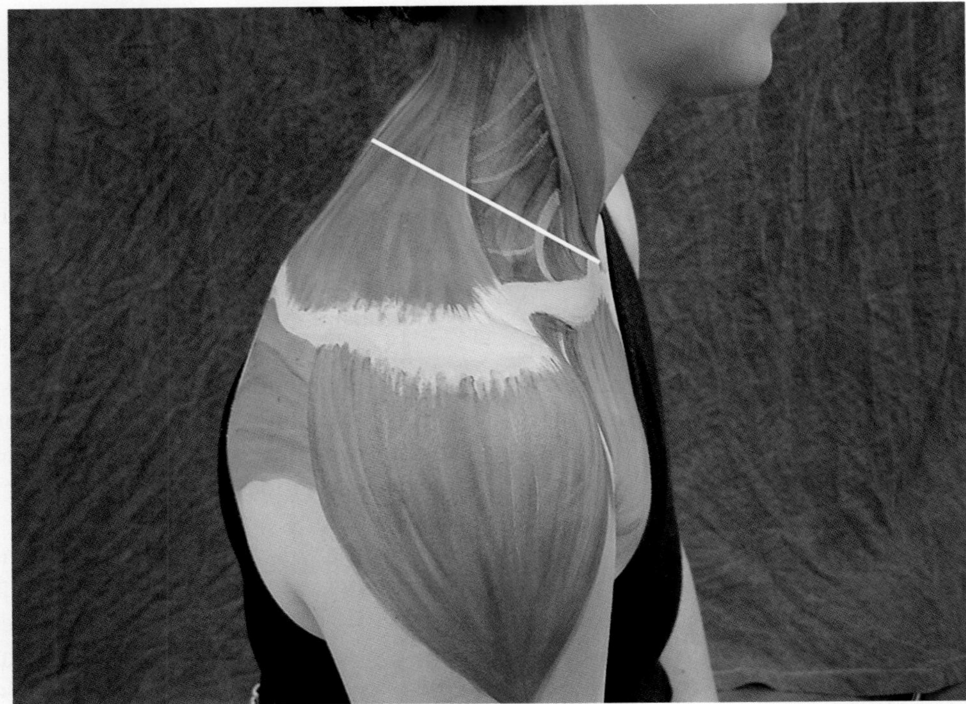

FIGURE 1-22 Lateral view of the neck indicating the surface anatomy of the cervical paravertebral block. The line joins the dorsal spine of C6 with the suprasternal notch.

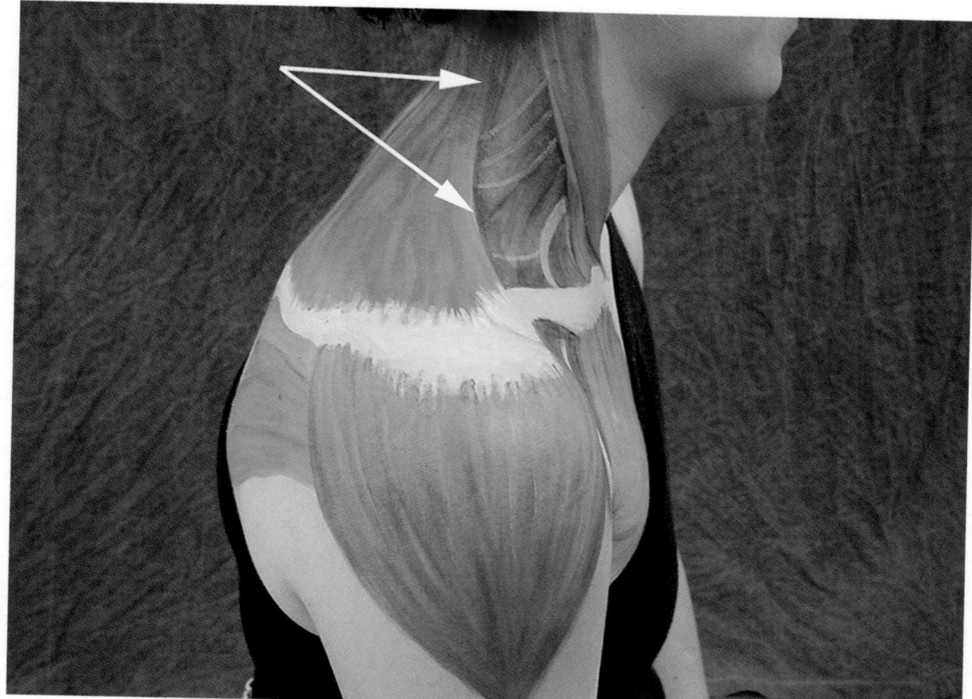

FIGURE 1-23 The *arrows* indicate the anterior border of the trapezius muscle.

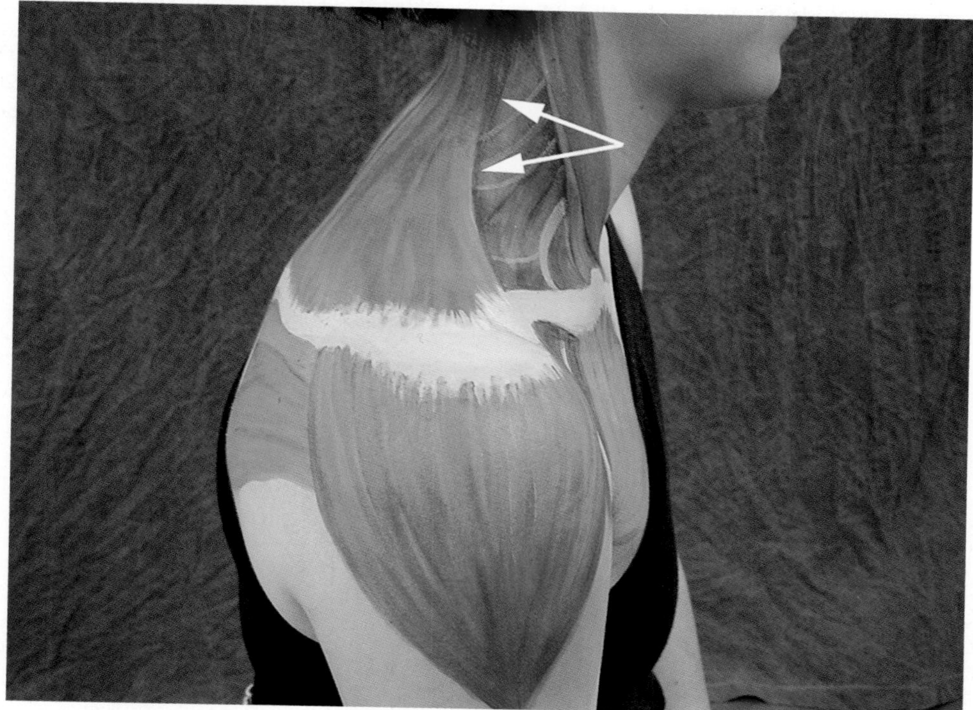

FIGURE 1-24 The *arrows* indicate the posterior border of the levator scapulae muscle.

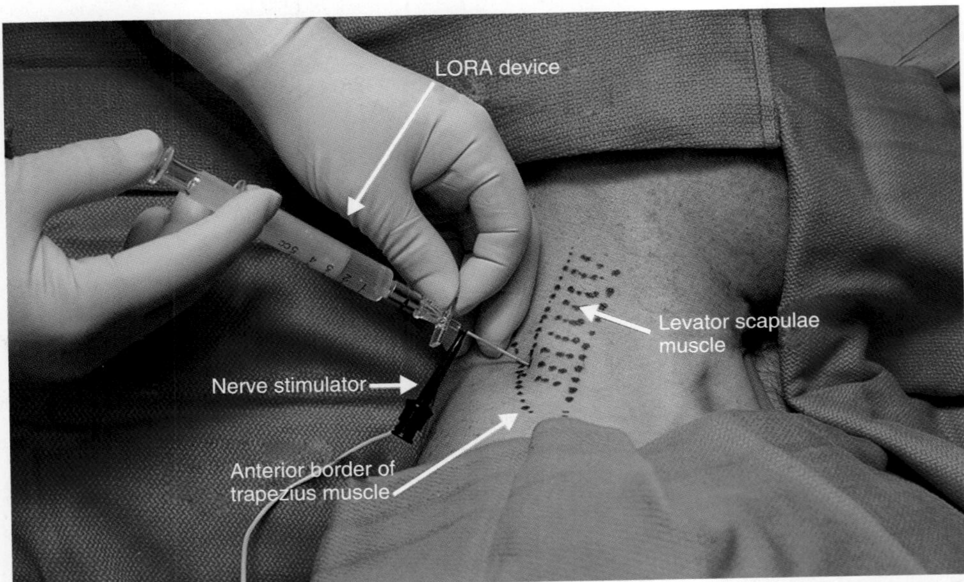

FIGURE 1-25 Needle entry is in the apex of the "V" formed by the anterior border of the trapezius muscle and the posterior border of the levator scapulae muscle. The needle is aimed at the suprasternal notch. A loss–of–resistance-to-air syringe and nerve stimulator are applied to the needle.

SUGGESTED FURTHER READING

1. Gray's Anatomy: The Anatomical Basis of Clinical Practice, 39th ed. Philadelphia, Elsevier, 2005.
2. Netter FH: Atlas of Human Anatomy, 2nd ed. East Hanover, NJ, Novartis, 1997.
3. Abrahams PH, Marks SC Jr, Hutchings RT: McMinn's Color Atlas of Human Anatomy, 5th ed. Philadelphia, Elsevier Mosby, 2003.
4. Boezaart AP: Anesthesia and Orthopaedic Surgery. New York, McGraw-Hill, 2006.
5. Hadzic A, Vloka JD: Peripheral Nerve Blocks: Principles and Practice. New York, McGraw-Hill, 2004.
6. Rathmell JP, Neal JM, Viscomi CM: Regional Anesthesia: The Requisites in Anesthesia. Philadelphia, Elsevier Mosby, 2004.
7. Brown DL: Atlas of Regional Anesthesia, 3rd ed. Philadelphia, Elsevier, 2006.
8. Barret J, Harmon D, Loughnane B, et al: Peripheral Nerve Blocks and Peri-operative Pain Relief. Philadelphia, WB Saunders, 2004.
9. Meier G, Büttner J: Atlas der peripheren Regionalanästhesie. Stuttgart, Georg Thieme Verlag, 2004.
10. Hahn MB, McQuillan PM, Sheplock GJ: Regional Anesthesia: An Atlas of Anatomy and Technique. St. Louis, Mosby, 1996.

Chapter 2

Interscalene Blocks

- Single-Injection Interscalene Block
- Continuous Interscalene Block

SINGLE-INJECTION INTERSCALENE BLOCK

Introduction

Single-injection interscalene block is done almost entirely for pain associated with shoulder surgery. This block usually is not indicated for surgery of the upper extremity distal to the shoulder joint. The approach used in this description is the longitudinal approach or lateral approach (1-3). This approach is used to avoid possible entry into the vertebral neuroforamina.

It is important to realize that continuous pain, paresthesia, and dysesthesia distal to the elbow are almost never symptoms of bona fide shoulder disease (4) (see Chapter 19). These symptoms almost always indicate an existing brachial plexopathy, and care should be taken in patients presenting with shoulder pain who also have pain distal to the elbow. Special care should be taken in patients presenting with primary frozen shoulder or "adhesive capsulitis". This condition is a fibromatosis like Dupuytren's disease, which in itself should not be painful if it is not in the acute phase. The pain of primary frozen shoulder is possibly caused by traction on the brachial plexus due to rotation of the scapula (see Chapter 19).

The clinician should be cautious of the patient scheduled for subacromial decompression without a clear diagnosis. The exact diagnosis of the shoulder lesion is often unclear in patients with existing brachial plexopathy. Interscalene block can potentially aggravate this condition (see Chapter 19).

Specific Anatomic Considerations

The osteotomes included in this block are illustrated in Figure 2-1. When studying this illustration, it should be clear that the inferior part of the glenoid, as well as the distal part of the ulna and the bones of the fourth and fifth fingers, are usually not included by interscalene block unless large volumes of local anesthetic agent are used. Also compare this figure with Figure 1-3, and note that the cephalad part of the clavicle is innervated by the C8-T1 osteotomes.

The C5, C6, and C7 dermatomes are usually included in interscalene block, but the C8 and T1 dermatomes usually are not included (Fig. 2-2).

The neurotomes involved in interscalene block include the neurotomes of the axillary, radial, musculocutaneous, and the median nerves (Fig. 2-3). The ulnar nerve and brachial and antebrachial cutaneous nerves are usually not included. Similarly, the intercostal brachial nerves are excluded.

Technique

The patient is placed in the supine position with the head slightly turned away from the operative side, and the patient's hand on the operative side is placed on the abdomen (Fig. 2-4).

The posterior border of the sternocleidomastoid muscle, the external jugular vein (*dotted line*), and the clavicle are marked (Fig. 2-5).

Before the skin is penetrated with the needle, all the nerves in the posterior triangle of the neck can be mapped transcutaneously (1,5). This can be done with a special probe (Fig. 2-6A) or with the tip of the needle (Fig. 2-6B). The nerve stimulator is typically set at 5 to 10 mA for this nerve mapping (5). The operator stands at the head, facing the patient's feet.

The clavicle forms the caudal border or base of the posterior triangle of the neck, and the circled area in Figure 2-7 indicates the position of the superficial cervical plexus.

After disinfecting the skin with an antiseptic agent, the superficial cervical plexus is blocked just behind the midpoint of the sternocleidomastoid muscle (Fig. 2-7).

The anesthesiologist stands at the head of the table facing the patient's feet. The interscalene groove is palpated with the index and middle fingers in the area of Winnie's point (Fig. 2-8).

These two fingers are now split, leaving the middle finger in the interscalene groove (Fig. 2-9). This causes congestion of the external jugular vein, which makes it easy to identify, and the index finger applies traction to tighten the skin for easy needle penetration.

The needle enters behind the sternocleidomastoid muscle approximately midway between the clavicle and the mastoid process, and is aimed at the brachial plexus, which is deep to the middle finger of the operator's left hand (Fig. 2-10). The needle enters longitudinally and is typically aimed approximately at the nipple on the ipsilateral side or at the midpoint of the clavicle.

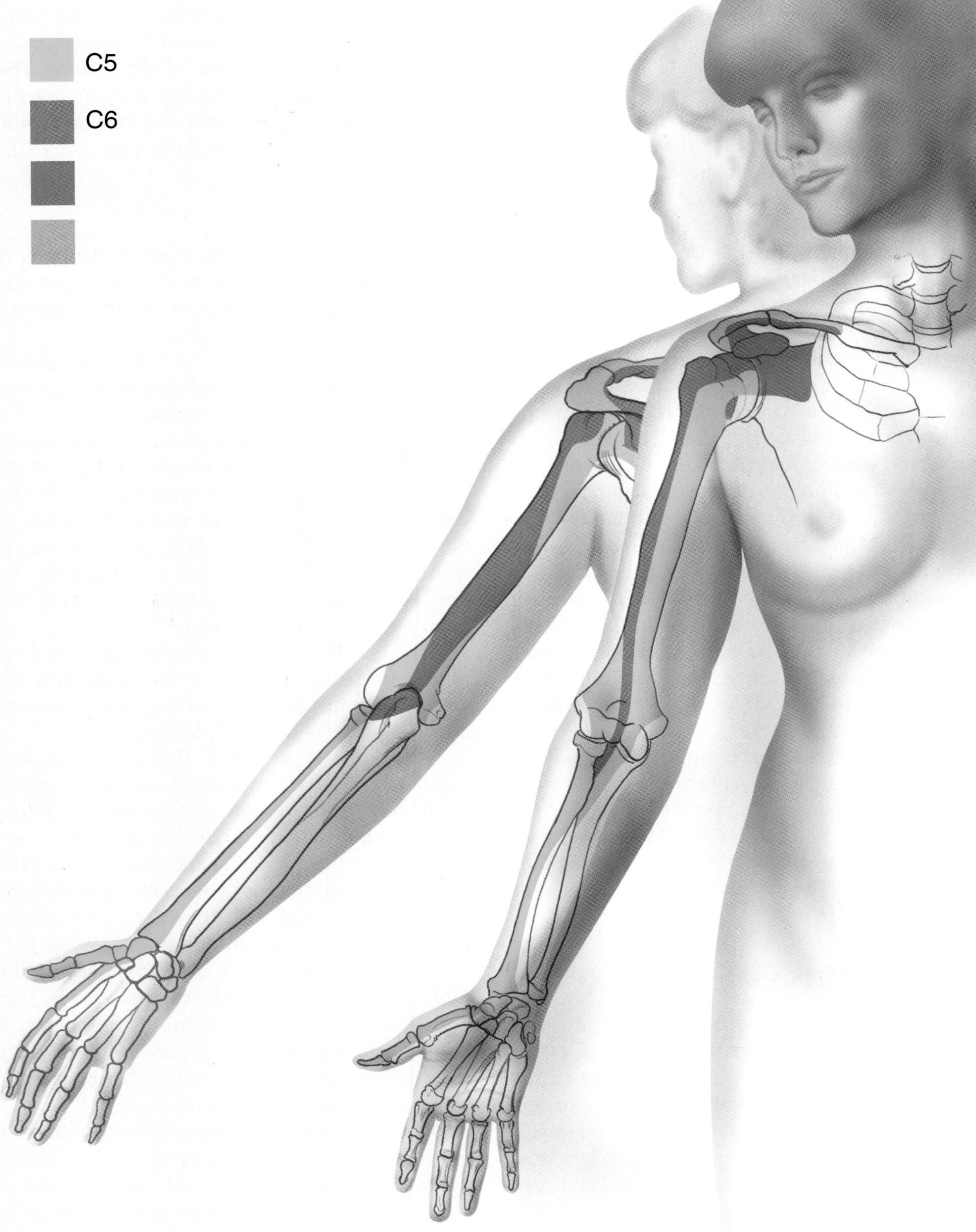

FIGURE 2-1 Osteotomes blocked by the interscalene block.

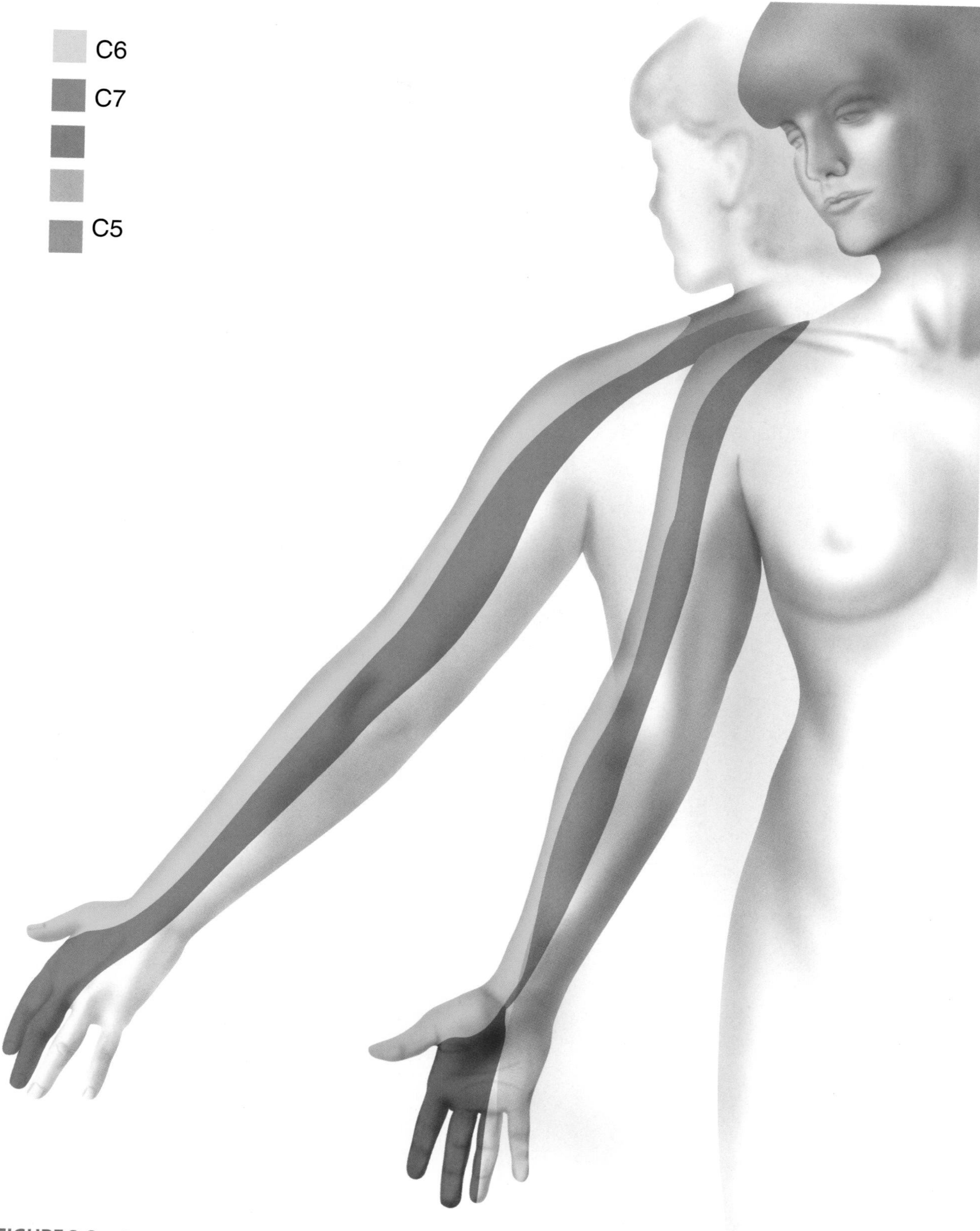

FIGURE 2-2 Dermatomes blocked by the interscalene block.

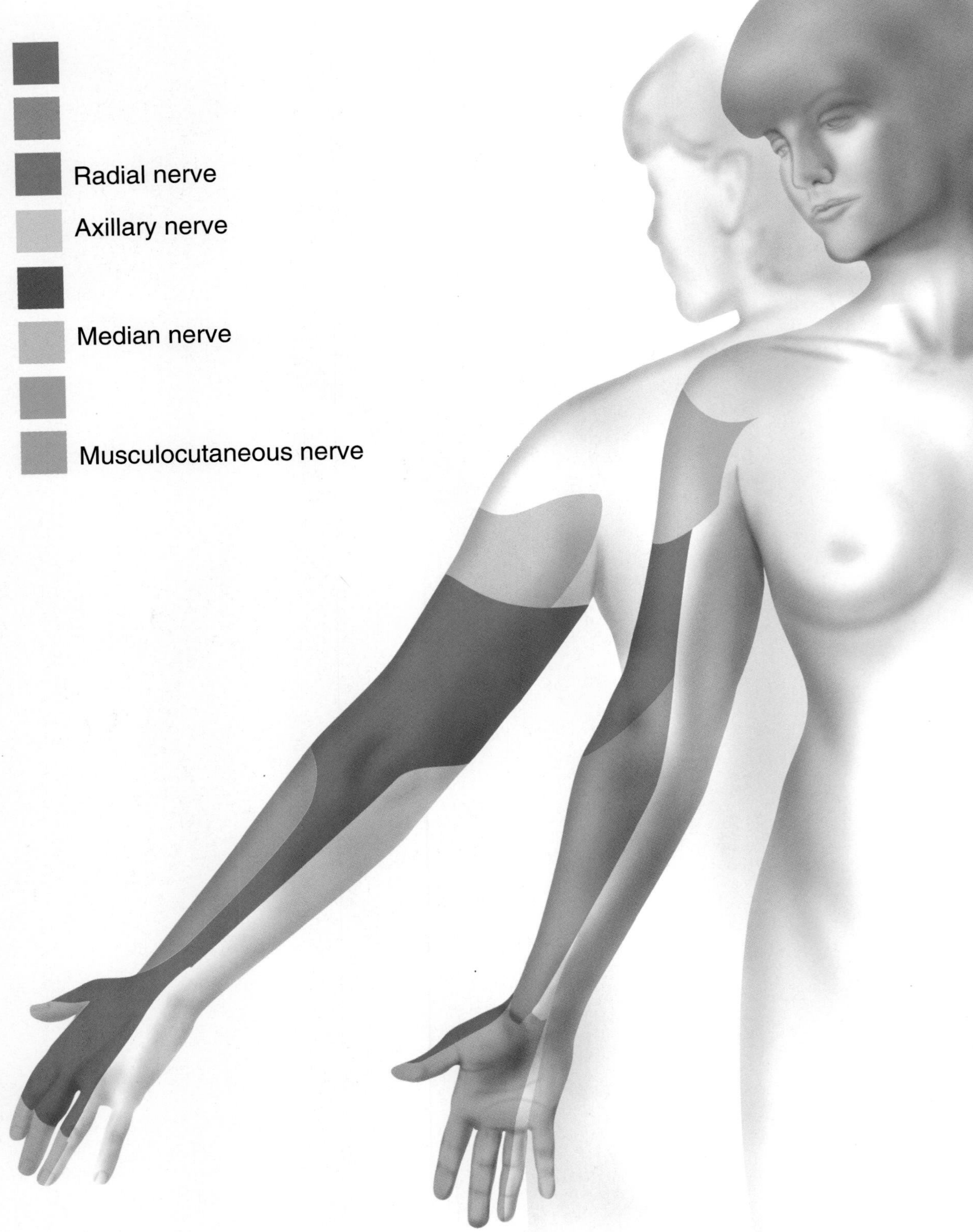

FIGURE 2-3 Neurotomes blocked by the interscalene block.

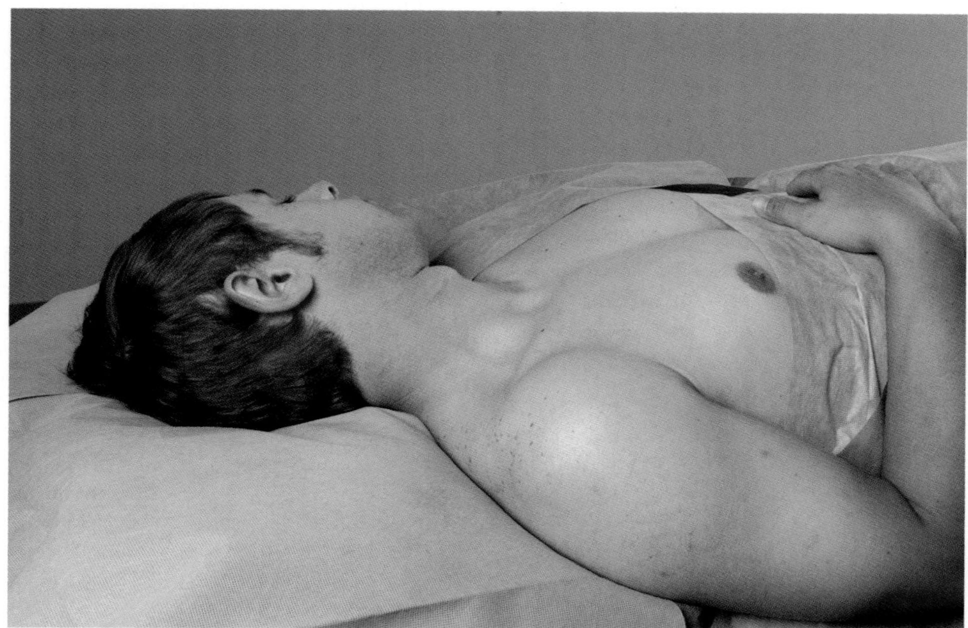

FIGURE 2-4 The patient is positioned in the supine position with the head turned slightly away from the operative side.

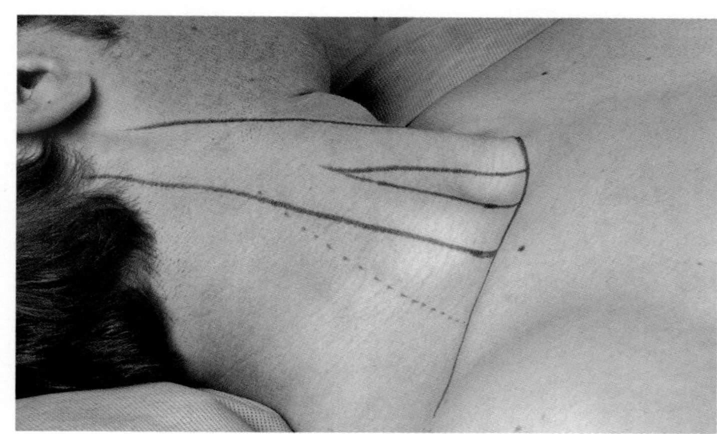

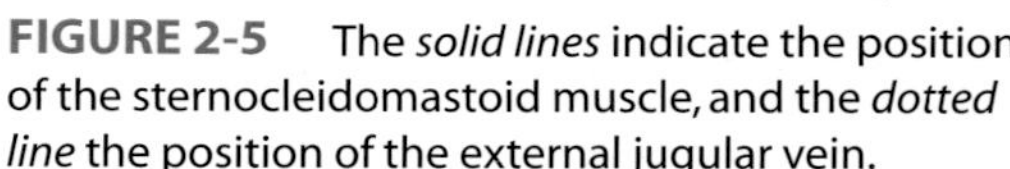

FIGURE 2-5 The *solid lines* indicate the position of the sternocleidomastoid muscle, and the *dotted line* the position of the external jugular vein.

If the needle is aimed too anterior, the phrenic nerve will be stimulated and an unmistakable diaphragmatic motor response will be noticed.

The nerve stimulator is typically set at 1 to 2 mA, 2 Hz, and a 100- to 300-μsec pulse width at this stage.

Contact with the brachial plexus will cause either a triceps or biceps motor response as the proximal (triceps) or distal (biceps) aspect of the superior trunk of the brachial plexus is encountered. If the phrenic nerve is encountered, there will be an unmistakable motor response of the abdomen as the diaphragm contracts, and the needle must be withdrawn slightly and redirected approximately 0.5 to 1 cm more posteriorly. If, on the other hand, the rhomboid muscles contract, the dorsal scapular nerve has been stimulated and the needle must, after slight withdrawal, be moved approximately 0.5 to 1 cm more anteriorly.

When the brachial plexus is stimulated and a brisk biceps or triceps motor response is demonstrated, the nerve stimulator is turned down to approximately 0.3 to 0.5 mA, and the brisk motor response should still be seen in the biceps or triceps muscle. If this brisk motor response is still present at 0.2 mA, it may indicate intraneural

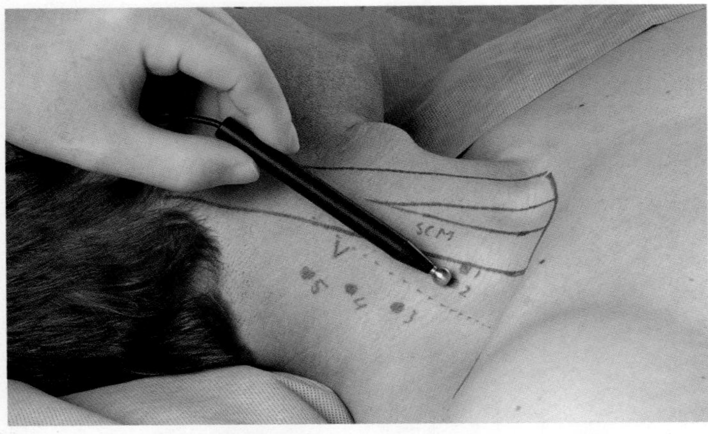

A

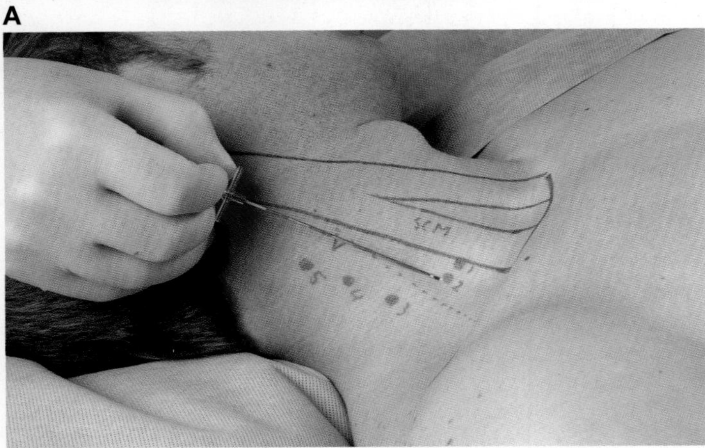

B

FIGURE 2-6 **A,** A dedicated probe is used to stimulate the nerves in the posterior triangle of the neck transcutaneously. SCM, sternocleidomastoid muscle; V, jugular vein; 1, position of the phrenic nerve; 2, brachial plexus; 3, position of the dorsal scapular nerve; 4, position of the nerve to the levator scapulae; 5, position of the accessory nerve. **B,** The needle can also be used for transcutaneous stimulation or mapping of the nerves in the posterior triangle of the neck.

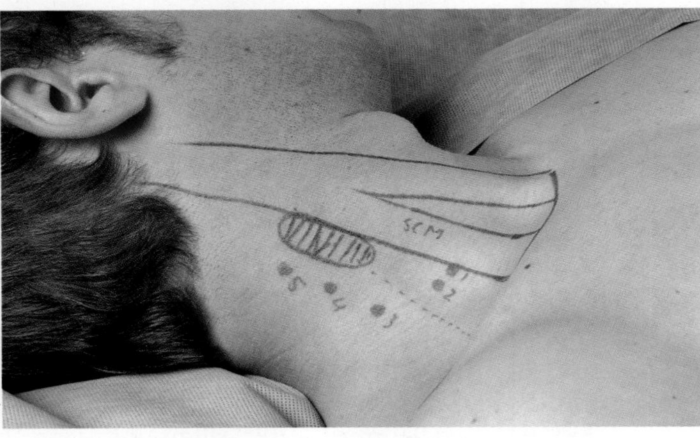

FIGURE 2-7 The *oval* indicates the position of the superficial cervical plexus as it exits behind the midpoint of the clavicular head of the sternocleidomastoid muscle.

needle placement and the needle should be withdrawn 1 or 2 mm. Brisk muscle twitches should ideally be seen at a nerve stimulator output setting of 0.3 to 0.5 mA. A motor response of the hand flexors or extensors or deltoid or pectoral muscles may also be accepted.

A positive Raj test is obtained when the motor response immediately ceases after injection of the local anesthetic agent or normal saline. This block is also ideally suited to the use of ultrasound (Figure 2-11).

Local Anesthetic Agent Choice

Amounts ranging from 15 to 60 mL of all known regional anesthetic agents have been used for

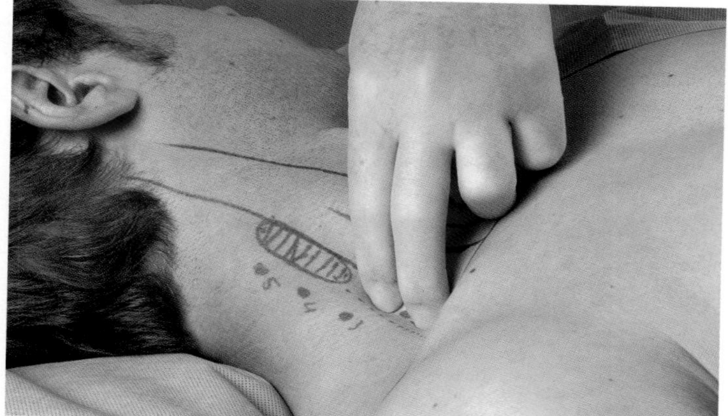

FIGURE 2-8 The groove between the anterior and middle scalene muscle is palpated.

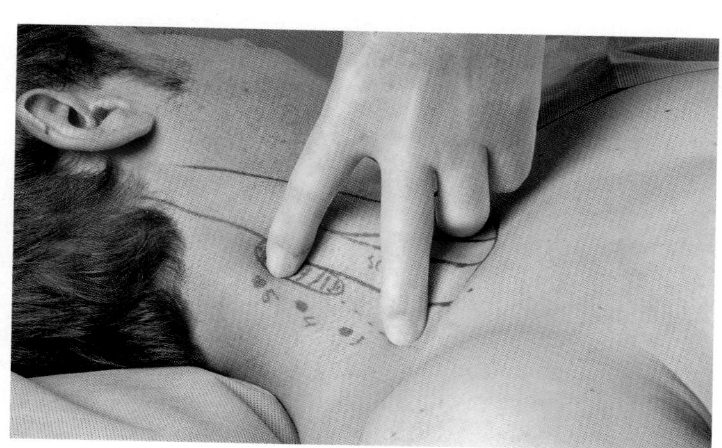

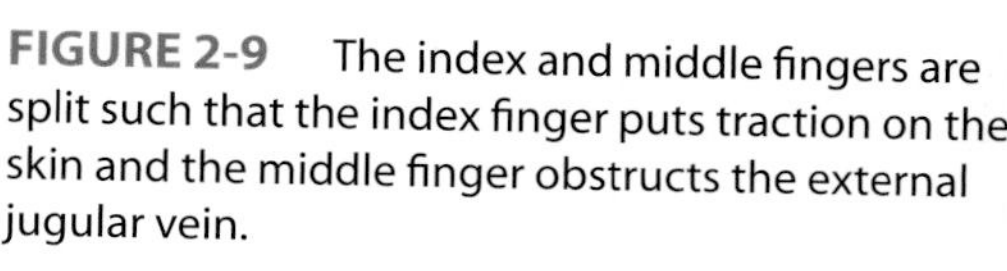

FIGURE 2-9 The index and middle fingers are split such that the index finger puts traction on the skin and the middle finger obstructs the external jugular vein.

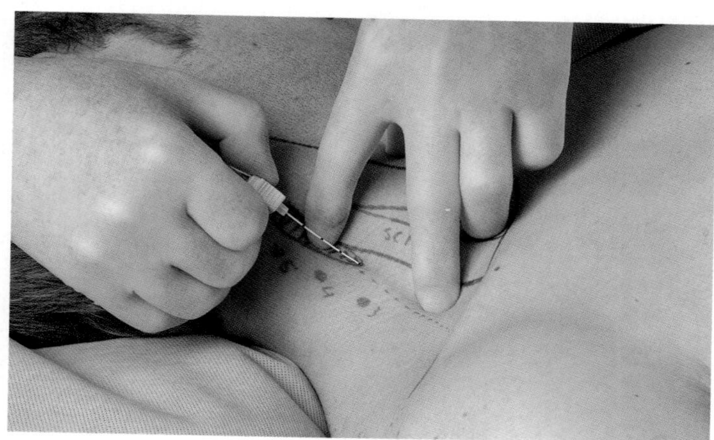

FIGURE 2-10 A 22-gauge stimulating needle, attached to a nerve stimulator, enters the skin, avoiding the jugular vein, and is aimed at the brachial plexus deep to the operator's middle finger.

single-injection interscalene block. The choice of this author is 20 to 40 mL of ropivacaine 0.5% to 0.75% or 20 to 40 mL bupivacaine 0.5%. The addition of buprenorphine may increase the block's duration of action up to threefold (6), but if a long-lasting block is required, it is advisable to place a catheter for continuous infusion (1).

(See single-injection interscalene block movie on DVD.)

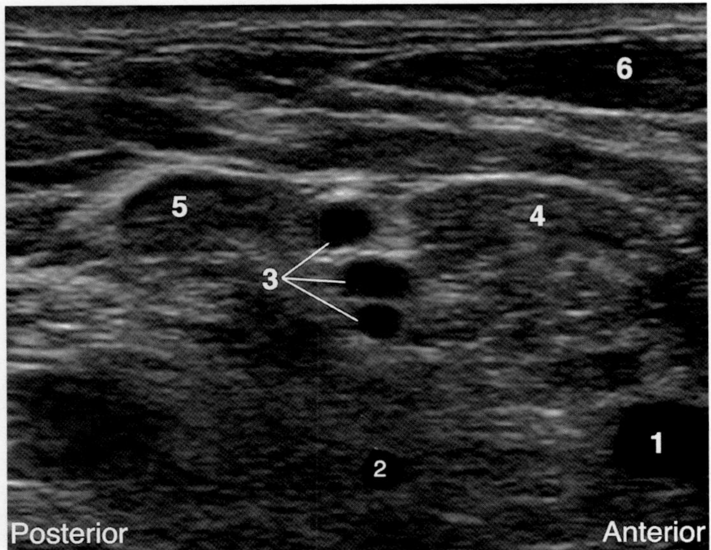

FIGURE 2-11 Transverse sonogram of the interscalene area: 1. Subclavian artery; 2. Vertebral artery; 3. Trunks of the brachial plexus; 4. Anterior scalene muscle; 5. Middle scalene muscle; 6. Sternocleidomastoid muscle.

CONTINUOUS INTERSCALENE BLOCK

Introduction

The continuous interscalene block is indicated for intraoperative and postoperative pain management in major shoulder surgery (1-3) such as shoulder arthroplasty and rotator cuff repair. This block should be used with caution in patients with frozen shoulder and is not indicated for conditions that are not painful for an extended period, such as arthroscopic subacromial decompression (4) (see Chapter 19). The same concerns regarding existing brachial plexopathy that were discussed for single-injection interscalene block apply for continuous interscalene block, and great care should be taken to protect other threatened nerves in the insensate arm. Nerves commonly injured by pressure (e.g., on the bed in the supine position) or poorly fitted arm slings are the ulnar nerve at the elbow or the radial nerve as it curls around the elbow. The use of an arm sling is important to prevent traction injury to the brachial plexus.

Specific Anatomic Considerations

The osteotomes (see Fig. 2-1), dermatomes (see Fig. 2-2), and neurotomes (see Fig. 2-3) shown for the single-injection interscalene block are similar to those for the continuous interscalene block. It should, however, be noted that although a wider spread of local anesthetic will be present during high-volume initial bolus injections, the area of block coverage will be smaller and more nerve-specific during the infusion of a smaller volume of a more dilute regional anesthetic agent.

Technique

The positioning of the patient (see Fig. 2-4), surface anatomy, and skin markings (see Fig. 2-5) are similar to those for a single-injection interscalene nerve block.

The area is covered with a fenestrated, clear, sterile plastic drape after skin preparation (Fig. 2-12).

For continuous interscalene nerve block, perform a superficial cervical plexus block (Fig. 2-13A) and anesthetize the path intended for subcutaneous tunneling (Fig. 2-13B). In this case, the path is toward the suprasternal notch. Make sure not to injure the external jugular vein with the needle.

The nerve stimulator, set at a current output of 5 to 10 mA, a frequency of 2 Hz, and a pulse width of 200 to 300 μsec, is clipped to the proximal end of an insulated 17-gauge Tuohy needle. The position of the brachial plexus and all the other nerves in the posterior triangle of the neck can now be confirmed by transcutaneous stimulation using the flat side of the tip of the Tuohy needle, or a specially manufactured probe as illustrated in Figure 2-6A. Once nerve positions are confirmed, the nerve stimulator is turned down to 1 to 2 mA.

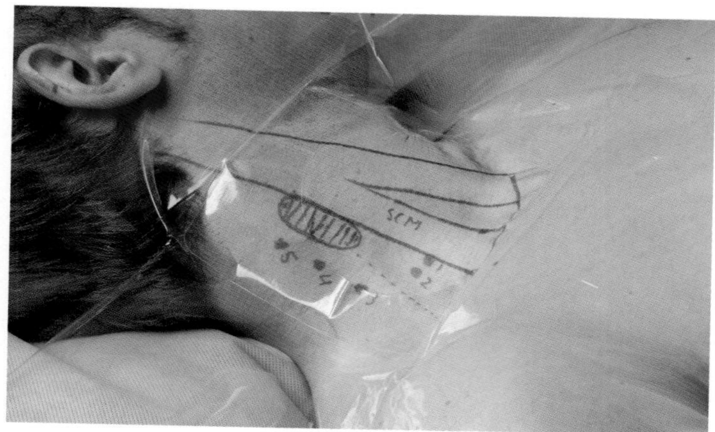

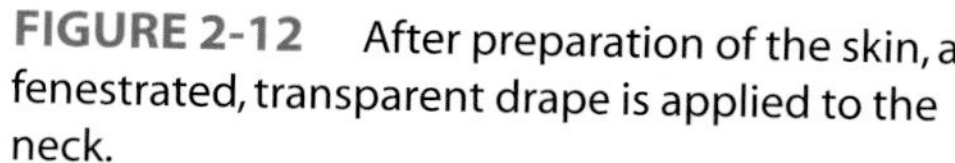

FIGURE 2-12 After preparation of the skin, a fenestrated, transparent drape is applied to the neck.

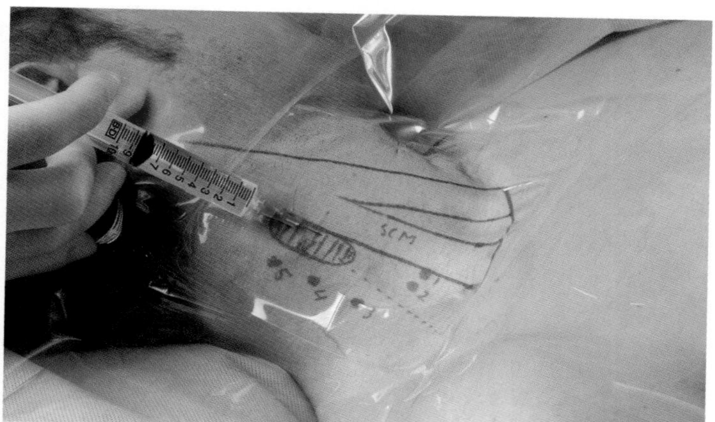

A

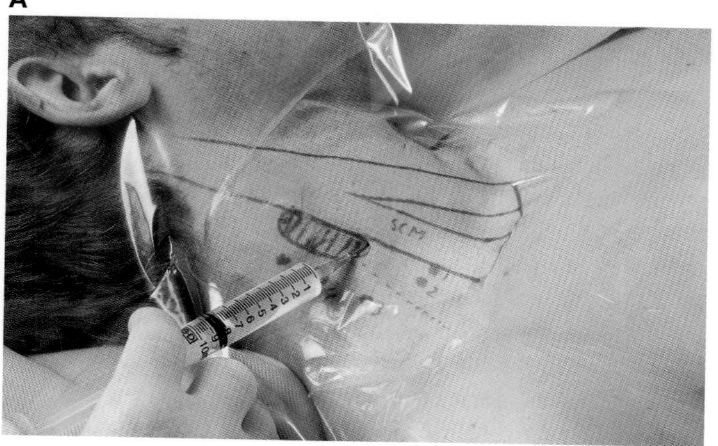

B

FIGURE 2-13 **A,** The superficial cervical plexus is blocked. **B,** The intended path for tunneling of the catheter is also anesthetized, taking care not to injure the external jugular vein.

The interscalene groove is palpated with the middle and index fingers and the fingers are split to put traction on the skin, leaving the middle finger in the interscalene groove (Fig. 2-14).

Needle entry is from behind the sternocleidomastoid muscle, halfway from the clavicle to the mastoid (Fig. 2-15). Ultrasound imaging can also be used (see Fig. 2-11). The needle entry is longitudinal, aiming toward the brachial plexus just deep to where the left-hand middle finger is placed. This is generally in the direction of the midpoint of the ipsilateral clavicle.

The phrenic nerve may be encountered, which causes unmistakable abdominal twitches

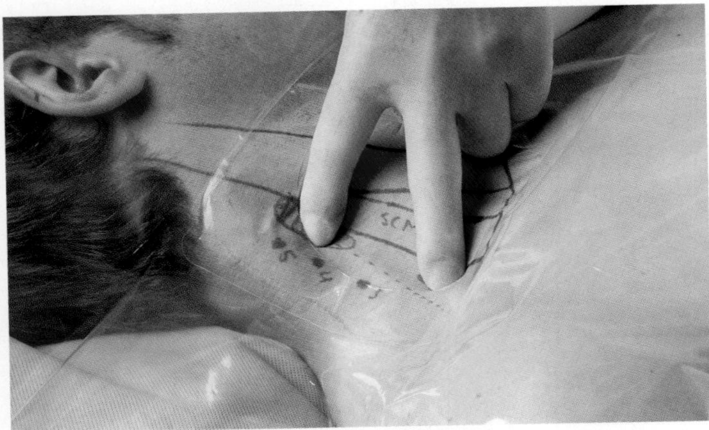

FIGURE 2-14 The index and middle fingers of the nonoperative hand palpate the groove between the anterior and middle scalene muscles, and the fingers are split such that the index finger applies traction to the skin and the middle finger remains in the groove between the two scalene muscles.

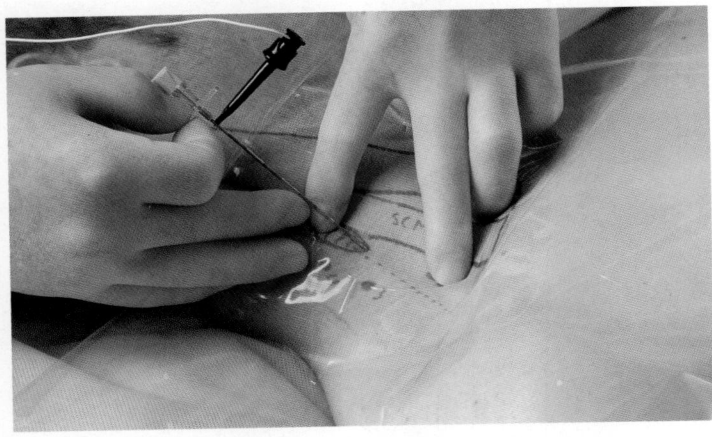

FIGURE 2-15 Needle entry is caudal to the external jugular vein and aimed at the brachial plexus deep to the operator's middle finger. The nerve stimulator is attached to the Tuohy needle.

because of a diaphragm motor response. The needle is then withdrawn slightly and moved approximately 0.5 to 1 cm posteriorly until the biceps or triceps muscle is twitching, which indicates stimulation of the superior or middle trunk of the brachial plexus. The nerve stimulator can then be turned down and a clear, brisk motor response should still be present at 0.3 to 0.5 mA. This indicates correct needle placement. It is essential that no saline or local anesthetic agent be injected through the needle at this stage because this will make later nerve stimulation through the catheter impossible or very difficult. If the anesthesiologist does subscribe to the notion that fluid "opens up the space," 5% dextrose in water can be used (7). This fluid, unlike normal saline, does not conduct electricity and therefore will not obliterate the electrical nerve stimulation response by dispersing the current density, as saline does.

If the needle tip is placed too far posterior, the dorsal scapular nerve will be encountered. This is indicated by contractions of the rhomboid muscles, which can easily be mistaken for deltoid muscle contractions.

Once the brachial plexus is identified with the needle, the stylet of the needle is removed (Fig. 2-16), the nerve stimulator is attached to the proximal end of the stimulating catheter, and the distal end of the catheter is placed inside the needle shaft (Fig. 2-17).

The special mark on the catheter, in this case a broad black mark, situated at the needle hub indicates that the catheter's tip is now situated at the tip of the needle (Fig. 2-18).

The catheter is advanced beyond the needle tip (Fig. 2-19).

If the motor response stops or decreases, carefully withdraw the catheter to inside the needle shaft again (Fig. 2-20).

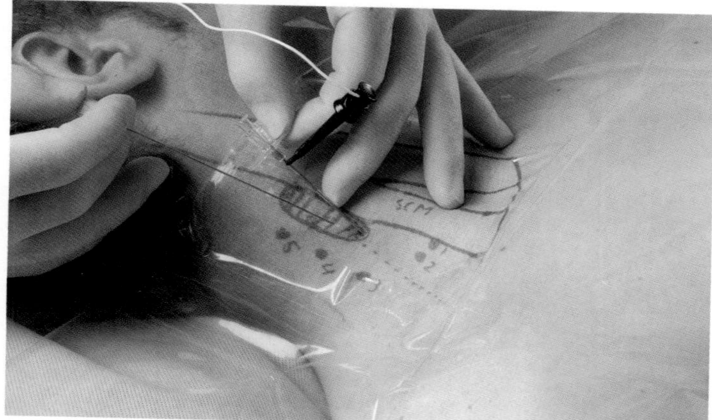

FIGURE 2-16 After an optimal motor response is obtained, the stylet is removed from the needle.

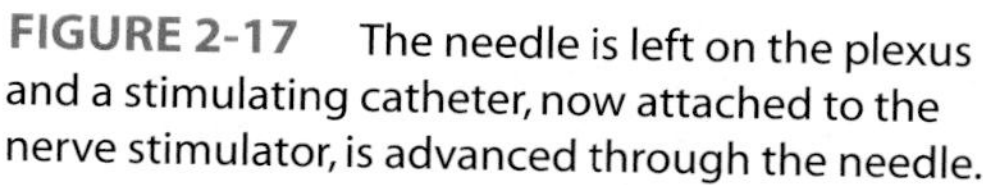
FIGURE 2-17 The needle is left on the plexus and a stimulating catheter, now attached to the nerve stimulator, is advanced through the needle.

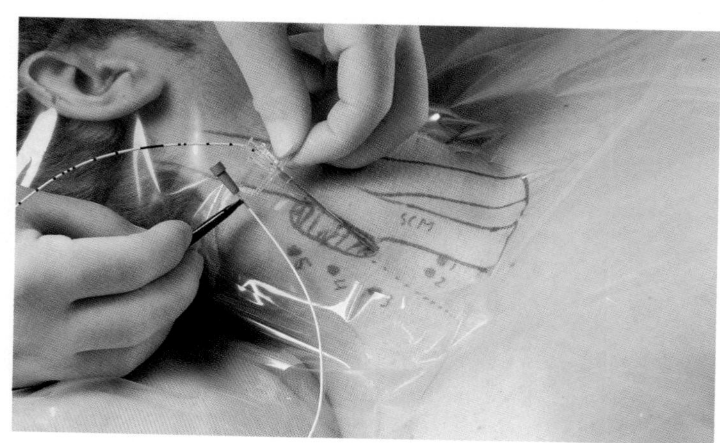

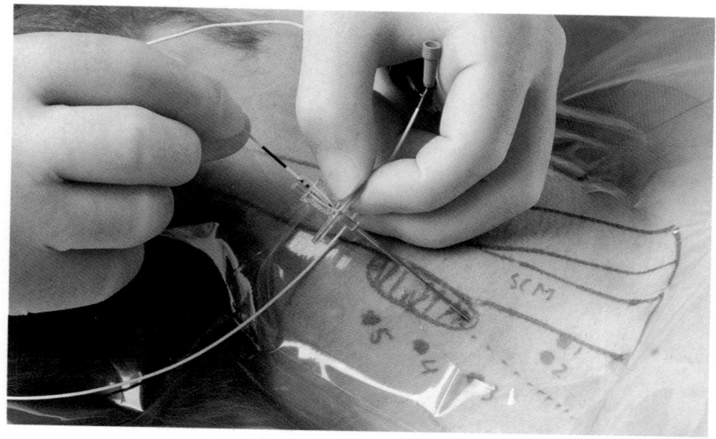

FIGURE 2-18 The special marking on the catheter indicates whether the tip of the catheter protrudes beyond the needle tip. Note that the nerve stimulator and proximal end of the catheter are held in the palm of the operator's left hand.

Rotate the needle a quarter of a turn clockwise or counterclockwise and advance the catheter again. If the motor response again disappears, withdraw the catheter again (Fig. 2-21), turn the needle in the opposite direction, and try again. Repeat this maneuver by rotating the needle, withdrawing the needle slightly, or advancing the needle slightly, until the motor response remains constant and brisk during advancement of the catheter.

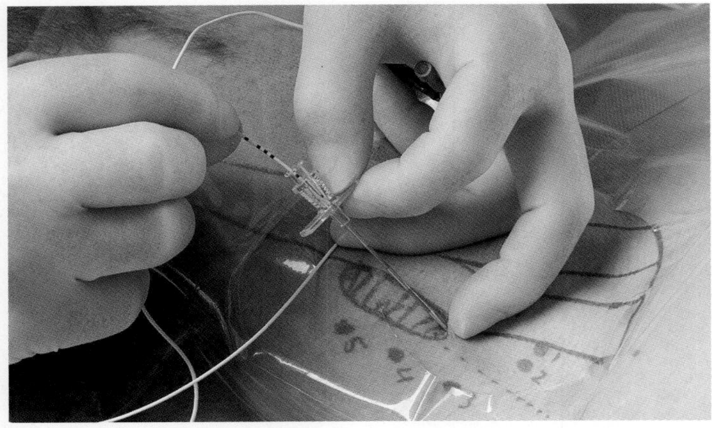

FIGURE 2-19 If the catheter is advanced so that the special mark on the catheter can no longer be seen, it means that the tip of the catheter has been advanced beyond the tip of the needle.

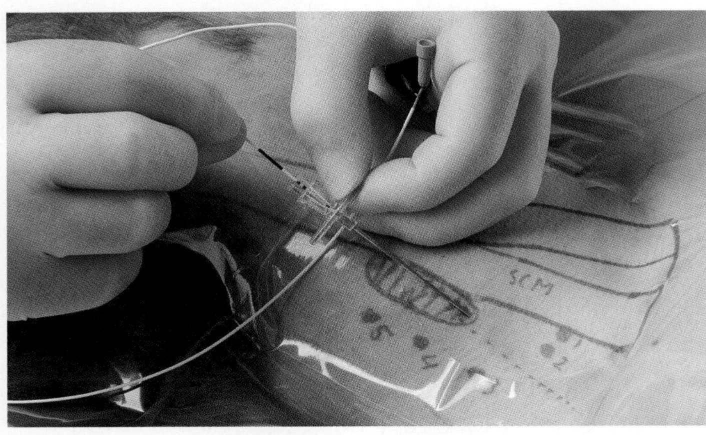

FIGURE 2-20 Should the motor response disappear, the catheter is carefully withdrawn until the special mark on the catheter is visible again. This means that the tip of the catheter is now inside the needle shaft and the needle can be safely manipulated.

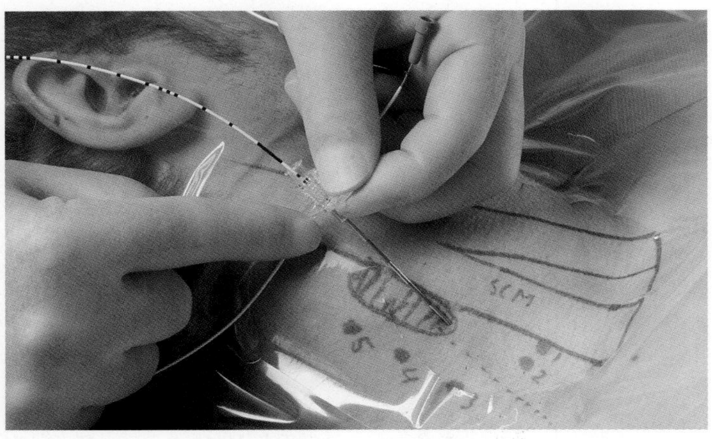

FIGURE 2-21 With the special mark on the catheter visible, the needle is now manipulated—in this case, turned a quarter turn clockwise—and the catheter is advanced again.

Make sure that the catheter is always withdrawn to inside the needle shaft before the needle is manipulated. Figure 2-22A shows the special marking on the catheter visible, which indicates that the tip of the catheter does not protrude beyond the needle tip. Figure 2-22B illustrates the catheter protruding beyond the needle tip, and the special marking on the catheter is no longer visible. This is an important concept because maneuvering the catheter while it protrudes

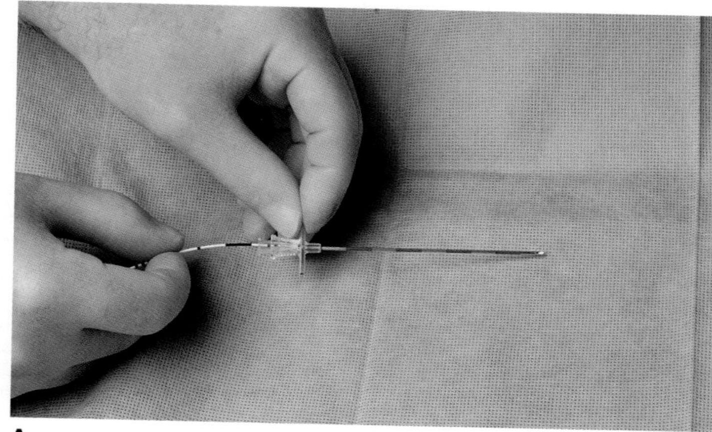
A

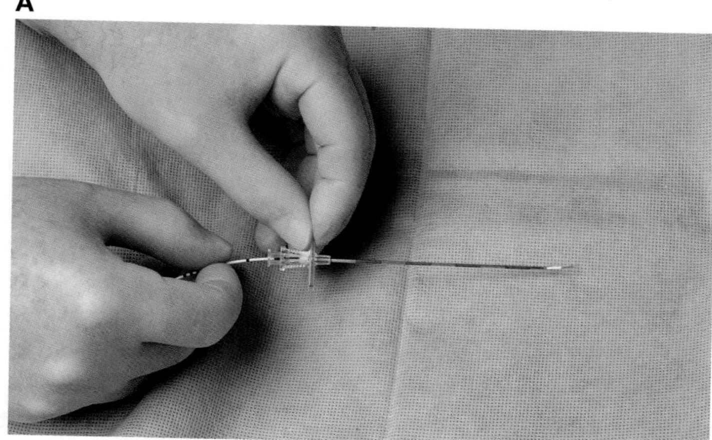
B

FIGURE 2-22 **A,** When the special mark on the catheter is visible outside the hub of the needle, the tip of the catheter has not yet reached the needle tip. **B,** If the special mark on the catheter disappears within the hub of the needle, it indicates that the catheter is now protruding beyond the tip of the needle.

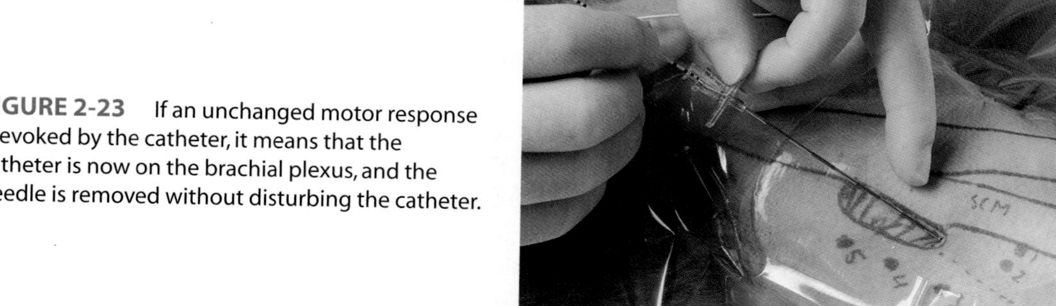

FIGURE 2-23 If an unchanged motor response is evoked by the catheter, it means that the catheter is now on the brachial plexus, and the needle is removed without disturbing the catheter.

beyond the needle tip can lead to shearing of the catheter. All makes of stimulating catheters have a marking indicating when the catheter tip leaves the needle tip.

The needle is removed without disturbing the catheter, similar to epidural catheterization (Fig. 2-23).

The catheter can now be tested again by attaching the nerve stimulator to its proximal end (Fig. 2-24). It should then be tunneled subcutaneously to prevent catheter dislodgement.

As illustrated in Chapter 12, the inner stylet of the needle is placed subcutaneously from a point approximately 1 to 2 mm from the catheter

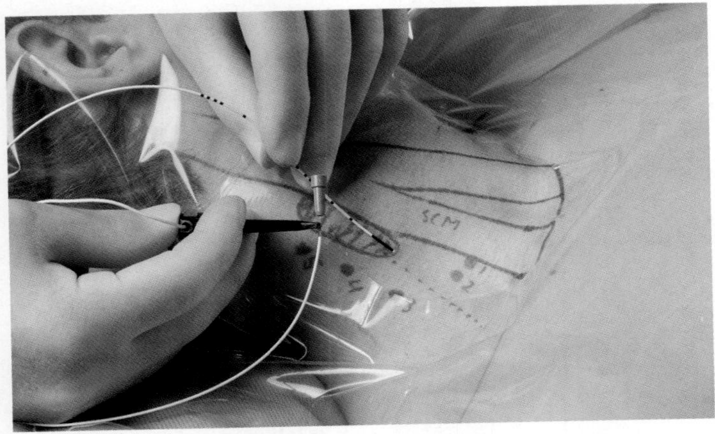

FIGURE 2-24 After removal of the needle, the position of the catheter can be tested again by attaching its proximal end to the nerve stimulator.

exit site toward the suprasternal notch, taking care not to puncture the external jugular vein by going deep to it. If a skin bridge is not required, the stylet of the needle enters through the same catheter exit site, taking care not to damage the catheter.

The needle is then "railroaded" back over the stylet while still taking special care not to disturb or damage the catheter.

The catheter is advanced retrograde through the needle and the needle is removed, leaving a loop of catheter at the original catheter exit site. The catheter is situated deep to the external jugular vein and exits in the area of the suprasternal notch.

Place the piece of silicone tubing that protected the catheter tip while it was packaged in the loop to protect the skin bridge (see Chapter 12).The skin bridge makes removal of the catheter easier.

If a skin bridge is not used, the catheter is "buried" under the skin.

Place the Luer lock connecting device on the proximal end of the catheter and attach the nerve stimulator and the syringe with the local anesthetic agent to the connecting device (Fig. 2-25). The nerve stimulator is set to an output of zero and then slowly turned up until a motor response can just be seen.

The motor response ceases immediately after the injection is started. This constitutes a positive Raj test, which further ensures that the secondary block through the catheter as well as the primary block will be successful.

Place the connecting device and catheter in the fixation device (see Chapter 18) or similar device, and place this on the contralateral shoulder of the patient in a convenient location.

Cover the catheter with a transparent adhesive dressing to enable daily inspection of the catheter exit site.

Local Anesthetic Agent and Infusion Choice

Most authors use 20 to 40 mL ropivacaine 0.5% to 0.75%, bupivacaine 0.5%, or levobupivacaine 0.5% for intraoperative analgesia, and an infusion of 0.2% of the same drug is usually used for the management of postoperative pain. There are various infusion strategies, but it should be successful to start with 0.2% ropivacaine or 0.25% bupivacaine at 5 mL/hour. Additional patient-controlled regional anesthesia consisting of 2- to 10-mL boluses at a lockout time of 30 to 60 minutes can be used.

There is a spectrum of infusion strategies, and which is used depends on the desired effect. For example, the infusion strategy for a rotator cuff repair, in which motor function is undesirable initially, would use a high volume and high concentration of local anesthetic drug initially, followed by a high infusion rate of a relatively high concentration of drug and zero or a small volume of patient-controlled boluses.

Adhesive capsulitis or frozen shoulder, on the other hand, would require a small volume and low concentration of the initial bolus drug

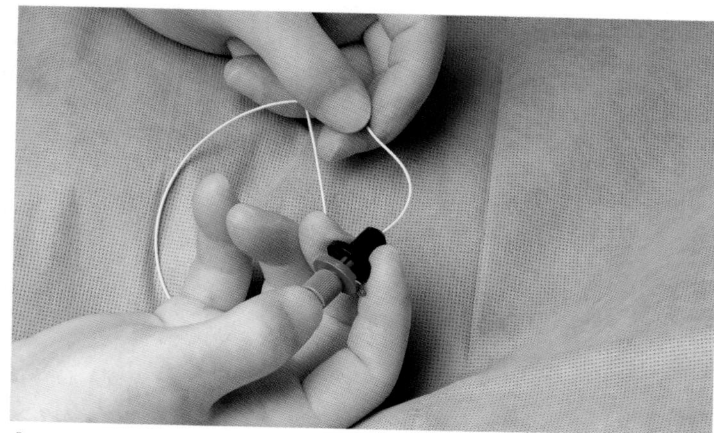

A

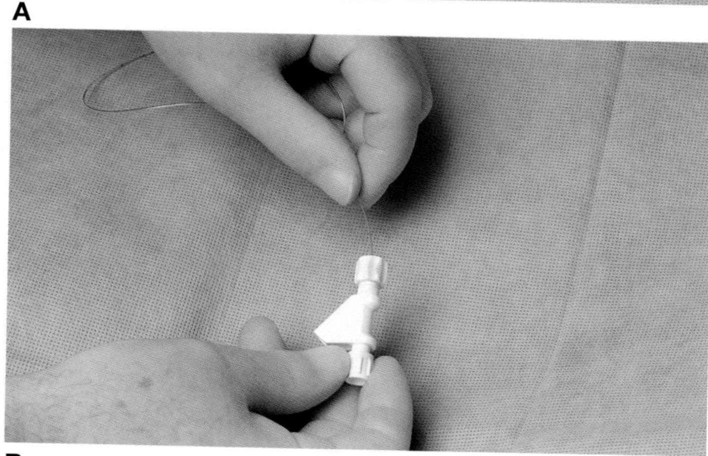

B

FIGURE 2-25 **A** and **B,** The Luer lock connecting device is attached to the proximal end of the catheter.

because motor function and patient participation in physical therapy are desirable, followed by a low infusion volume of a low-concentration drug, but a higher volume and concentration of patient-controlled boluses for physical therapy sessions. Ropivacaine is probably the drug of choice because of its motor-sparing properties. It may also be desirable to provide a higher infusion volume at nighttime so that patient-controlled boluses are unnecessary, thus ensuring that the patient has a good night's rest; a lower infusion rate and higher patient-controlled boluses can be reinstituted during the daytime.

Catheter Removal

Removal of the catheter is a sterile procedure (see Chapter 12).

Clean the skin bridge area with a suitable disinfectant. Hold the proximal part of the catheter with the left hand, fold the silicone tubing skin bridge around the catheter with the right hand, and remove the distal end of the catheter. Inspect the tip of the catheter for completeness, keep this part sterile, and with the left hand remove the entire catheter.

(See continuous interscalene block movie on DVD.)

REFERENCES

1. Boezaart AP, de Beer JF, du Toit C, et al: A new technique of continuous interscalene nerve block. Can J Anesth 1999;46:275-281.
2. Meier G, Bauereis Ch, Heinrich Ch: Der interscalenäre Plexuskatheter zur Anästhesie und postoperativen Schmerztherapie: Erfahrungen mit einer modifizierten Technik. Anaesthetist 1997;46:715-719.
3. Borgeat A, Ekatodramis G: Anaesthesia for shoulder surgery. Best Pract Res Anaesthesiol 2002;16:211-225.
4. Boezaart AP, Franco CD: Blocks above the clavicle. In: Boezaart AP (ed): Anesthesia and Orthopaedic Surgery. New York, McGraw-Hill, 2006, pp 291-309.

5. Bösenberg AT, Raw RM, Boezaart AP: Surface mapping of peripheral nerves in children with a nerve stimulator. Paediatr Anaesth 2002;12:398-403.
6. Candido KD, Winnie AP, Ghaleb AH, et al: Buprenorphine added to the local anesthetic for axillary brachial plexus block prolongs postoperative analgesia. Reg Anesth Pain Med 2002;27:162-167.
7. Tsui BC, Wagner A, Finucane B: Electrophysiologic effect of injectates on peripheral nerve stimulation. Reg Anesth Pain Med 2004;29:189-193.

Chapter 3

Cervical Paravertebral Block

- Single-Injection and Continuous Cervical Paravertebral Blocks

SINGLE-INJECTION AND CONTINUOUS CERVICAL PARAVERTEBRAL BLOCKS

Introduction

The cervical paravertebral block (CPVB) is indicated for painful conditions of the entire upper limb (1-4). It is specifically indicated for major shoulder, major elbow, and major wrist surgery, provides a more sensory than motor block, and has a wider distribution than the interscalene block because it is performed at the root level of the brachial plexus. It should not be done for minor surgery and relatively painless conditions. It is possible to place the cervical paravertebral after surgery using the loss-of-resistance-to-air or ultrasound technique without nerve stimulation. The techniques and equipment for single-injection CPVB and continuous CPVB are identical except for the placement of the catheter in the latter (4).

Specific Anatomic Considerations

The anatomic considerations for this block are discussed in Chapter 1.

The osteotomes included with this block are illustrated in Figure 3-1, while the dermatomes are illustrated in Figure 3-2, and the neurotomes in Figure 3-3 (see also Chapter 1).

Technique

The patient is positioned in the lateral decubitus or sitting position for this block (1-4). A line is drawn from the dorsal spine of C6 to the suprasternal notch (Fig. 3-4).

Needle entry is in the apex of the "V" formed by the trapezius and levator scapulae muscles and on the line drawn from the C6 dorsal spine to the suprasternal notch. First, identify the wide groove between the levator scapulae and trapezius muscles at the base of the skull (Fig. 3-5A). The circled number "7" on Figure 3-5A indicates the position of the dorsal spine of C7, and the "6" the dorsal spine of C6.

Then, while keeping the fingers in the groove, move downward (caudad; Fig. 3-5B) until the line connecting the dorsal spine and the suprasternal notch is reached (Fig. 3-5C). The solid line runs from the dorsal spine of C6 to the suprasternal notch, and the groove between the levator scapulae and trapezius muscles can be palpated. Make sure that this groove is not the groove anterior to the levator scapulae muscle, between the latter and the posterior scalene muscle. The correct groove is usually not more that 5 cm from the midline, but usually approximately 4 cm. If it were more than 5 cm, it would be wise to reassess the landmarks. The Pippa approach (5) is for single-injection CPVB and does not seek to avoid penetration of the extensor muscles of the neck. In the Pippa approach, needle entry is 3 cm from the midline, but this approach cannot be used for catheter placement for continuous nerve block. The needle entry point used by Sandefo and colleagues (5) and the use by Rettig and coworkers (6) of thin, sharp needles for paravertebral blocks have been criticized (7,8). For catheter placement, needle entry should be in the groove on the line between the front and middle finger on Figure 3-5C, as shown in Figure 3-5D. This is to avoid penetration of the often-tender extensor muscles of the neck. Penetration of these muscles for single-injection CPVB does not seem to cause pain and seems to be acceptable (5,6).

After skin preparation, the area is covered with a sterile, fenestrated, clear plastic drape (Fig. 3-6). The fingers of the nonoperative hand separate the muscles and a 25-gauge needle is used to anesthetize the skin and subcutaneous tissue. This needle remains on the plane of the line drawn between the C6 spinal process and the suprasternal notch.

The subcutaneous tissue is anesthetized liberally, but after direct subcutaneous injection, as a safety measure, no local anesthetic agent is injected until contact with the bony pars intervertebralis, articular column, or short transverse process of C6 is made. Only after contact with the bone should local anesthetic agent be injected, and only on withdrawal of the needle. This is done to prevent the theoretical possibility of intramedullary or subdural injection if the bony structures are missed and the needle is accidentally aimed too medially, or numbing of the plexus if the bony structures are missed laterally.

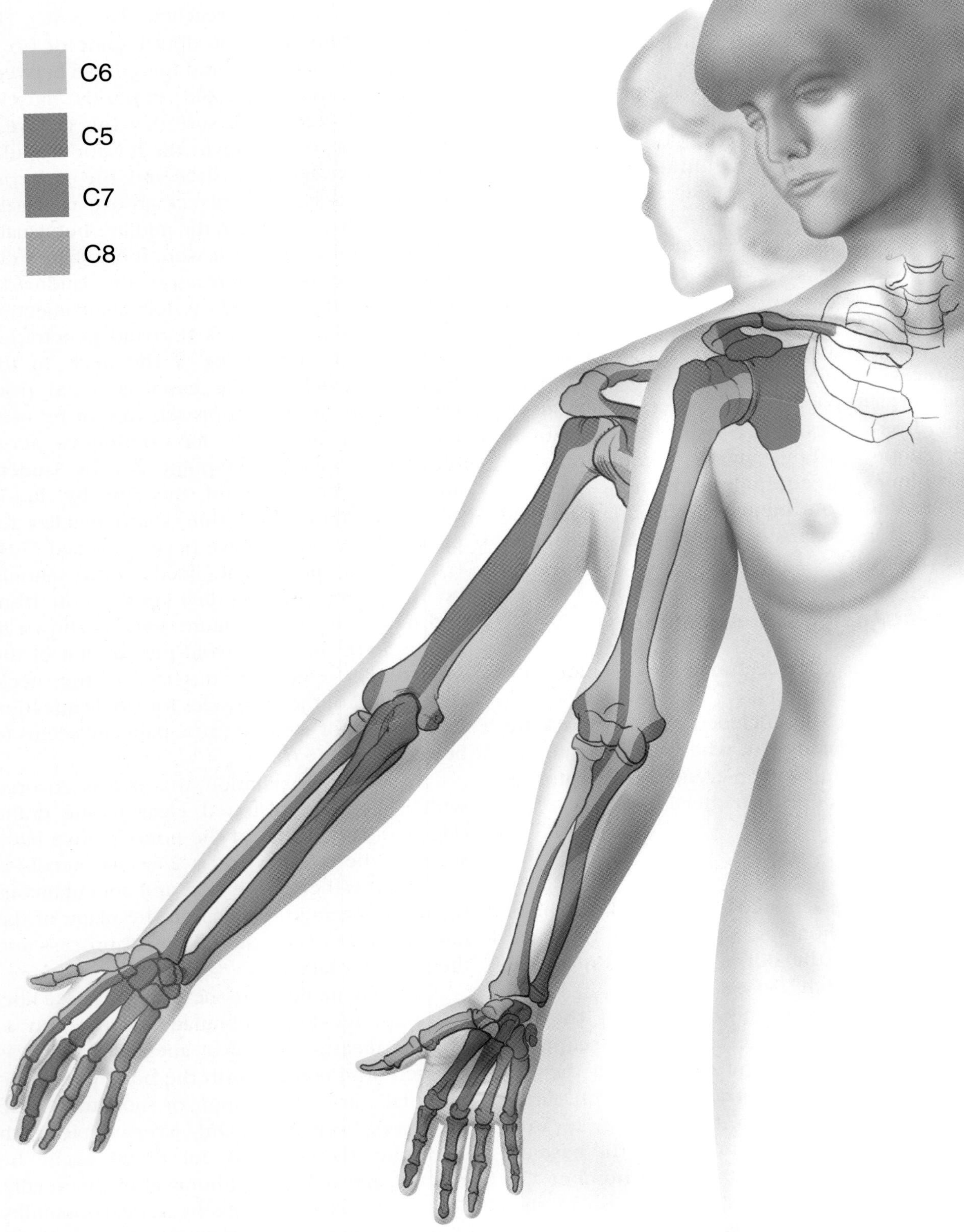

FIGURE 3-1 The osteotomes included in the brachial plexus root block.

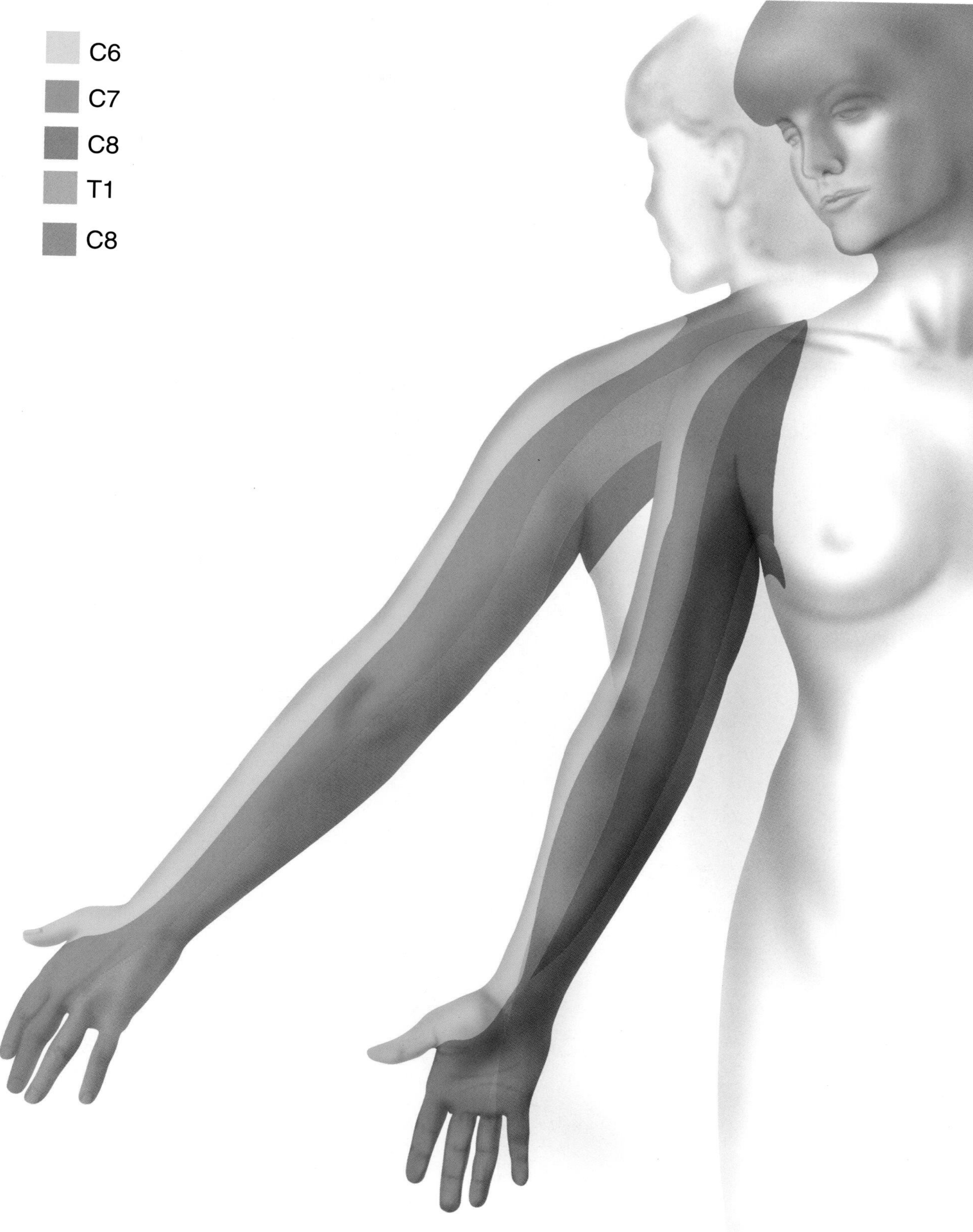

FIGURE 3-2 The dermatomes included in the brachial plexus root block.

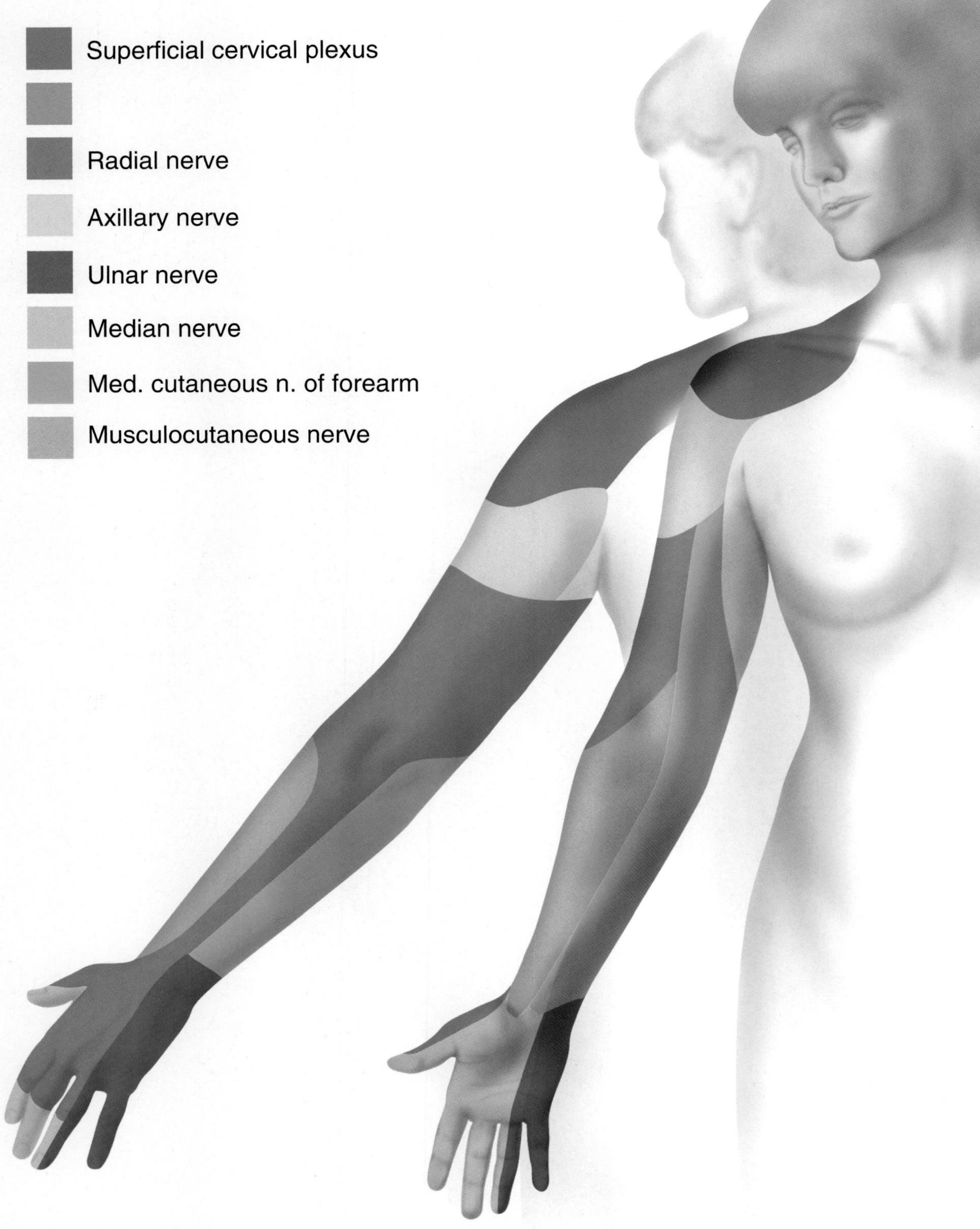

FIGURE 3-3 The neurotomes included in the brachial plexus root block.

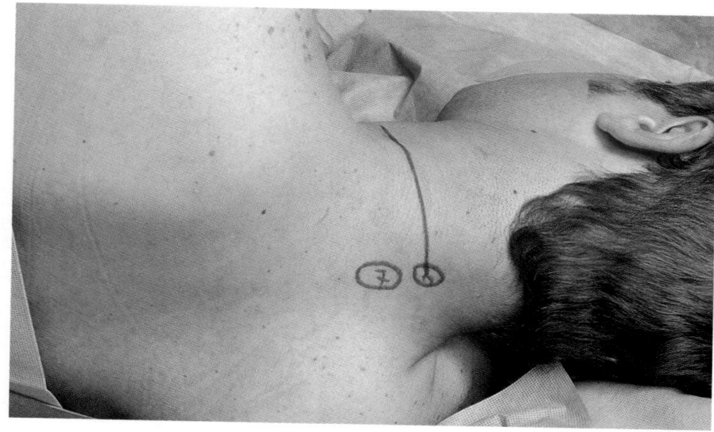

FIGURE 3-4 In this instance, the patient is placed in the lateral position. The "7" indicates the dorsal spine of C7, and "6" the dorsal spine of C6. The *solid line* joins the dorsal spine of C6 with the suprasternal notch.

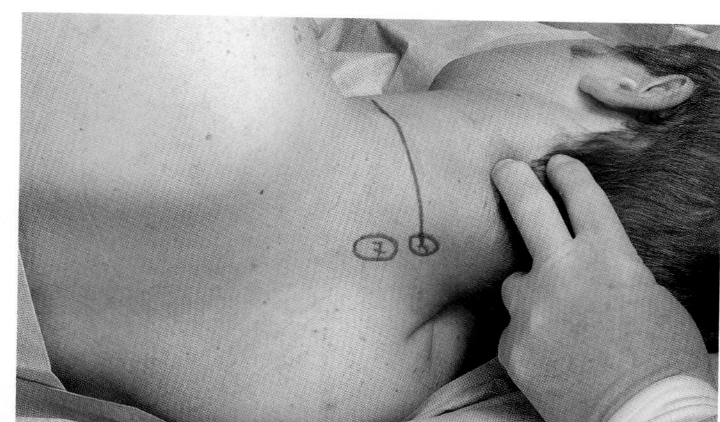

A

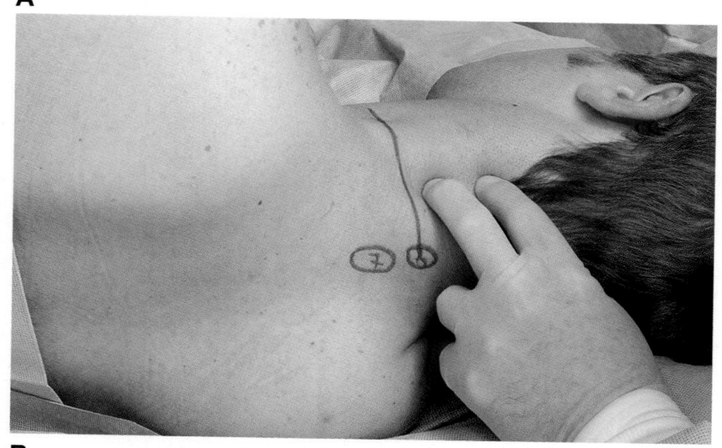

B

FIGURE 3-5 **A,** Feel for the groove between the trapezius and levator scapulae muscles in the occipital area, where this groove is widest and easiest to palpate. **B,** Move the palpating fingers caudad.

The subcutaneous path intended for tunneling of the catheter is also adequately anesthetized (Fig. 3-7).

The trapezius and levator scapulae muscles are again separated with the fingers of the nonoperative hand and a 17- or 18-gauge insulated Tuohy needle, which is attached to a nerve stimulator set to a current output of 1 to 3 mA, a frequency of 2 Hz, and a pulse width of 100 to 300 μsec, is advanced aiming toward the suprasternal notch until contact with the bony structures is made (Fig. 3-8). Notice that this needle always remains on the plane of the line drawn from the C6 dorsal spine to the suprasternal notch.

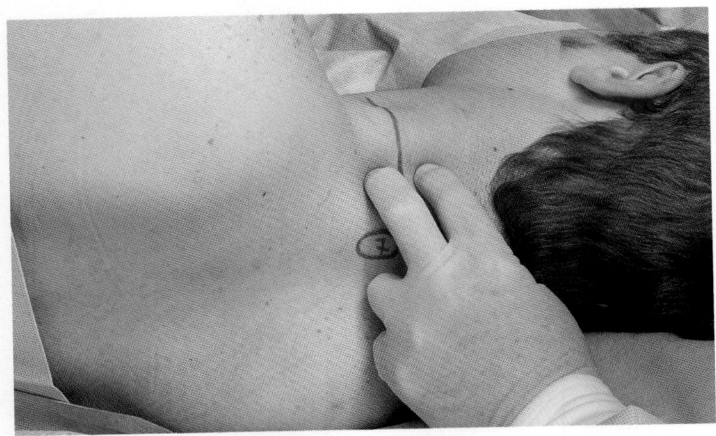

C

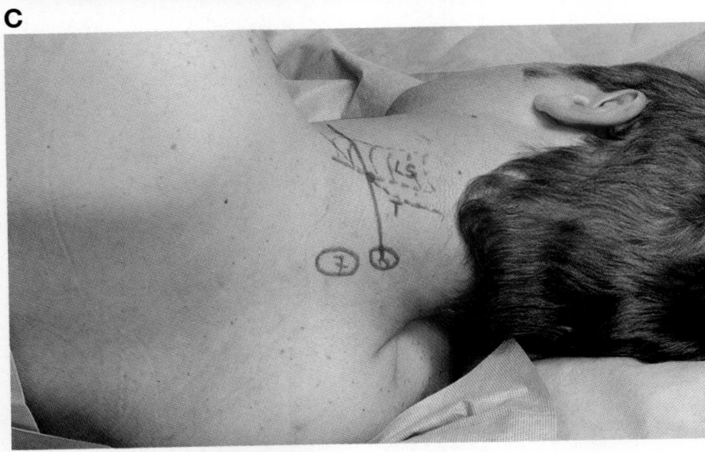

D

FIGURE 3-5 *(continued)* **C,** The palpating fingers are moved until the groove can be palpated at the level of C6. **D,** A *solid line* is drawn from the dorsal spine of C6 to the suprasternal notch. 6, Dorsal spine of C6; 7, dorsal spine of C7; LS, levator scapular muscle; T, trapezius muscle. The dot in the apex of the "V" between these two muscles indicates the point of needle entry.

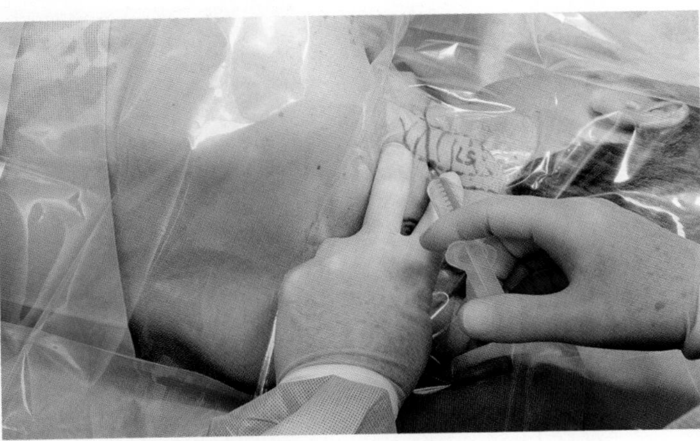

FIGURE 3-6 The levator scapulae and trapezius muscles are separated by the index and middle fingers of the nonoperative hand, and the skin and subcutaneous tissue are injected with a local anesthetic agent using a 25-gauge needle.

It is advisable to use a needle designed not to perforate the dura (i.e., a 17- or 18-gauge Tuohy needle) when any paravertebral block (cervical, thoracic, lumbar, or sacral) is performed (8). This is because the dural sleeve can follow well down the nerve roots to the area where the paravertebral block is done, essentially making all paravertebral block extradural, peridural, or epidural blocks. The same safety precautions required for epidural block should therefore be applied to paravertebral blocks (9,10) (Fig. 3-9).

After contact with the bone, the stylet of the needle is removed and a loss-of-resistance-to-air syringe is attached to the needle (Fig. 3-10). The

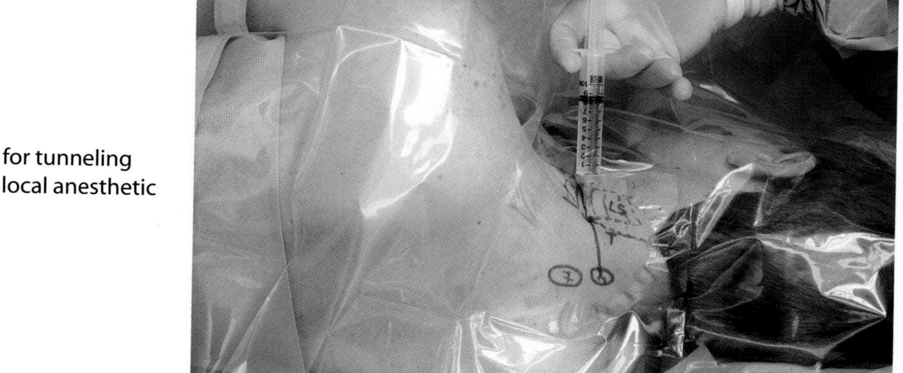

FIGURE 3-7 The intended path for tunneling of the catheter is also injected with local anesthetic agent.

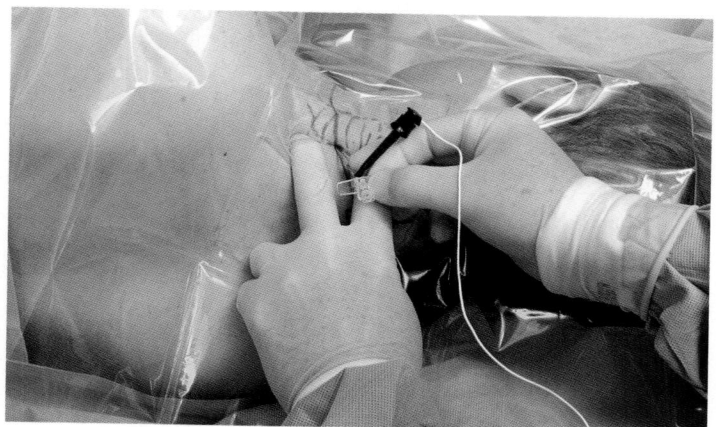

FIGURE 3-8 An 18-gauge insulated Tuohy needle is attached to a nerve stimulator and enters the skin in the apex of the "V" between levator scapulae and trapezius muscles. It is advanced anteromedially, aiming for the suprasternal notch, until the pars intervertebralis or articular column is encountered.

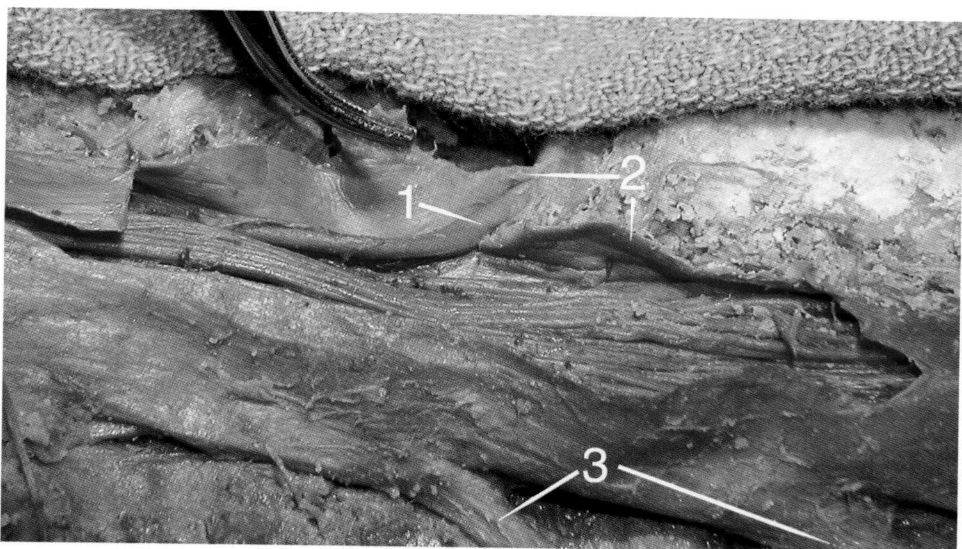

FIGURE 3-9 A dissection of the nerve root in the lumbar area shows the dura surrounding the nerve roots. This configuration is similar for the cervical, thoracic, lumbar, and sacral roots. 1, Nerve root; 2, dura; 3, nerve roots surrounded by dura. (Photograph courtesy of Carlos D. Franco, MD.)

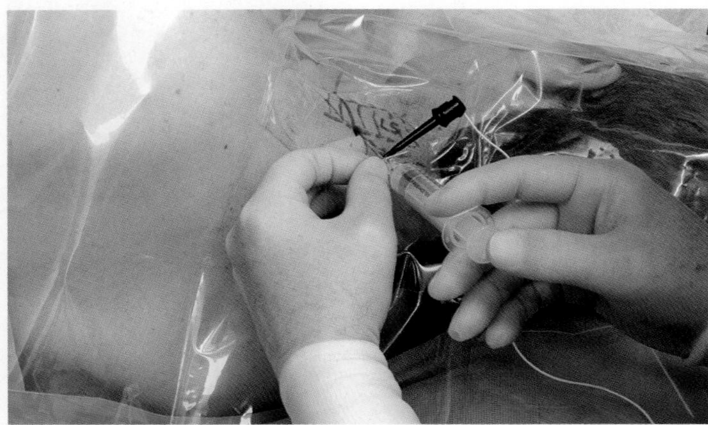

FIGURE 3-10 Once contact with the bony part is made, a loss–of–resistance-to-air syringe and nerve stimulator are attached to the insulated Tuohy needle.

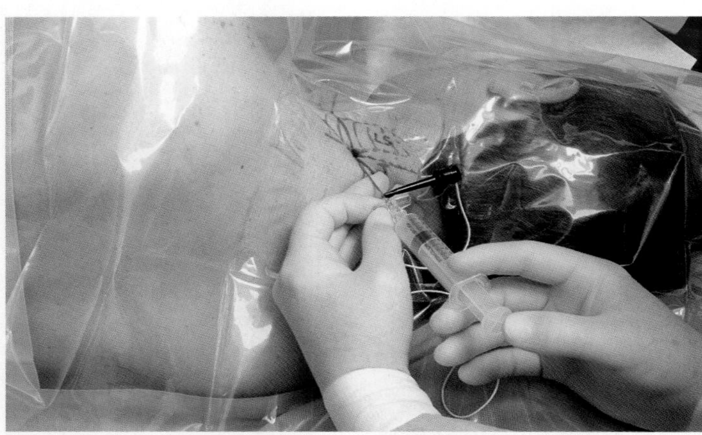

A

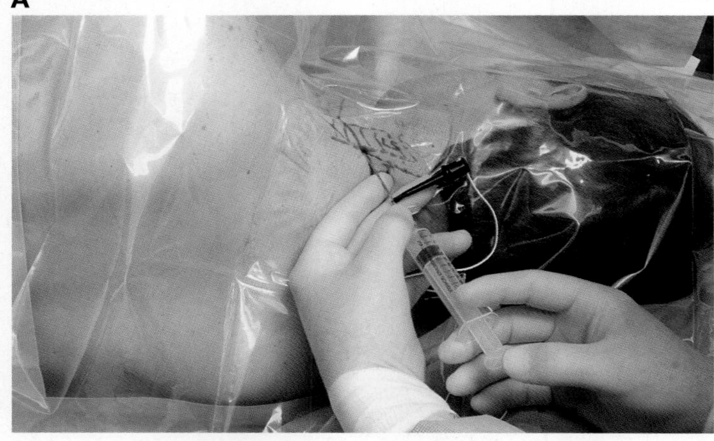

B

FIGURE 3-11 **A,** The needle is advanced by walking it off the bony process in a lateral direction. Notice the middle finger is placed under the shaft of the needle. **B,** An alternative technique of holding the needle to ensure that the needle is walked laterally off the bony process.

needle tip is now carefully walked off the bony structures in a lateral direction, remaining on the plane of the line drawn from the dorsal spine of C6 to the suprasternal notch.

At this stage, the tip of the needle should be against the "wall of bone" formed by the pars intervertebralis, articular column, or short transverse process of C6.

After walking off these bony structures, the needle is advanced carefully in an anterior direction, remaining on the plane of the line between the dorsal spine of C6 and the suprasternal notch. Note the middle finger (Fig. 3-11A) or index finger (Fig. 3-11B) under the shaft in these two needle-advancing techniques. Loss of resistance to air occurs simultaneously with a

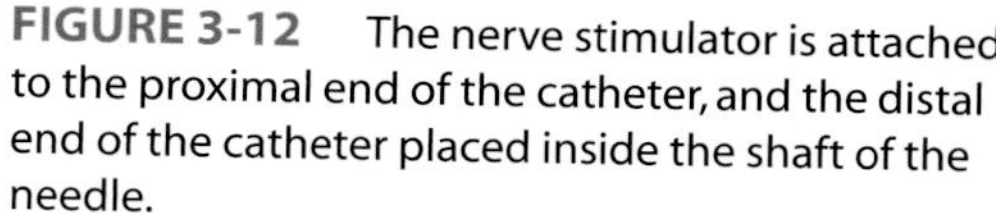

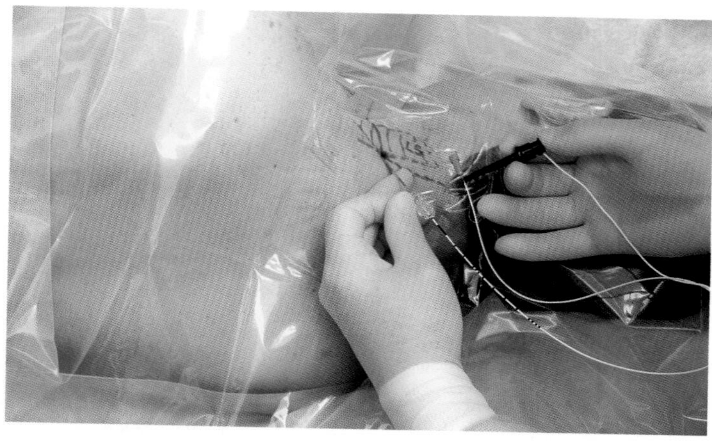

FIGURE 3-12 The nerve stimulator is attached to the proximal end of the catheter, and the distal end of the catheter placed inside the shaft of the needle.

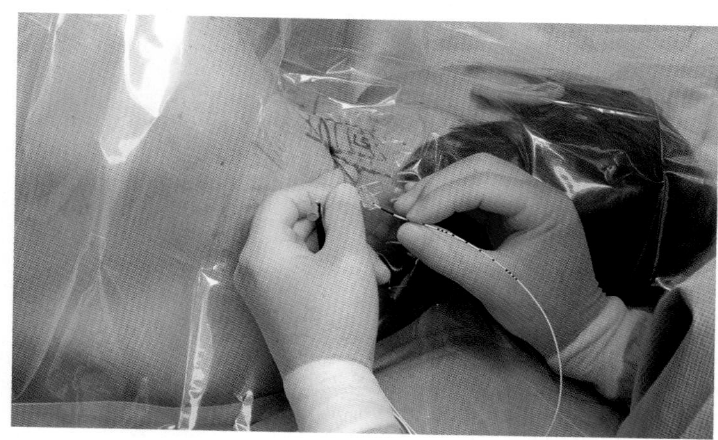

FIGURE 3-13 The catheter is advanced while an unchanged motor response is observed.

motor response. The muscles involved are usually the biceps, deltoid, or major pectoral muscles at the C5-C6 level. This is good if shoulder surgery is planned, but not for major wrist or elbow surgery. If major wrist or elbow surgery is planned, the needle should be withdrawn and slightly redirected caudad. This can be repeated until a triceps or hand motor response is seen, which indicates that the needle is now in the vicinity of the C7-C8 nerve roots—ideal for wrist and elbow surgery. Because the posterior aspect of the roots of the brachial plexus contains mainly sensory fibers, the patient may sometimes report a sensory pulsation just before the appearance of the motor response. This block is ideally suited to the use of ultrasound (Figure 3-17).

The recording on the associated DVD gives a posterior view of the loss of resistance to air and motor response appearing simultaneously. Observing the patient's mouth, it can be seen that the patient reports a sensory pulsation before the motor response appeared. This is more common in young patients. The tip of the needle is now situated between the anterior and middle scalene muscles and is in contact with the C6 root of the brachial plexus.

The nerve stimulator is removed from the needle and attached to the proximal end of the stimulating catheter, and the tip of the catheter is inserted into the needle shaft (Fig. 3-12).

Notice that the proximal part of the catheter and the nerve stimulator clip can be placed in the palm of the left hand, which also holds and manipulates the needle (Fig. 3-13). The right hand advances the catheter tip into the needle shaft and beyond. If ultrasound is used, an assistant holds the ultrasound probe (Figure 3-16).

The nerve stimulator is typically set at a current output of 1 mA or at an output that is comfortable for the patient. The motor response should be unchanged, and the broad black mark on the catheter indicates that the catheter tip is

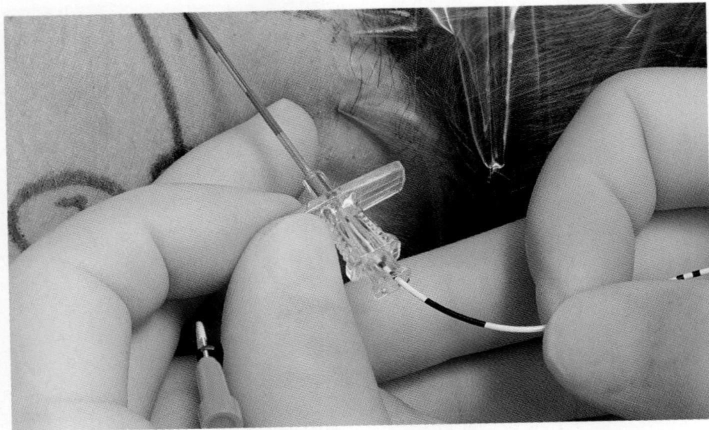

FIGURE 3-14 The special mark on the catheter at the hub of the needle indicates that the tip of the catheter has not yet protruded beyond the needle tip.

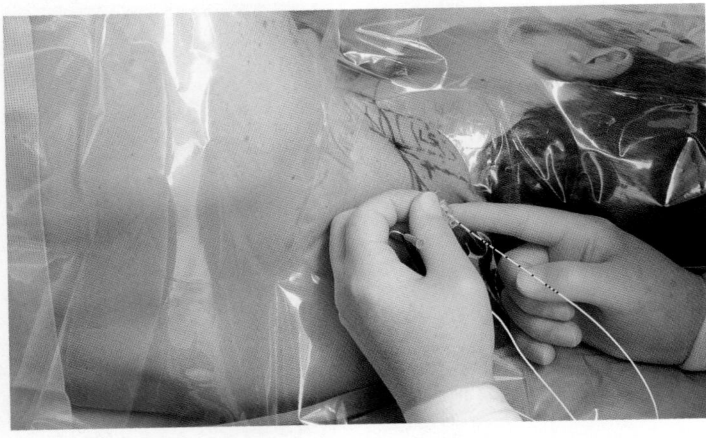

FIGURE 3-15 The needle should not be manipulated if the special mark on the catheter is not visible.

situated at the tip of the needle (Fig. 3-14). It is important not to manipulate the needle if the special mark is not completely visible.

Advance the catheter beyond the needle tip. If the motor response disappears, carefully withdraw the catheter tip to inside the needle shaft, make a small adjustment to the needle by rotating it clockwise or counterclockwise, advancing it slightly, or withdrawing it slightly. Repeat this maneuver until the muscle twitches remain unchanged during catheter advancement (Fig. 3-15). This indicates that the catheter tip is now situated on the nerve root. Advance the catheter approximately 3 to 5 cm beyond the needle tip, but never further than 5 cm.

It may be of considerable help to use ultrasonography to identify the pars intervertebralis and the nerve roots, as illustrated in Figure 3-16. The ultrasound probe is held anterior to the levator scapulae muscle and outside the sterile field. Figure 3-17 illustrates the pars intervertebralis (articular column), nerve roots, and subclavian artery.

Remove the needle without disturbing the catheter, and remove the inner stylet of the catheter (Fig. 3-18). The catheter position can now be reconfirmed by attaching the nerve stimulator to the catheter. The motor response should be unchanged.

The catheter will probably dislodge if it is not secured. The best method of securing the catheter is by subcutaneous tunneling, as illustrated in Chapter 12. This is done by first placing the inner stylet of the needle subcutaneously from a point approximately 1 to 2 mm from the catheter exit site, if a skin bridge is required, to where the tunneling is anticipated. If a skin bridge is not required, the needle stylet enters through the same site as the catheter, with care taken not to damage the catheter. This area has already been anesthetized.

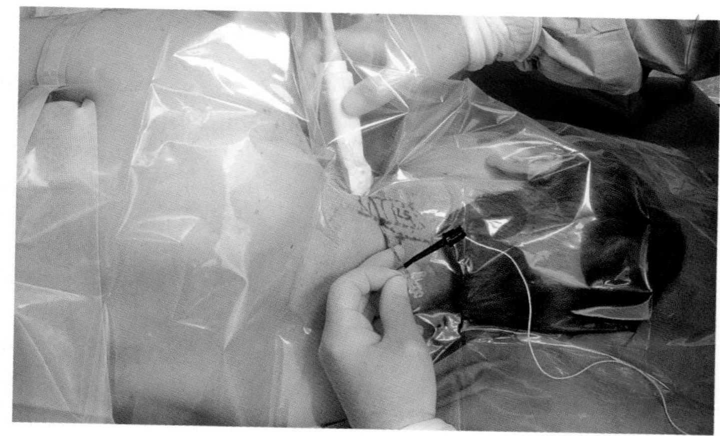

FIGURE 3-16 An ultrasound probe placed anterior to the levator scapulae muscle indicates the position of the needle relative to the bony pars intervertebralis and the nerves of the brachial plexus.

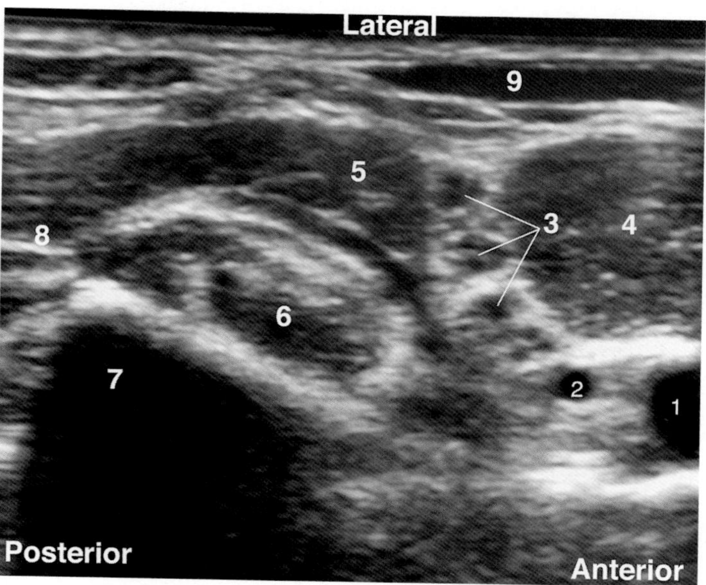

FIGURE 3-17 Ultrasonographic image of the lateral aspect of the neck: 1. Subclavian artery; 2. Vertebral artery; 3. Brachial plexus roots; 4. Anterior scalene muscle; 5. Middle scalene muscle; 6. Posterior scalene muscle; 7. Pars intervertebralis (articular column) of C6; 8. Needle entry from posterior.

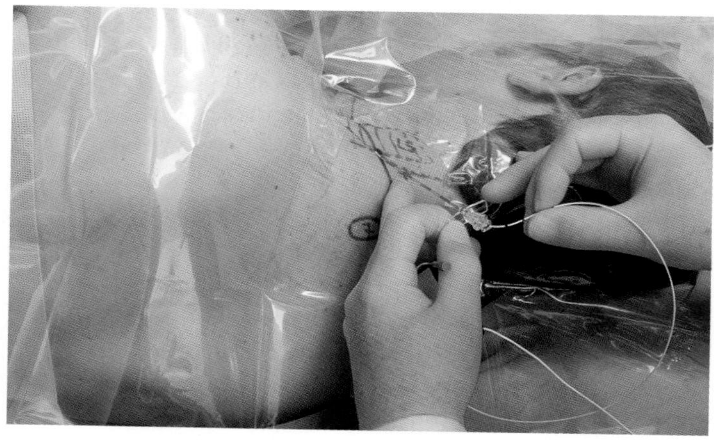

FIGURE 3-18 The needle is removed without disturbing the position of the catheter.

The needle is now "railroaded" back over the stylet and the stylet removed.

The proximal end of the catheter is fed through the needle and the needle is removed, leaving a loop of catheter.

The silicone tubing that protected the catheter tip during packaging is handy to use to protect the skin bridge. The proximal end of the catheter can also be looped through the skin bridge. The skin bridge makes removal of the catheter easier.

Attach the Luer lock connecting device to the catheter and attach the nerve stimulator to the connecting device.

The motor response should remain unchanged. Injection of local anesthetic agent or any other conductor of electricity (e.g., saline) that decreases and disperses the current density at the catheter tip will cause the motor response to stop immediately. This is a positive Raj test and gives final confirmation that the block will be successful.

The catheter is covered with a sterile transparent dressing and the connecting device is placed in the fixation device.

Local Anesthetic Agent and Infusion Choice

Fifteen to 40 mL of ropivacaine 0.5% to 0.75% is usually used for intraoperative analgesia, and an infusion of 0.2% at 3 to 10 mL/hour is used for postoperative pain management. Patient-controlled boluses of 5 to 10 mL with a lockout time of 30 to 120 minutes can be used if indicated.

The concentration of the infusion drug and the rate on infusion should be individualized depending on the clinical situation. If a motor and sensory block is required, such as for rotator cuff repair or total shoulder replacement the first few days after surgery, a relatively high concentration (0.2%) and a relatively high infusion rate (5 mL/hour) can be used. This, combined with patient-controlled boluses of 10 mL locked out at 120 minutes, should give good results. If, on the other hand, sensory block without motor block is required, a low concentration of the drug (e.g., 0.1%) can be used at a low infusion rate (3 to 5 mL/hour), and the patient-controlled boluses can be set at 10 mL and locked out at 60 minutes.

Another strategy is to use a drug concentration of 0.5%, infused at 5 mL/hour for the first 25 hours, which should provide a good motor and sensory block. If the reservoir is filled with 240 mL, an infusion of 5 mL/hour should leave 120 mL in the reservoir after 24 hours. If the reservoir is then filled with saline, the infusion concentration is halved to 0.25%, which should increase the motor function somewhat for the second day. After another 24 hours, there will again be 120 mL left in the reservoir, and it can again be filled with saline, which will now decrease the concentration of ropivacaine to 0.125%. This would allow the motor function to improve further. This process can be repeated until the block is no longer required. This infusion strategy allows for a solid motor block directly after surgery, followed by a gradual return to full motor function and sensation as the pain naturally decreases and requirements for motor function increase.

Catheter Removal

Catheter removal, when the patient no longer requires continuous nerve block and after full sensation has returned to the arm, is done by fixating the proximal end of the catheter and then removing the distal end before removing the entire catheter. The catheter removal technique is illustrated in Chapter 12.

(See continuous cervical paravertebral block movie on DVD.)

REFERENCES

1. Boezaart AP, Koorn R, Rosenquist RW: Paravertebral approach to the brachial plexus: an anatomic improvement in technique. Reg Anesth Pain Med 2003;28: 241-244.
2. Boezaart AP, De Beer JF, Nell ML: Early experience with continuous cervical paravertebral block using a stimulating catheter. Reg Anesth Pain Med 2003;28: 406-413.
3. Boezaart AP: Continuous interscalene block for ambulatory shoulder surgery. Best Pract Res Clin Anaesthesiol 2002;16:295-310.
4. Boezaart AP, Franco CD: Blocks above the clavicle. In: Boezaart AP (ed): Anesthesia and Orthopaedic Surgery. New York, McGraw-Hill, 2006, pp 291-309.
5. Sandefo I, Iohom G, Van Elstraete A, et al: Clinical efficacy of the brachial plexus via the posterior approach. Reg Anesth Pain Med 2005;30:238-242.
6. Rettig HC, Gielen MJM, Jack NTM, et al: A comparison of the lateral and posterior approach for brachial plexus block. Reg Anesth Pain Med 2006;31:119-126.

7. Boezaart AP, Raw RM: Sleeping beauty or big bad wolf [editorial]. Reg Anesth Pain Med 2006;31:186-191.
8. Boezaart AP, Franco FC: Thin sharp needles around the dura. Reg Anesth Pain Med 2006;31:388-389.
9. Voermans NC, Crul BJ, De Bondt BJ, et al: Permanent loss of cerebral spinal cord function associated with the posterior approach. Anesth Analg 2006;102:330.
10. Boezaart AP: Please don't blame the block … [letter]. Anesth Analg 2007;104:211-212.

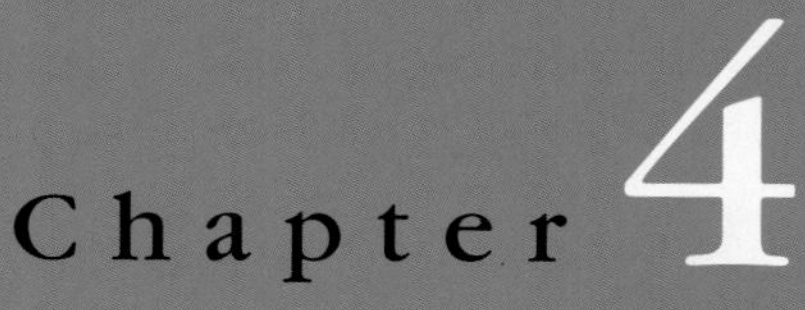

Chapter 4

Supraclavicular Block

- Single-Injection Supraclavicular Block

SINGLE-INJECTION SUPRACLAVICULAR BLOCK

Introduction

The supraclavicular approach to the brachial plexus is a technique usually associated with rapid-onset, predictable, and dense anesthesia (1,2). This is because the block is performed at the level of the plexus trunks, where the entire sensory, motor, and sympathetic innervation of the upper arm is carried in just three nerve structures confined to a small space between the first rib and the clavicle in the cephalocaudal axis, and the anterior and middle scalene muscles along the anteroposterior orientation.

The supraclavicular block can be used to provide anesthesia for any surgery on the upper extremity that does not involve the shoulder (1). It is a good choice for elbow, wrist, and hand surgery. The block is ideal for adult patients, but may be considered in pediatric patients older than 10 years of age on a case-by-case basis. This block is not performed bilaterally because of the potential risk of respiratory emergency from pneumothorax or phrenic nerve block (2). However, although this recommendation seems logical, it has not been substantiated in the published literature.

Specific Anatomic Considerations

The gross anatomy is described in detail in Chapter 1, but it is important to review the anatomy of the pleura as it relates to the supraclavicular block. There are two potential places where the pleura could be injured during performance of this block: the pleural dome and the first intercostal space (Figs. 4-1 and 4-2). The pleural dome is the apex of the parietal pleura (inside lining of the rib cage), circumscribed by the first rib. The first ribs are short, broad, flattened, "C"-shaped bones located on each side of the upper chest with their concavities facing medially toward each other. This concavity or medial border forms the outer boundary of the pleural dome. The anterior scalene muscle, by inserting in the medial border of the first rib, comes in contact medially with the pleural dome and becomes an important landmark to locate it. There is no pleural dome lateral to the anterior scalene muscle. Because the anterior scalene is located in almost the same parasagittal plane as the sternocleidomastoid muscle, the parasagittal plane of the lateral insertion of this muscle on the clavicle can be used as a landmark to locate the lateral boundary of the pleural dome in the neck.

The used of ultrasound for this block has effectively eliminated the potential danger of pneumothorax.

Technique

The patient is positioned supine or semi-sitting with the head turned slightly away from the side to be blocked. The ipsilateral elbow is flexed and the forearm is placed on the patient's lap or held in the anesthesiologist's nonoperative hand. If possible, the patient's wrist is supinated so the fingers are not leaning against the patient and are free to move (Fig. 4-3).

The point at which the lateral border of the sternocleidomastoid muscle meets the clavicle is marked as shown in Figure 4-4 (*medial arrow*). The point of needle entry is approximately 2.5 cm lateral to the insertion of the sternocleidomastoid muscle to the clavicle or the width of the clavicular head of the patient's sternocleidomastoid muscle (see Fig. 4-4, *lateral arrow*), and approximately 1 cm above the clavicle (see Fig. 4-4, *dot*).

A 50-mm, short-bevel, 22-gauge insulated needle is used. After a small skin wheal is raised, the stimulating needle is inserted perpendicular to the skin (Fig. 4-5).

The needle is advanced for a few millimeters, then turned caudad, remaining in the parasagittal plain in a direction parallel to the patient's midline. The nerve stimulator is initially set at a current output of 0.8 mA, a pulse width of 100 to 300 μsec, and a frequency of 1 Hz (3).

Good results with this block may be obtained when a flexion or extension motor response in the fingers is elicited (1-3). When this motor response in the fingers is observed, the injection is started without decreasing the nerve stimulator output (3).

If needle repositioning is necessary, it is redirected either anterior or posterior but in exactly the same original parasagittal plane (parallel to the midline of the patient). The tip of the needle is kept above the clavicle.

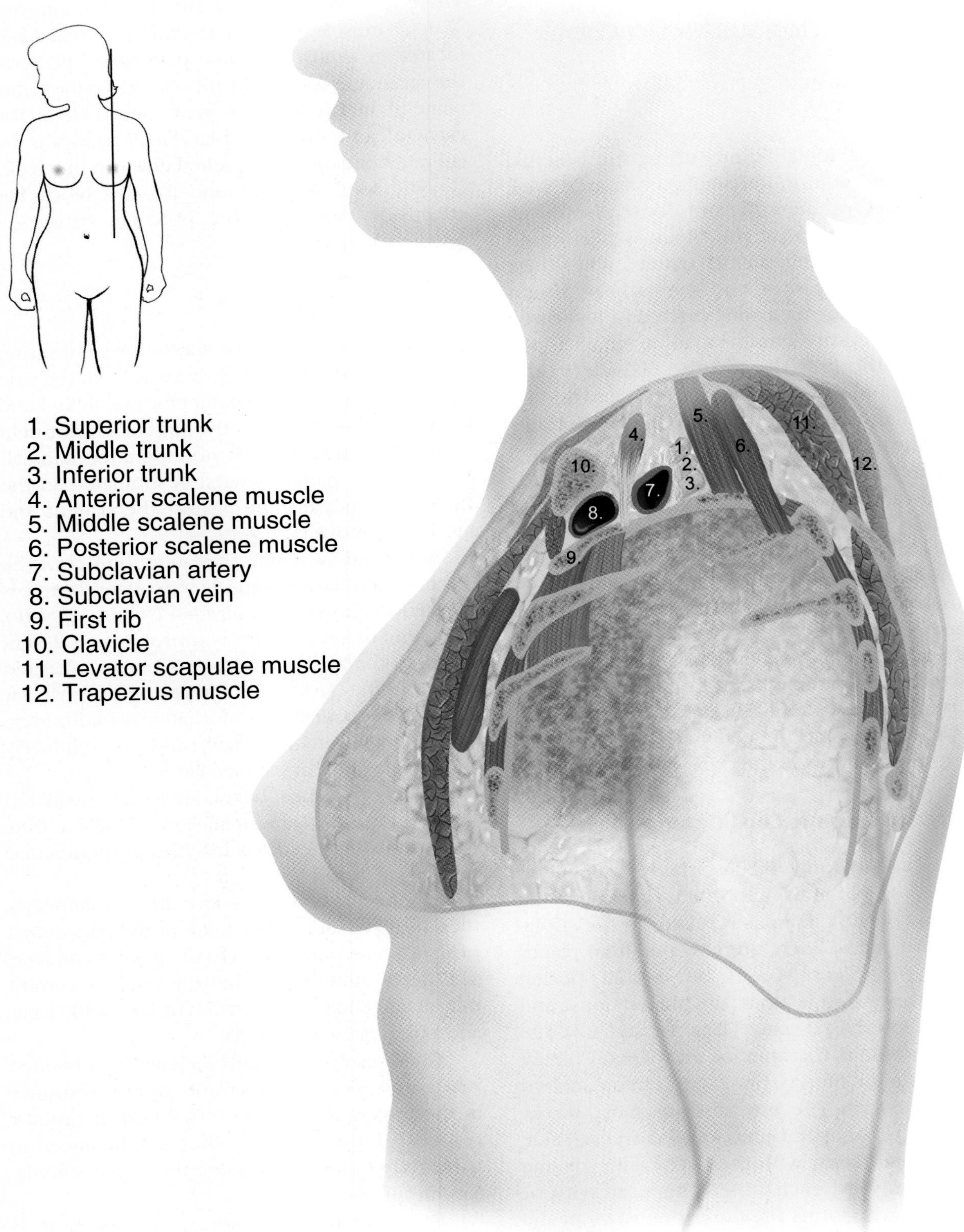

FIGURE 4-1 Section through the mid-clavicular line.

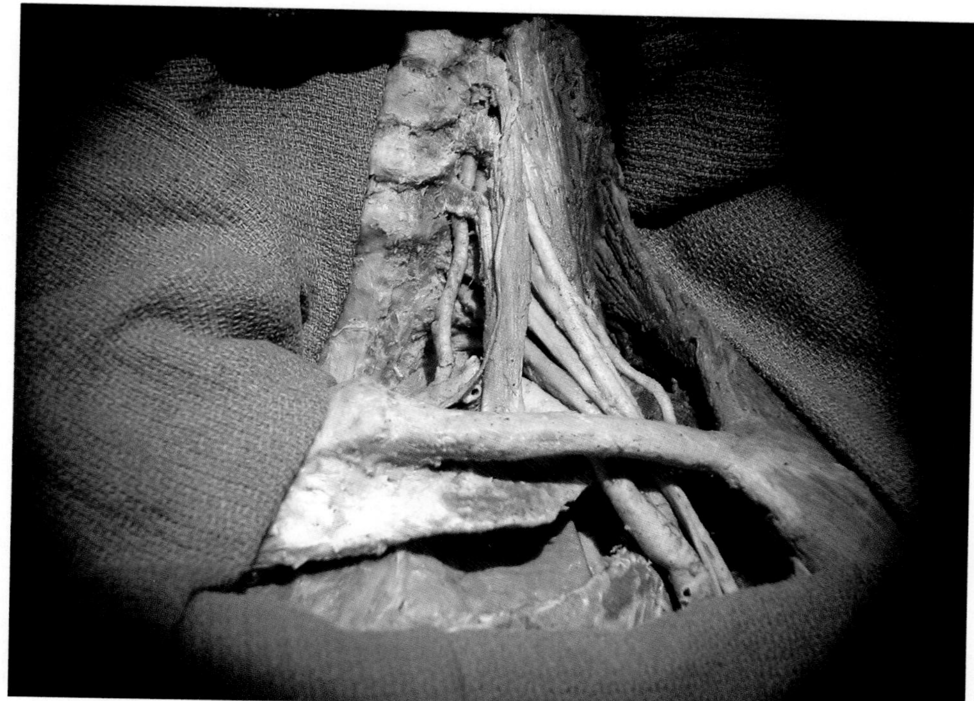

FIGURE 4-2 Dissection of the supraclavicular area showing the relationship between the lung and the brachial plexus at this level. (Photograph courtesy of Carlos D. Franco, MD.)

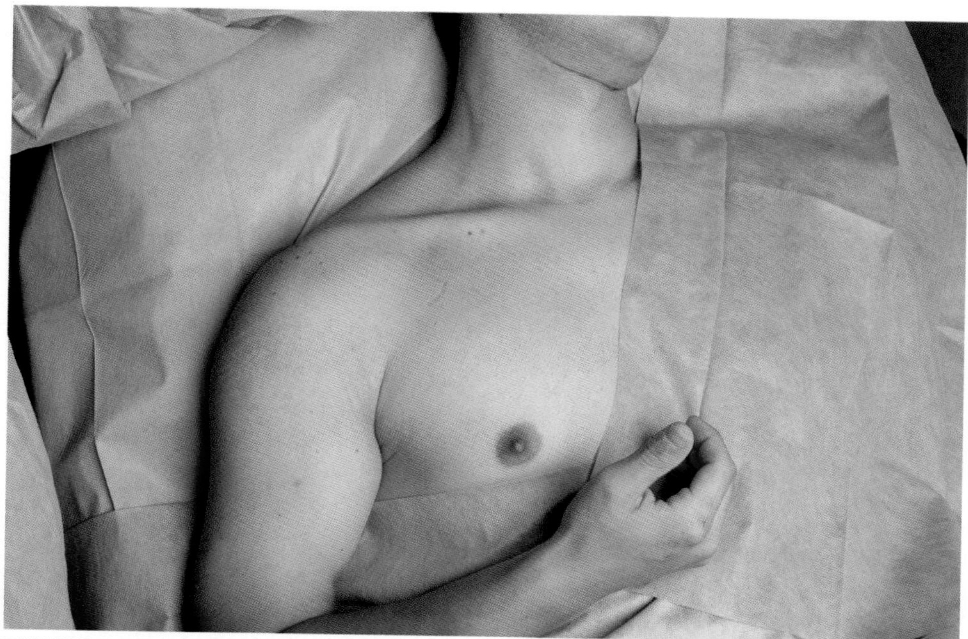

FIGURE 4-3 The patient is placed in a supine or semi-sitting position.

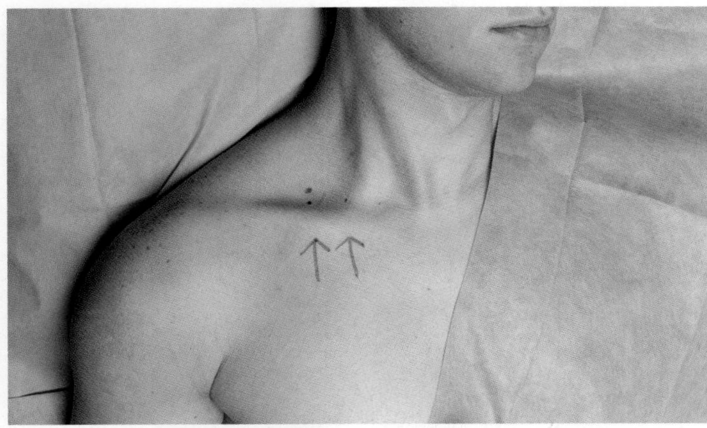

FIGURE 4-4 The *medial arrow* indicates the position of the clavicular head of the sternocleidomastoid muscle, and the *lateral arrow* is 2.5 cm lateral to the medial arrow. The uppermost lateral *dot* indicates the point of needle entry.

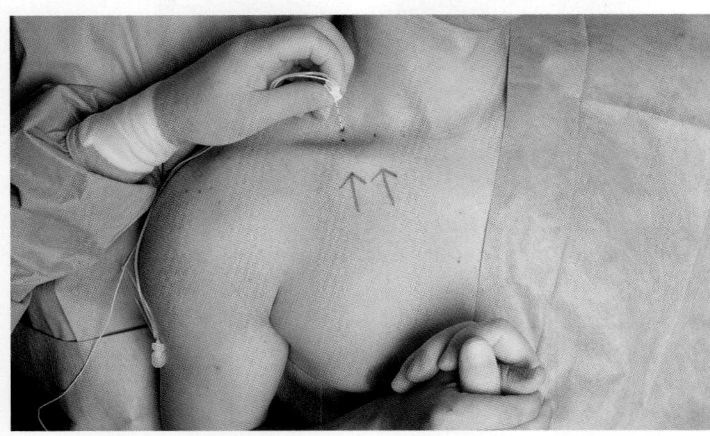

FIGURE 4-5 The needle is now aimed perpendicular to the skin.

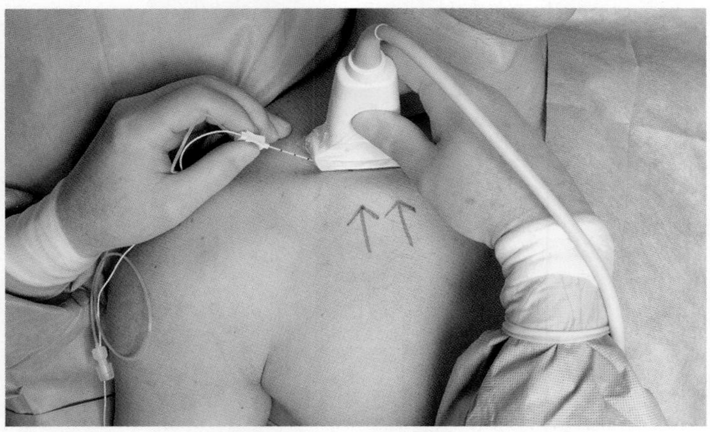

FIGURE 4-6 Position of the ultrasound probe relative to the needle.

Ultrasonography is a very useful addition to this block. The probe is placed supraclavicularly, and the needle enters as shown in Figure 4-6.

Local Anesthetic Agent Choice

Twenty to 40 mL (1.5%) mepivacaine with 1:200,000 epinephrine is commonly used. This provides approximately 3 to 4 hours of surgical anesthesia. The same anesthetic solution without epinephrine provides about 2 to 3 hours of surgical anesthesia. Other local anesthetic agents, such as ropivacaine (0.5% to 0.75%), bupivacaine (0.5%), and levobupivacaine (0.625%), are also commonly used. These drugs provide good anesthesia lasting 5 to 8 hours.

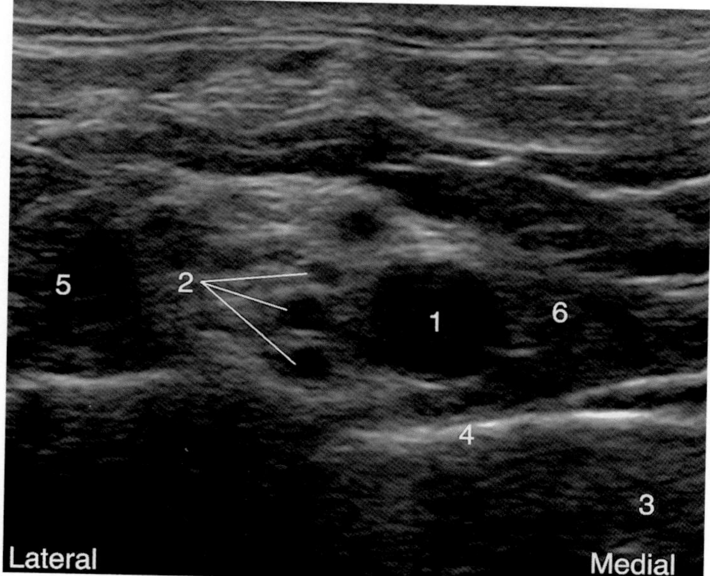

FIGURE 4-7 Ultrasonogragh of the supraclavicular area: 1. Subclavian artery; 2. Brachial plexus trunks; 3. Lung; 4. First rib; 5. Middle scalene muscle; 6. Anterior scalene muscle.

REFERENCES

1. Boezaart AP, Franco CD: Blocks above the clavicle. In Boezaart AP (ed): Anesthesia and Orthopaedic Surgery. New York, McGraw-Hill, 2006, pp 291-309.
2. Franco CD, Gloss FJ, Voronov G, et al: Supraclavicular block in the obese population: An analysis of 2020 blocks. Anesth Analg 2006;102:1252-1254.
3. Franco CD, Domashevich V, Voronov G, et al: The supraclavicular block with a nerve stimulator: To decrease or not to decrease, that is the question. Anesth Analg 2004;98:1167-1171.

Chapter 5

Distal Brachial Plexus: Applied Anatomy

- Brachial Plexus Cords

BRACHIAL PLEXUS CORDS

The cords of the brachial plexus are referred to as posterior (see Fig. 1-1, [13]), medial (see Fig. 1-1, [14]), and lateral (see Fig. 1-1, [12]), according to their relationship with the axillary artery. The three cords originate from the divisions and terminate in the branches of the brachial plexus.

As can be seen from Figure 5-1, the cords are close to the coracoid process (*arrow*), to which the minor pectoral muscle is attached. Furthermore, the large vessels to the arm separate the brachial plexus from the dome of the rib cage. The subclavian vein and artery are seen and the brachial plexus cords are superolateral to the vascular structures.

The *top arrows* in Figure 5-2 indicate the border of the deltoid muscle, whereas the two *lower arrows* indicate the border of the major pectoral muscle. Needle entry for infraclavicular block is either 1.5 to 2 cm from the midpoint of the coracoid process (indicated by the *lines*), or, using the superior approach, through the deltopectoral trough.

Lateral Cord

The lateral cord stems mainly from the C5, C6, and C7 roots and gives rise to the musculocutaneous nerve and lateral head of the median nerve.

The musculocutaneous nerve supplies the coracobrachialis, biceps, and brachialis muscles—all flexors of the upper arm (Fig. 5-3). The median nerve has no branches in the upper arm and, in the forearm, supplies the pronator of the forearm and superficial flexor muscles of the medial two fingers and deep flexors of the lateral fingers. It also supplies the abductor of the thumb and the first and second lumbrical muscles. Therefore, electrical stimulation of the lateral cord results in flexion at the elbow, pronation of the forearm, and flexion in the hand. The net effect of this is that the fifth digit (the little finger) moves laterally, toward the cord being stimulated (i.e., the lateral cord; see Chapter 6).

(See lateral cord movie on DVD.)

Figure 5-4 shows the sensory distribution of the lateral cord.

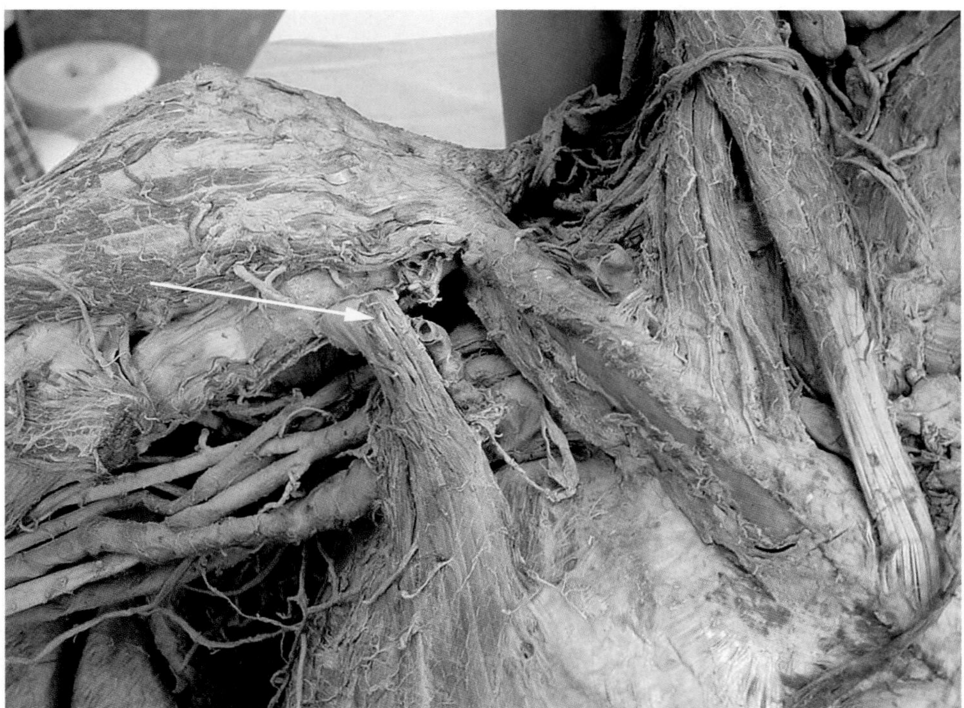

FIGURE 5-1 Dissection of the right subclavian area. *Arrow* indicates implantation of the minor pectoral muscle on the coracoid process.

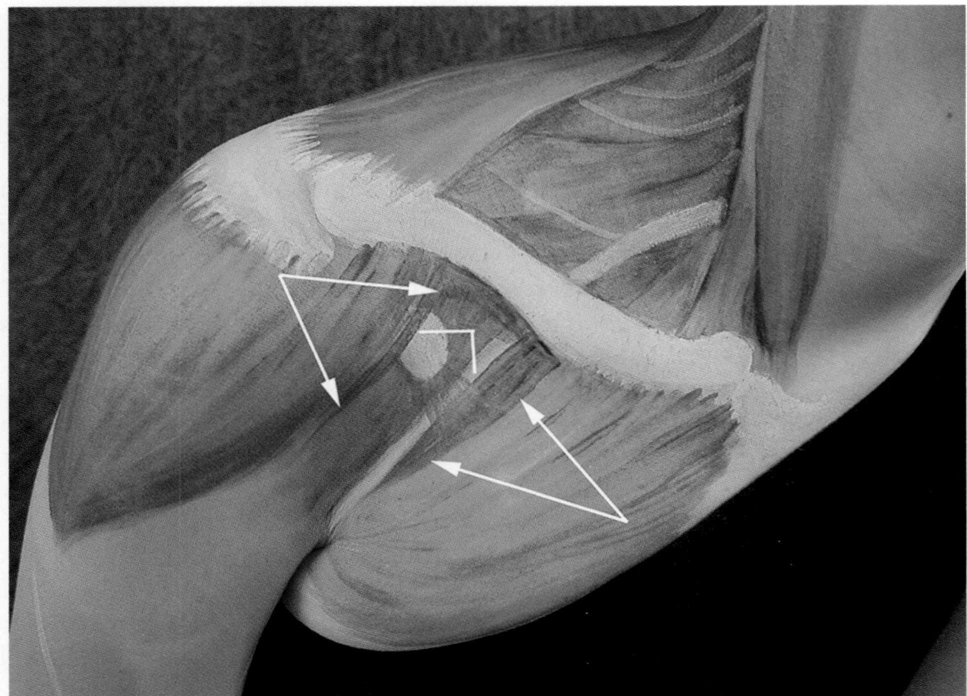

FIGURE 5-2 The *upper arrows* indicate the medial border of the deltoid muscle and the *lower arrows* indicate the lateral border of the major pectoral muscle. Note the deltopectoral trough, the position of the coracoid process, and the surface anatomy of the cords.

Medial Cord

The medial cord stems mainly from the C8 and T1 roots and gives rise to the ulnar nerve and medial head of the median nerve (Fig. 5-5).

The ulnar nerve supplies the deep flexors of the forearm, the abductor, flexor, and opponens of the fifth digit, the abductor of the thumb, and the third and fourth lumbricals of the hand (Fig. 5-6). The median nerve has no branches in the upper arm. It supplies the pronator of the forearm, superficial flexors of the medial two fingers, and deep flexors of the lateral fingers. It also supplies the abductor of the thumb and the first and second lumbrical muscles. Therefore, electrical stimulation of the medial cord results in flexion of the fingers and flexion and ulnar deviation of the wrist.

With the arm in the anatomic position, the fifth digit moves medially when the medial cord is stimulated (see Chapter 6), which results from flexion of the fingers and ulnar deviation of the wrist.

(See medial cord movie on DVD.)

Figure 5-7 shows the sensory distribution of the medial cord.

Posterior Cord

The posterior cord stems mainly from the C6, C7, and C8 roots and gives rise to the axillary and radial nerves.

The axillary nerve supplies the deltoid muscle, whereas the radial nerve supplies the extensor muscles of the arm, forearm, wrist, and hand (Fig. 5-8). Electrical stimulation of the posterior cord therefore results in extension of the elbow, wrist, and hand.

The fifth digit (little finger) moves posteriorly because of extension of the elbow and fingers when the posterior cord is stimulated (see Chapter 6). It should now be obvious that the fifth digit moves "toward" the cord that is being stimulated.

(See posterior cord movie on DVD.)

Figure 5-9 shows the sensory distribution of the posterior cord.

Text continued on page 74

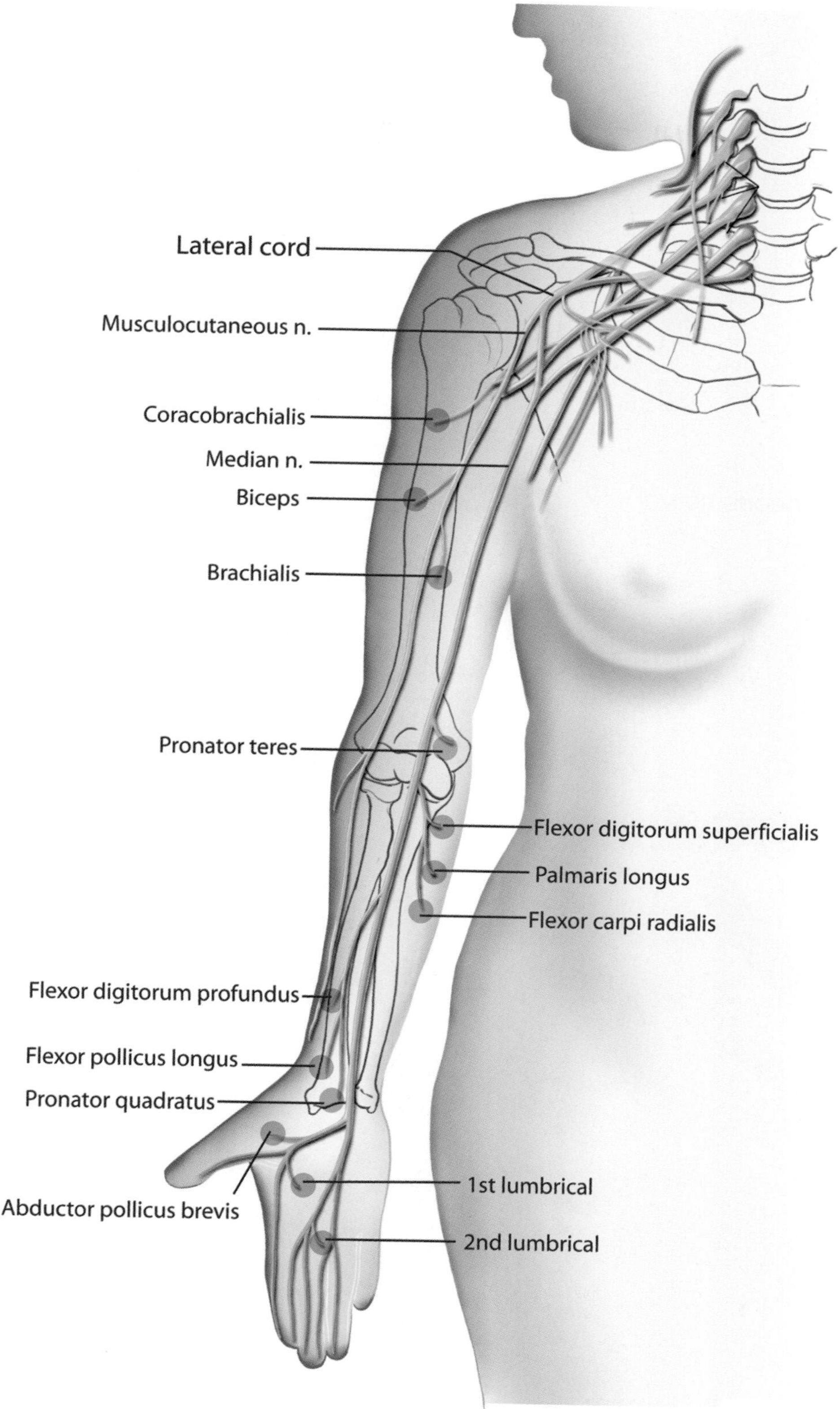

FIGURE 5-3 Muscles innervated by the nerves from the lateral cord of the brachial plexus.

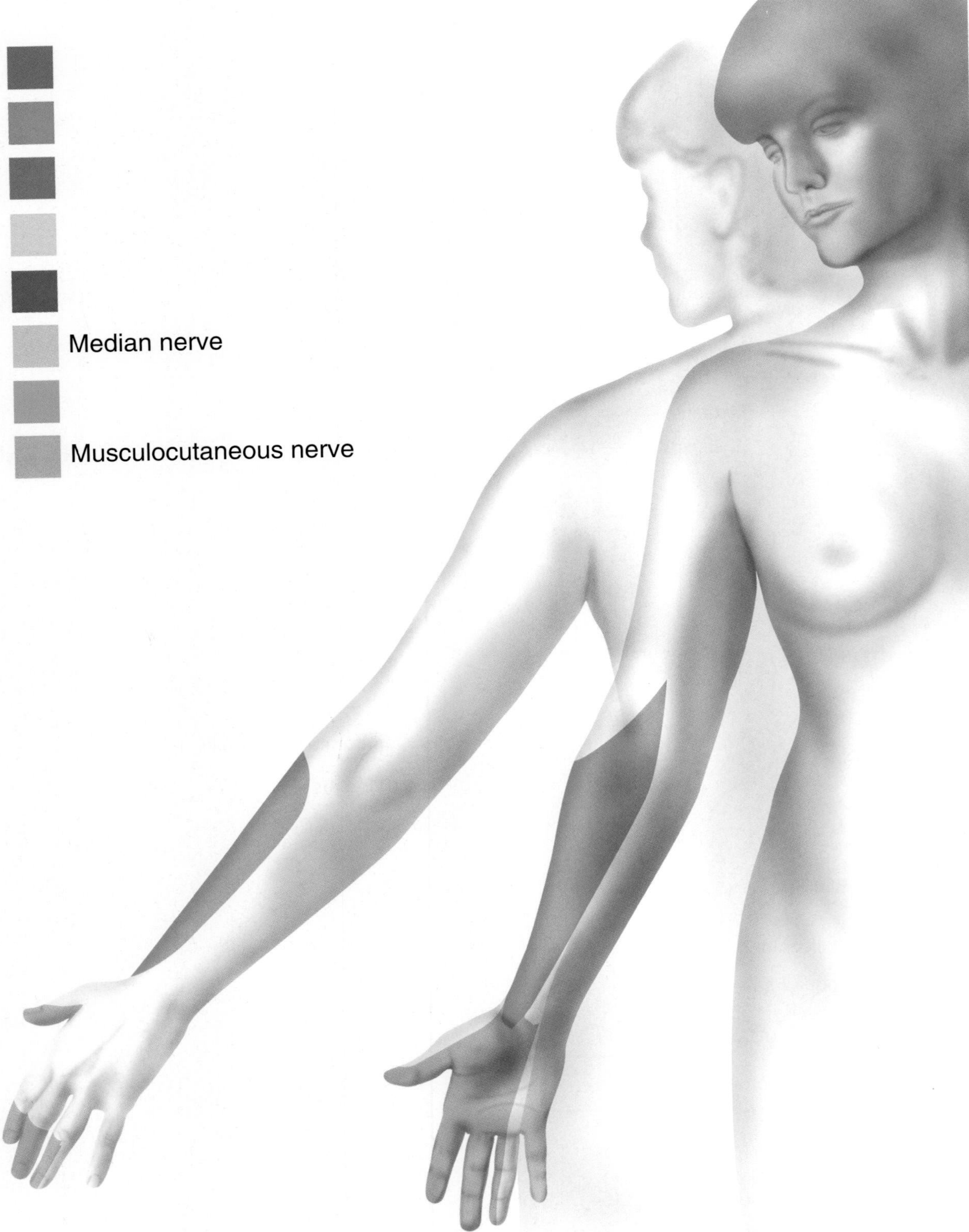

FIGURE 5-4 Sensory neurotomes innervated by the nerves of the lateral cord of the brachial plexus.

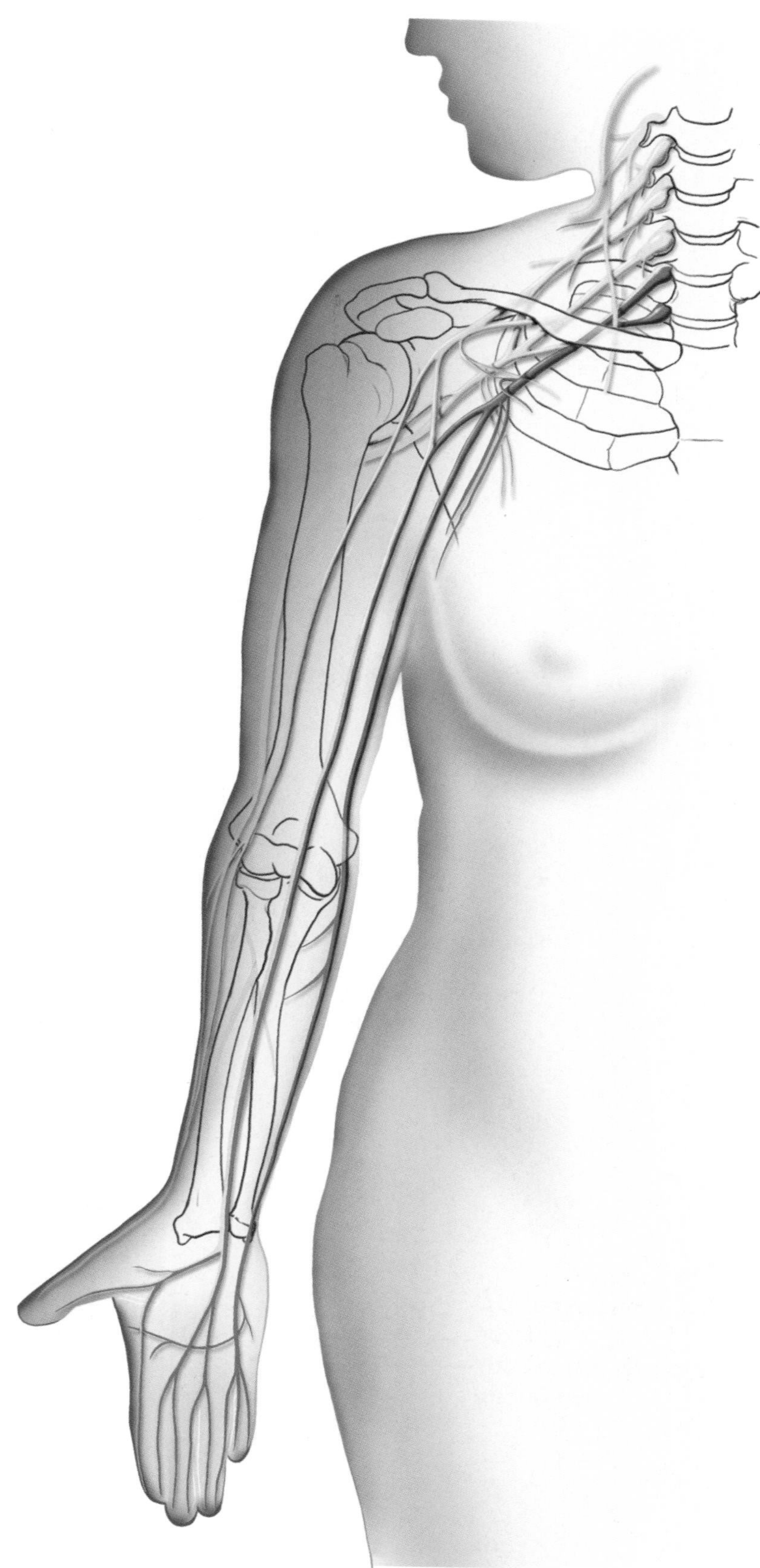

FIGURE 5-5 The medial cord of the brachial plexus.

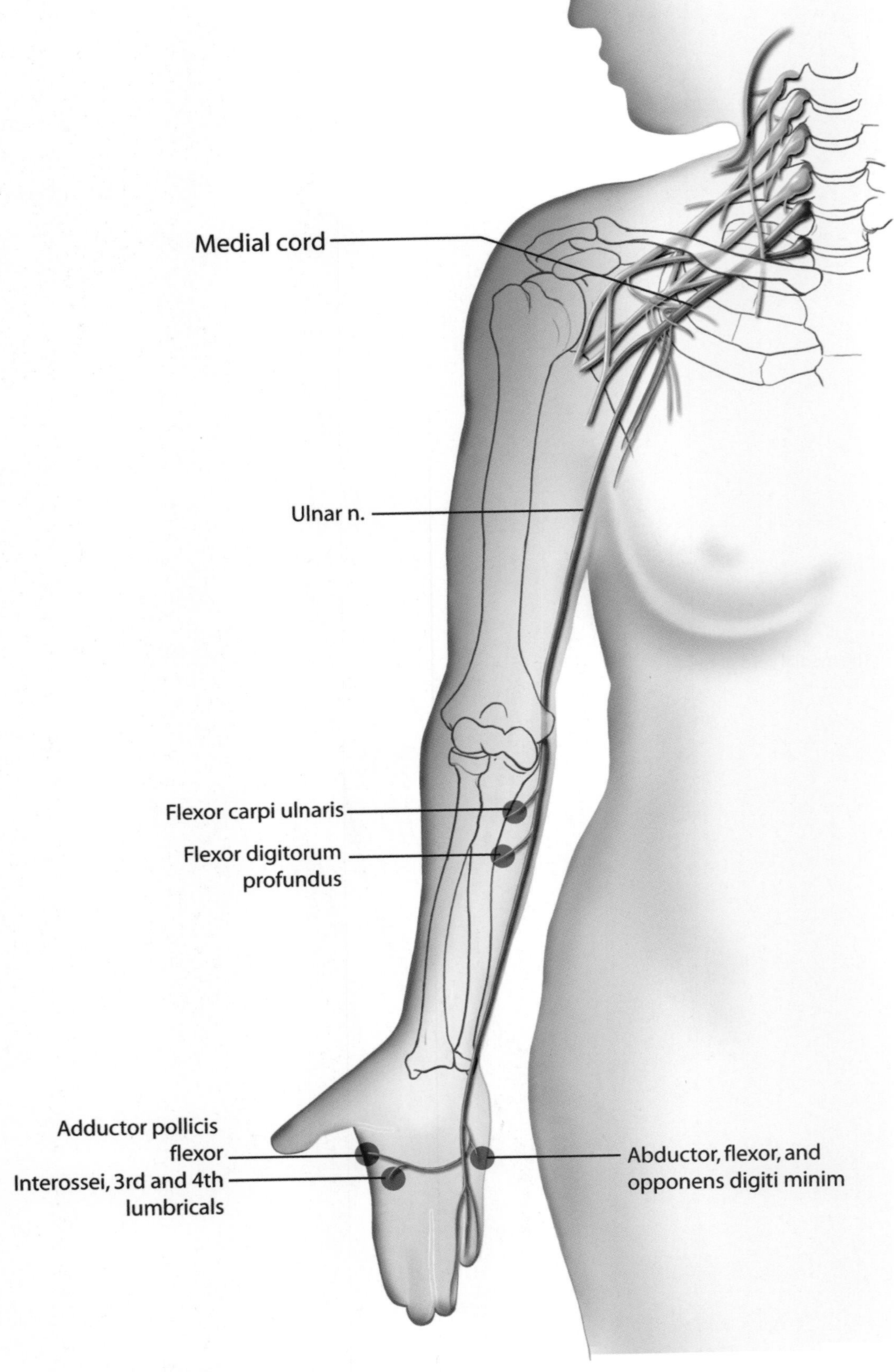

FIGURE 5-6 Muscles innervated by the medial cord of the brachial plexus.

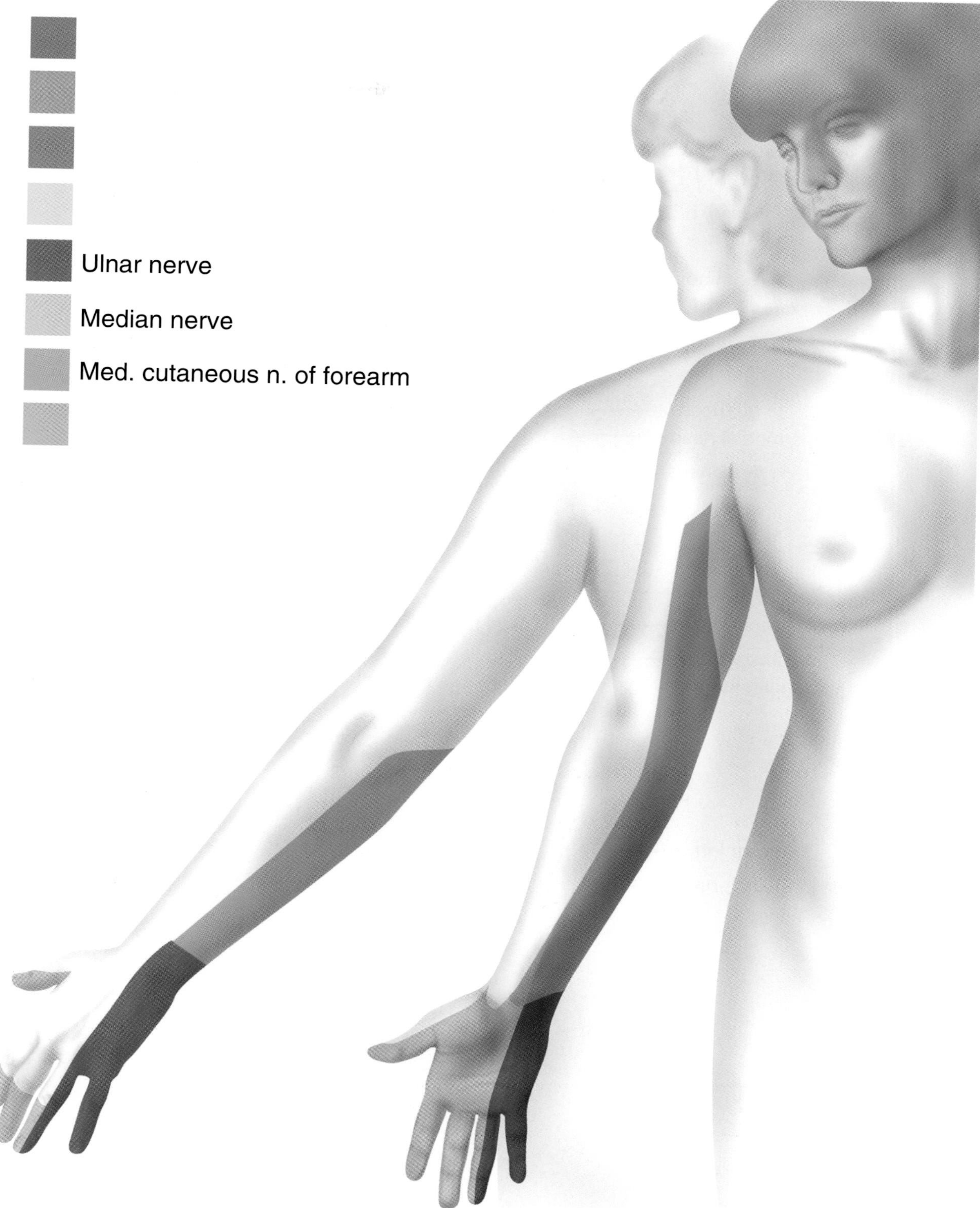

FIGURE 5-7 Sensory neurotomes innervated by the nerves of the medial cord of the brachial plexus.

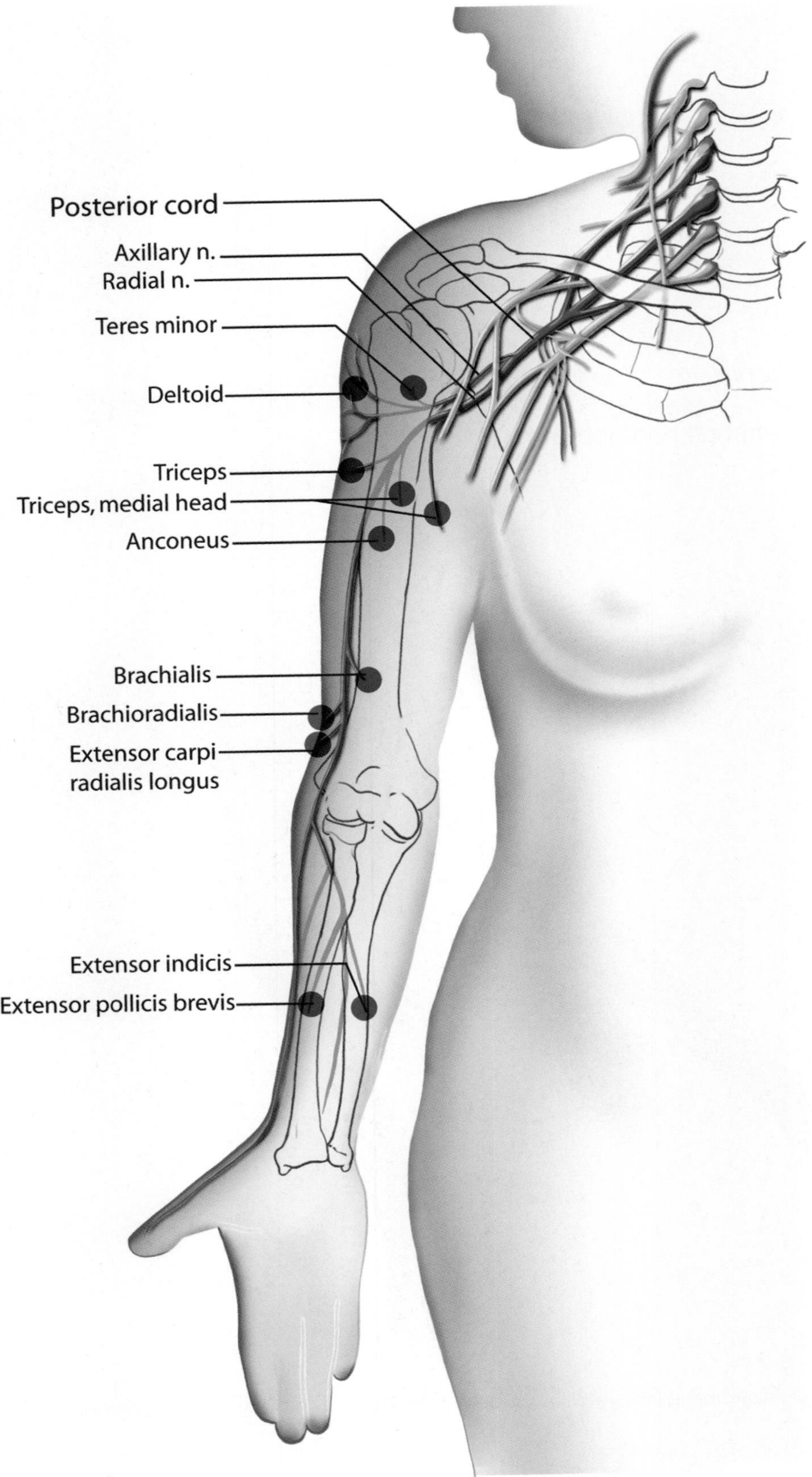

FIGURE 5-8 Muscles innervated by the posterior cord of the brachial plexus.

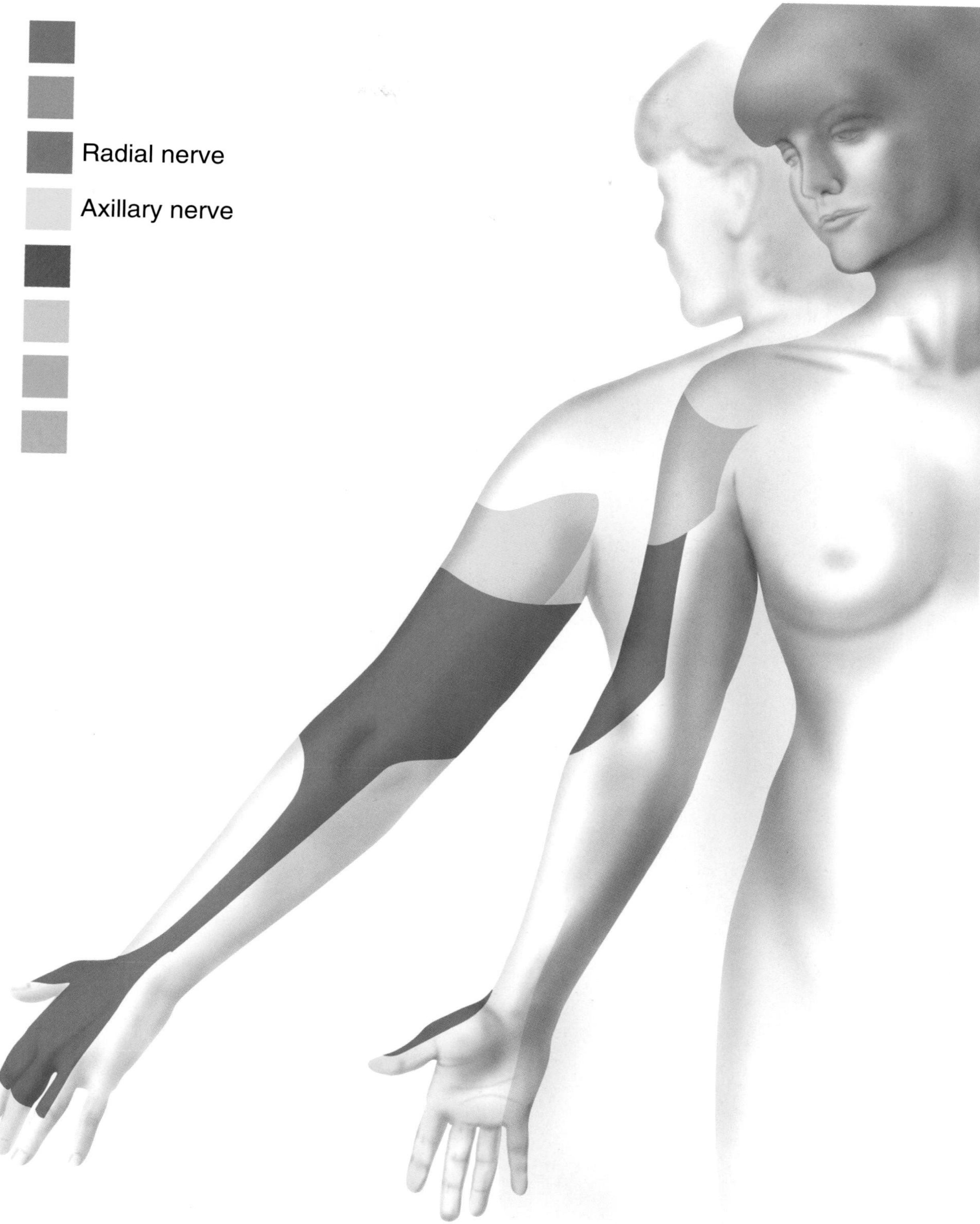

FIGURE 5-9 Sensory neurotomes innervated by the nerves of the posterior cord of the brachial plexus.

SUGGESTED FURTHER READING

1. Gray's Anatomy: The Anatomical Basis of Clinical Practice, 39th ed. Philadelphia, Elsevier, 2005.
2. Netter FH: Atlas of Human Anatomy, 2nd ed. East Hanover, NJ, Novartis, 1997.
3. Abrahams PH, Marks SC Jr, Hutchings RT: McMinn's Color Atlas of Human Anatomy, 5th ed. Philadelphia, Elsevier Mosby, 2003.
4. Boezaart AP: Anesthesia and Orthopaedic Surgery. New York, McGraw-Hill, 2006.
5. Hadzic A, Vloka JD: Peripheral Nerve Blocks: Principles and Practice. New York, McGraw-Hill, 2004.
6. Rathmell JP, Neal JM, Viscomi CM: Regional Anesthesia: The Requisites in Anesthesia. Philadelphia, Elsevier Mosby, 2004.
7. Brown DL: Atlas of Regional Anesthesia, 3rd ed. Philadelphia, Elsevier, 2006.
8. Barret J, Harmon D, Loughnane B, et al: Peripheral Nerve Blocks and Peri-operative Pain Relief. Philadelphia, WB Saunders, 2004.
9. Meier G, Büttner J: Atlas der peripheren Regionalanästhesie. Stuttgart, Georg Thieme Verlag, 2004.
10. Hahn MB, McQuillan PM, Sheplock GJ: Regional Anesthesia: An Atlas of Anatomy and Technique. St. Louis, Mosby, 1996.
11. Borene S, Edwards JN, Boezaart AP: At the chords, the pinkie towards: Interpreting infraclavicular motor response to neurostimulation. Reg Anesth Pain Med 2004;29:125-129.

Chapter 6

Infraclavicular Block

- **Single-Injection Infraclavicular Block**
- **Continuous Infraclavicular Block**

SINGLE-INJECTION INFRACLAVICULAR BLOCK

Introduction

This block is commonly used for single-injection regional anesthesia for hand, wrist, arm, and elbow surgery (1). This block is performed at the level of the cords of the brachial plexus; it is easy to perform, has a short onset time, and covers all the nerves distal to the shoulder joint.

All the neurotomes distal to the shoulder joints are typically incorporated in this block; unless the suprascapular nerve is specifically blocked separately, this block is not suitable for shoulder surgery.

Technique

A point approximately 2.5 cm (1 inch) medial and 2.5 cm (1 inch) caudal from the midpoint of the coracoid process marks the point of needle entry if the pericoracoid technique is used (2) (Fig. 6-1). The *dotted line* in Figure 6-1 indicates the midline of the clavicle, and a point 1 cm caudal on this line marks the point of needle entry in the vertical infraclavicular plexus (VIP) block technique, which is popular in Europe (3). The "superior" approach is described here (1,4,5).

The patient is placed in the supine or semi-sitting position to decrease venous congestion in the infraclavicular area. The hand is placed on the patient's abdomen or held in the anesthesiologist's hand (Fig. 6-1 and 6-2).

After skin preparation, the skin and subcutaneous tissue is anesthetized in the coracodeltoid trough with a local anesthetic agent, as indicated in Figure 6-3. Only a superficial skin wheal is required for this block.

A 50- to 100-mm, shallow-bevel insulated needle is used (Fig. 6-4). It is connected to a nerve

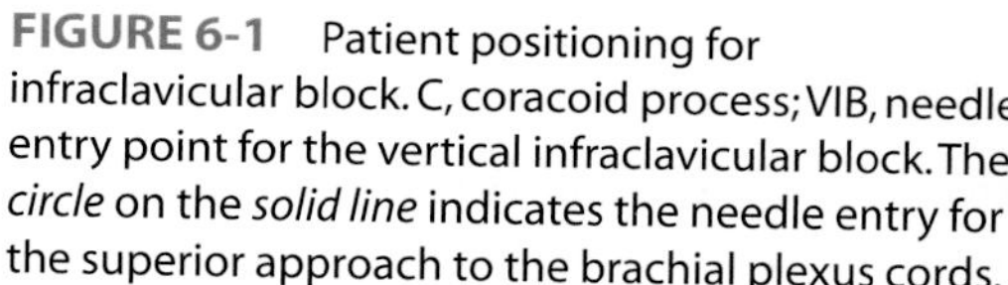

FIGURE 6-1 Patient positioning for infraclavicular block. C, coracoid process; VIB, needle entry point for the vertical infraclavicular block. The *circle* on the *solid line* indicates the needle entry for the superior approach to the brachial plexus cords.

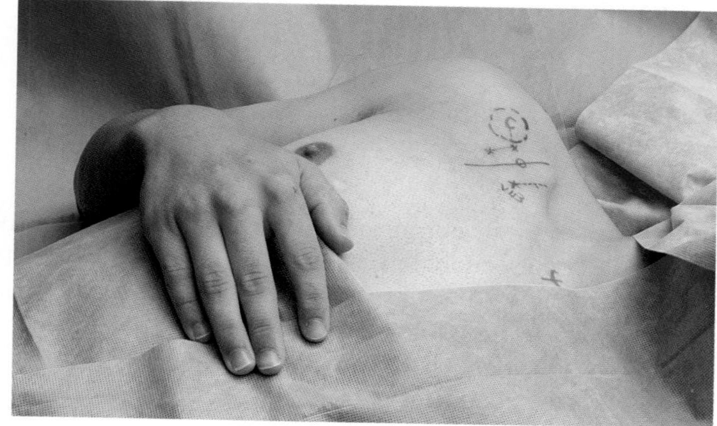

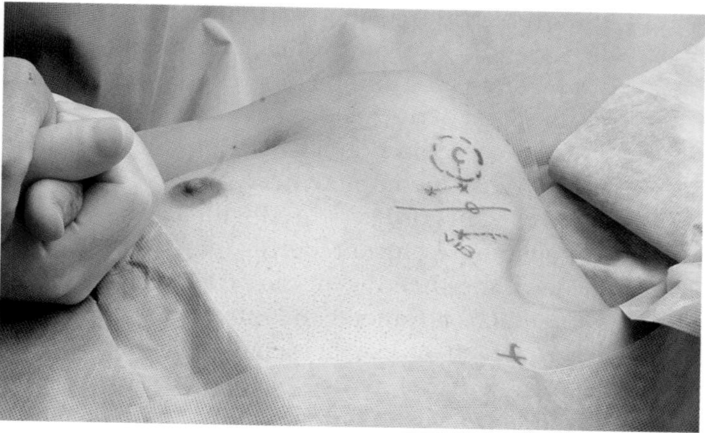

FIGURE 6-2 The patient's hand can be held in the anesthesiologist's nonoperative hand or can be placed on the abdomen.

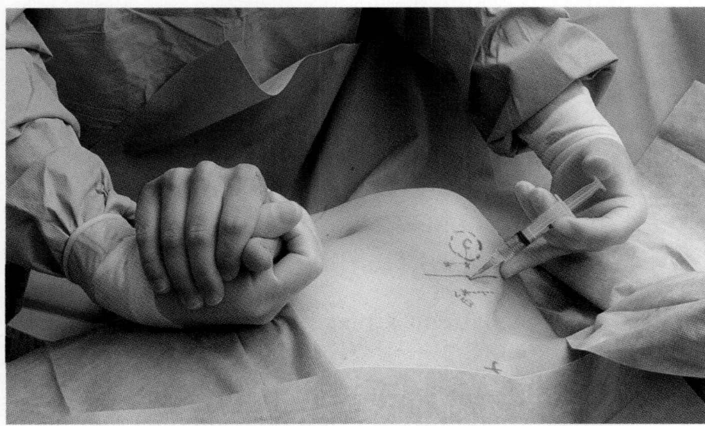

FIGURE 6-3 A small skin wheal is raised in the deltopectoral trough.

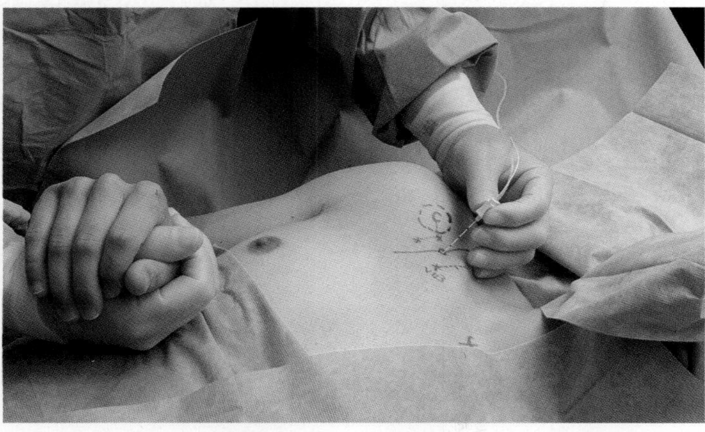

FIGURE 6-4 A 50-mm stimulating needle enters at 45 degrees to the coronal plane while remaining in the parasagittal plane.

stimulator, set to an output of 1 to 1.5 mA, 100- to 300-μsec pulse duration, and a frequency of 2 Hz. Needle entry is close to the clavicle in the coracoclavicular trough, aimed posteriorly at an angle of 15 degrees to the coronal plane. The needle is advanced until arm muscle motor responses are observed.

It is important that the needle should remain within the parasagittal plane, without medial or lateral deviation. Medial misdirection of the needle can result in lung and pleura penetration. Lateral misdirection of the needle may place it on the base of the coracoid bone, which, although harmless, may cause incomplete nerve block.

After the correct cord is located with a brisk motor response at a current output of 0.3 to 0.5 mA, the local anesthetic agent can be injected.

As the needle is advanced, the musculocutaneous nerve, which is usually separated from the lateral cord of the brachial plexus, may be encountered. This causes unmistakable biceps contractions without hand flexion or pronation, and it should be ignored at this stage of the block. Similarly, the axillary nerve may be encountered, which causes a deltoid muscle motor response. This response should also be ignored at this stage of the block.

Ultrasonography may be very helpful in performing the single-injection infraclavicular block (6). Hold the probe in the coracopectoral trough and identify the axillary artery (Fig. 6-5). Inject local anesthetic agent approximately at the same point described previously for the superior approach to anesthetize the skin. Because muscles are not penetrated with this approach, only a small skin wheal is required.

Place a 50–90 mm, shallow-beveled stimulating needle through the skin and, under ultrasonographic guidance, behind the artery—between the artery and the cords—and inject local anesthetic to "push" the nerves away from the artery (Fig. 6-6). The "doughnut" sign can be seen as the local

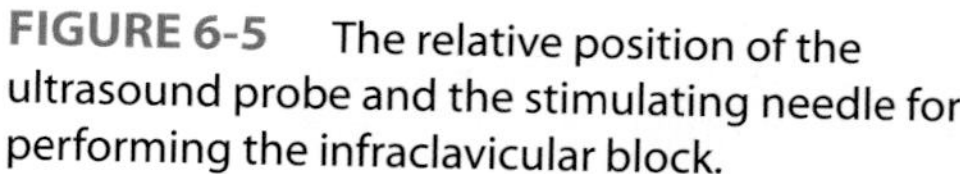

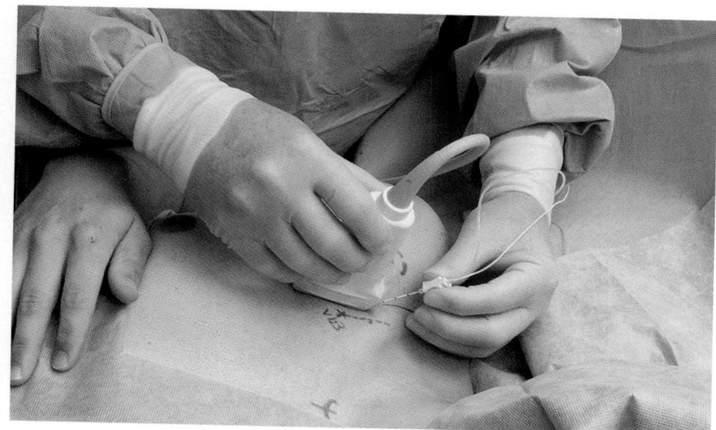

FIGURE 6-5 The relative position of the ultrasound probe and the stimulating needle for performing the infraclavicular block.

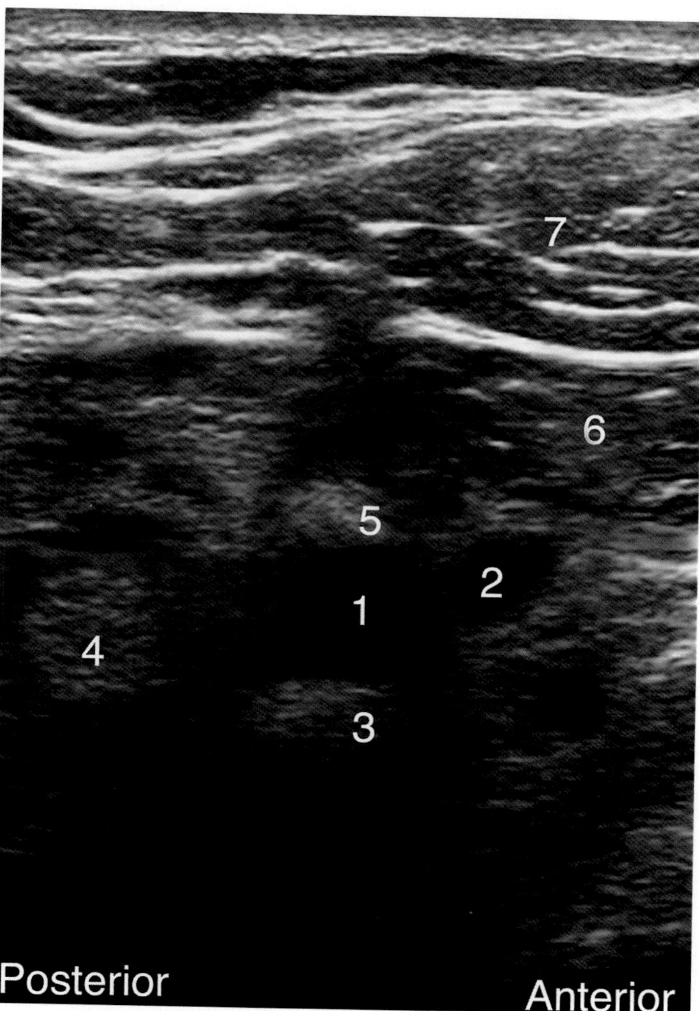

FIGURE 6-6 Ultrasonograph of the infraclavicular area: 1. Axillary artery; 2. Axillary vein; 3. Medial cord of the brachial plexus; 4. Posterior cord of the brachial plexus; 5. Lateral cord of the brachial plexus; 6. Minor pectoral muscle; 7. Major pectoral muscle.

anesthetic agent spreads around the brachial plexus cords.

Flexion of the fingers and ulnar deviation at the wrist indicate medial cord stimulation—the fifth digit (little finger) moves medially (7) (Fig. 6-7).

Pronation and hand flexion would indicate lateral cord stimulation, in which the fifth digit moves laterally (7) (Fig. 6-8).

Extension of the fingers (i.e., the fifth digit moves posteriorly) would indicate posterior

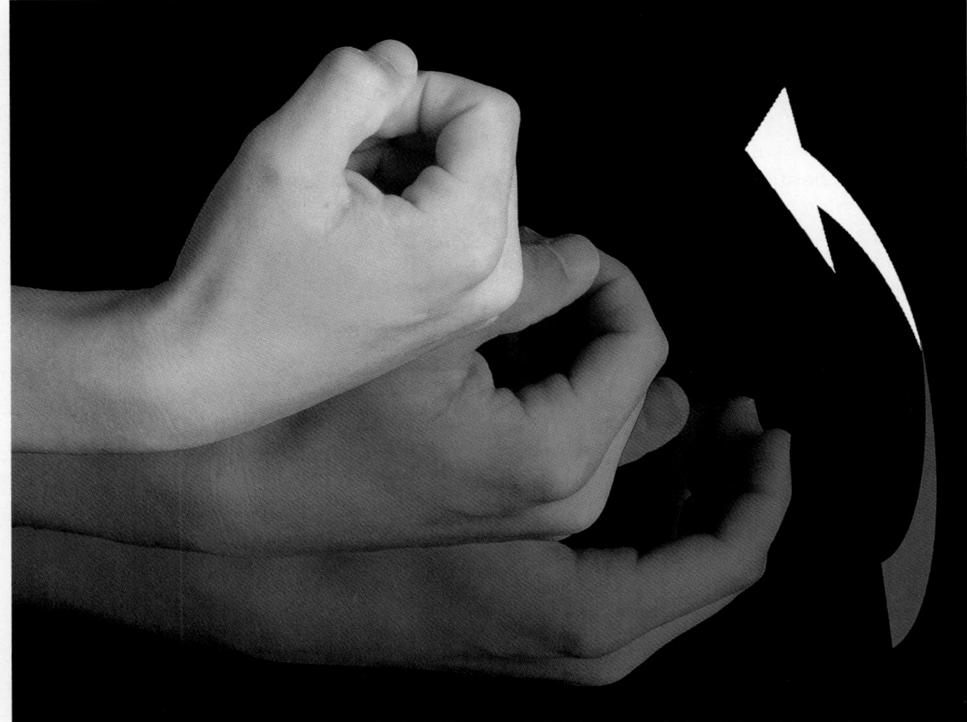

FIGURE 6-7 During medial cord stimulation, the fifth digit (little finger) moves medially.

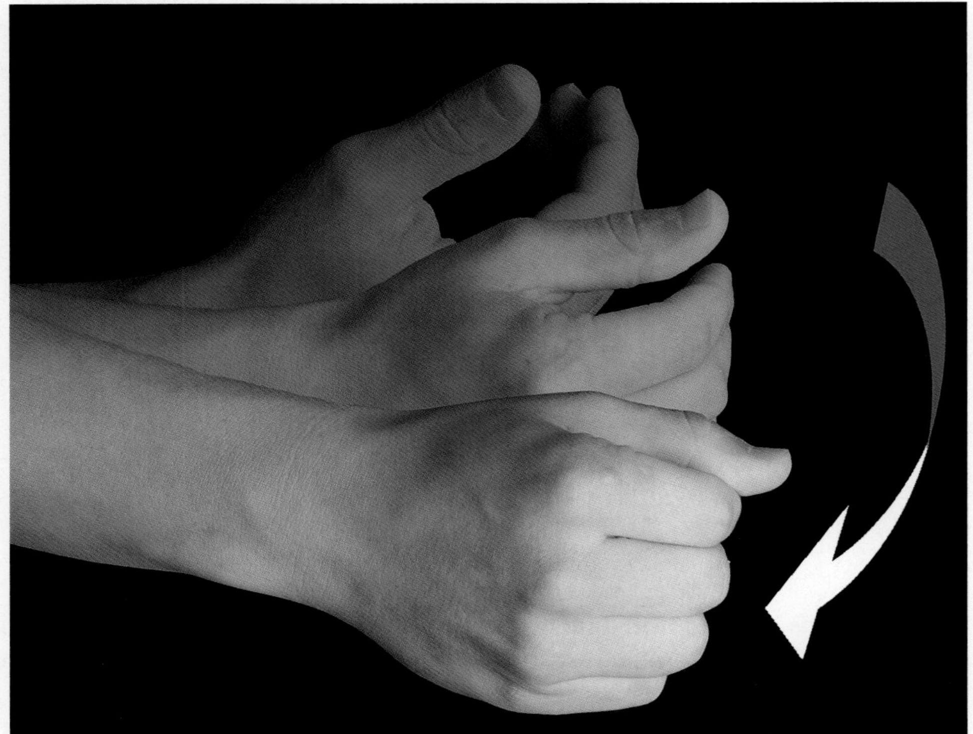

FIGURE 6-8 During lateral cord stimulation, the fifth digit (little finger) moves laterally.

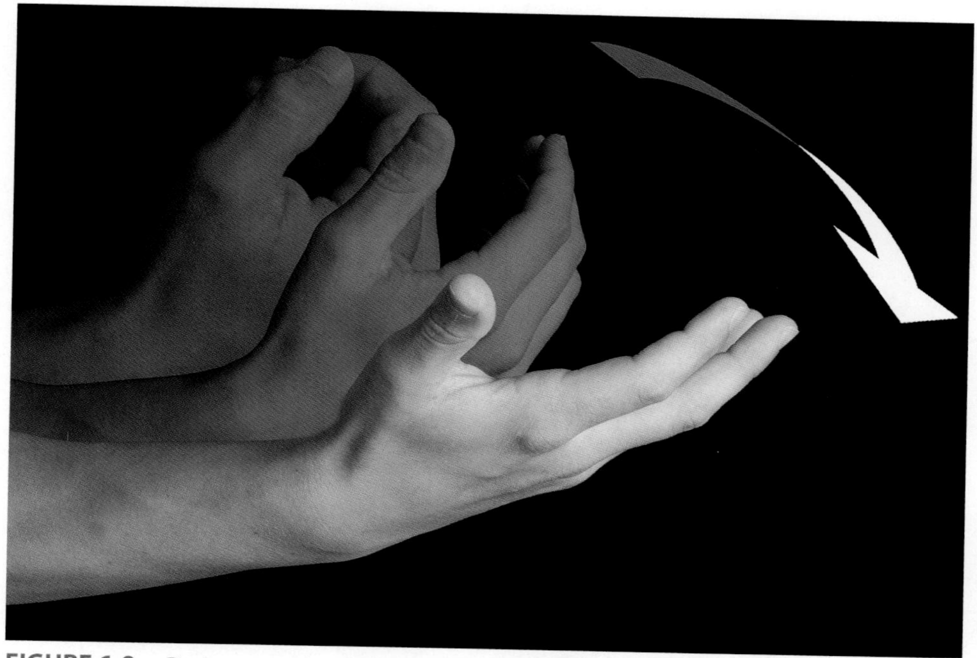

FIGURE 6-9 During posterior cord stimulation, the fifth digit (little finger) moves posteriorly.

cord stimulation (7) (Fig. 6-9). The fifth digit thus moves toward the cord that is being stimulated.

The current of the nerve stimulator is turned down until a brisk motor response of the muscles innervated by the most appropriate cord for the planned surgery can still be observed at 0.3 to 0.5 mA. Brisk motor twitches at an output of less than 0.2 mA may indicate intraneural placement, but this statement has not been verified by research.

While keeping the needle steady and observing the motor response, the operator injects the local anesthetic agent. The motor response stops immediately on injection. This constitutes a positive Raj test and is an indication that the block will be successful. Any solution that conducts electricity, such as normal saline, disperses the current density and causes a cessation of the motor response if the needle tip is in the same fascial plane as the nerve.

The other cords of the brachial plexus can now be sought and blocked, if appropriate. The best results are obtained if the posterior and medial cords are blocked.

Local Anesthetic Agent Choice

Most local anesthetic agents and combinations have been used for this block. Typically, 15 to 40 mL of ropivacaine 0.5% to 0.75% is used, of which 10 to 25 mL is injected onto the most appropriate cord and the remainder into at least one of the other cords. Adding buprenorphine 0.3 mg (8) to the mixture may lengthen the duration of action of the block, but if a long-acting block is required, it is best to place a continuous nerve block. The addition of dexamethasone 40 mg has been suggested to lengthen the duration of action of local anesthetic agents, but this needs to be verified by research.

(See pericoracoid approach for infraclavicular block movie on DVD.)

CONTINUOUS INFRACLAVICULAR BLOCK

Introduction

Like the single-injection infraclavicular block, the continuous infraclavicular block is used for surgery of the arm distal to the shoulder (9). This block has been inconsistent in clinical practice. Wrist and elbow surgery requires blockage of all three cords of the brachial plexus, as does postoperative pain management of these joints. However, with the continuous infraclavicular block, all three of the cords are blocked with the initial, relatively large-volume primary block, but

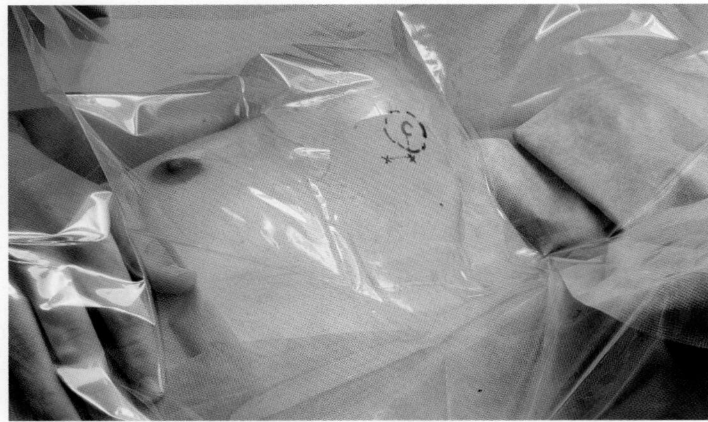

FIGURE 6-10 After skin preparation, a sterile, fenestrated drape is placed over the infraclavicular area.

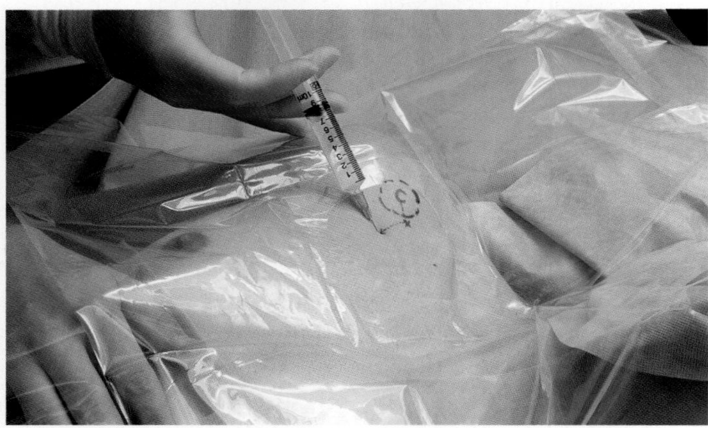

FIGURE 6-11 The skin and subcutaneous tissue are anesthetized.

only the cord on which the catheter has been placed seems to be affected by the smaller-volume continuous infusion. This sometimes leaves the other two cords unblocked, and relatively large-volume boluses are needed to recapture blockage of these cords.

Technique

The patient is positioned in the supine or semi-sitting position with the hand placed on the abdomen. After skin preparation, the area is covered with a sterile, fenestrated, transparent plastic drape (Fig. 6-10).

The surface landmarks are similar to those for the single injection pericoracoid infraclavicular block: 2.5 cm medial and 2.5 cm caudal from the coracoid process. Another approach is 1 cm caudal on a line from the midline of the clavicle. Many authors have different approaches to the infraclavicular block. Of note are the more medial-to-lateral approach used by Borgeat and colleagues (10), the more superior approach used by Klaastad and associates (4,5), and the pericoracoid approach used by Whiffler (11). The pericoracoid approach, in which the needle (and catheter) is aimed medially and cephalad, is described here. The needle and catheter are placed on the brachial plexus at the trunks in the vicinity of the first rib (1).

The skin, subcutaneous tissue, and the intended path of tunneling are thoroughly anesthetized with lidocaine and 1:200,000 epinephrine (Fig. 6-11). The epinephrine is added to reduce skin and subcutaneous bleeding.

An insulated 17- or 18-gauge Tuohy needle, attached to a nerve stimulator set to a current output of 1 to 2 mA, a frequency of 2 Hz, and a pulse width of 100 to 300 μsec, is aimed medially and cephalad towards the interscalene groove (Fig. 6-12). Penetration of the fascia surrounding the major pectoral muscle can usually be felt clearly.

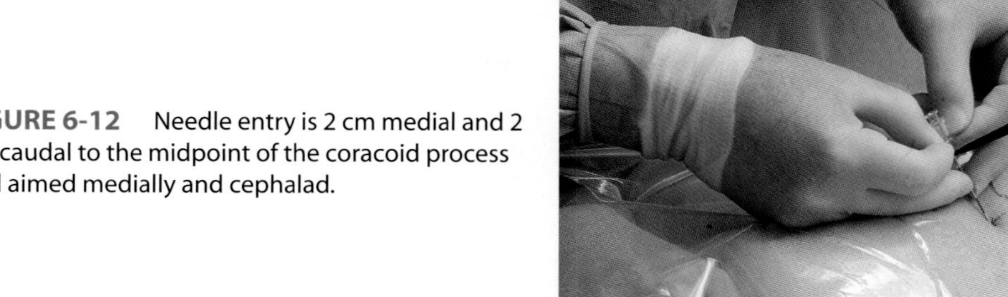

FIGURE 6-12 Needle entry is 2 cm medial and 2 cm caudal to the midpoint of the coracoid process and aimed medially and cephalad.

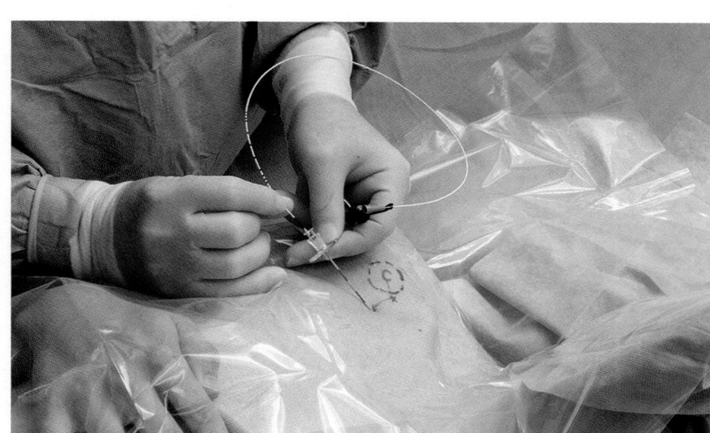

FIGURE 6-13 After the needle is placed on the appropriate cord, the nerve stimulator is attached to the proximal end of the catheter and the catheter advanced through the needle.

A more anteroposterior approach is often also used (9).

When the appropriate cord of the brachial plexus is encountered, the nerve stimulator output is turned down to 0.3 to 0.5 mA. This confirms accurate needle placement, but it does not guarantee accurate catheter placement. It is important not to inject any conducting fluid such as local anesthetic agent or normal saline through the needle at this point because this will render stimulating catheter placement impossible. If the anesthesiologist subscribes to the notion of "opening of the space," 5% dextrose and water can be used because saline will disperse the current and render further nerve stimulation with the catheter useless.

The bevel of the needle is pointed in the direction the catheter is intended to go. The needle is placed on the most appropriate cord of the brachial plexus for the planned surgery.

The nerve stimulator is set to 0.5 to 1 mA, or at a level that is comfortable for the patient, and attached to the proximal end of the stimulating catheter. Note the special mark on the catheter, which indicates that the catheter tip is situated at the tip of the needle. The catheter is advanced beyond the needle tip, and if the motor response disappears, it simply means that the catheter tip is moving away from the cord.

Withdraw the catheter tip carefully to inside the needle shaft, make a small adjustment to the needle such as turning it clockwise or counterclockwise or advancing or withdrawing it slightly, and advance the catheter again (Fig. 6-14). Repeat this maneuver until the motor response remains constant during catheter advancement. Advance the catheter 3 to 5 cm beyond the needle tip, but not more than 5 cm.

Remove the needle without disturbing the catheter (Fig. 6-15).

A special tunneling device can now be used to tunnel the catheter subcutaneously, or the

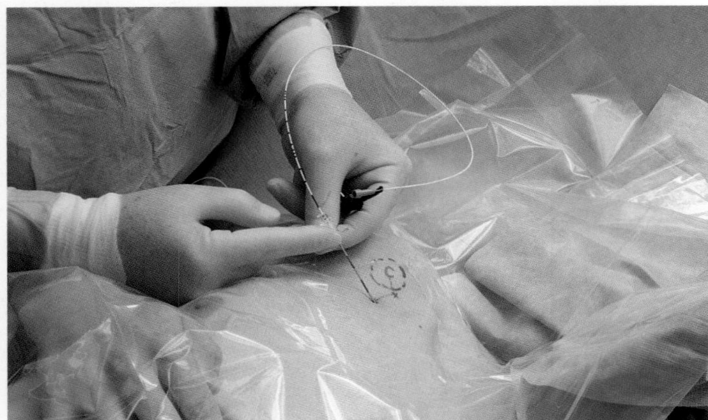

FIGURE 6-14 If the motor response is lost, the catheter is withdrawn and the needle manipulated. The catheter is advanced again.

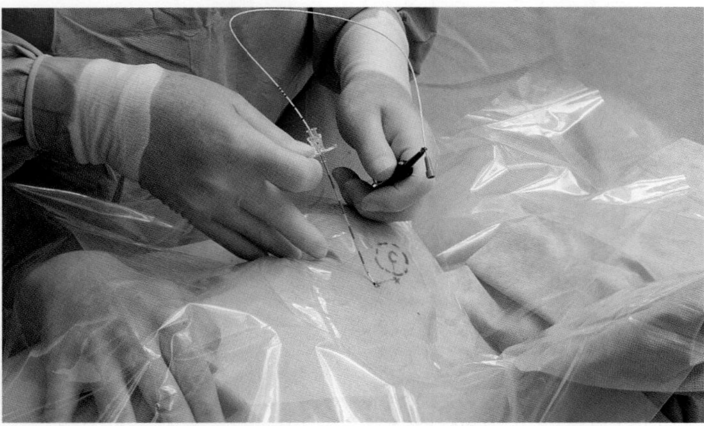

FIGURE 6-15 After the catheter is properly placed on the desired port, the needle is removed without disturbing the catheter.

Tuohy needle and its stylet can be used. Tunneling is essential to prevent catheter dislodgement (see Chapter 12). The skin bridge may be important for short- to medium-term catheter use because it can facilitate easy catheter removal. However, a skin bridge may be responsible for a higher incidence of leakage around the catheter. The risk of leakage may be offset against tunneling without a skin bridge, which in turn may make catheter removal more difficult.

The Luer lock connecting device is attached to the proximal end of the catheter. The nerve stimulator, set to an output of 0 mA, is attached to the connecting device and the nerve stimulator output is slowly turned up until a muscle twitch can just be seen. Local anesthetic agent or any conducting fluid, such as normal saline, can be injected and the muscle twitches will stop immediately once the injection is started. This constitutes a positive Raj test and gives further assurance that the secondary block will be successful. The catheter adaptation device and catheter are attached to the fixation device, which is attached to a convenient place on the opposite side of the patient's upper body.

Local Anesthetic and Infusion Choice

Most local anesthetic agents have been used for this block. Typically, 15 to 40 mL of ropivacaine 0.5% to 0.75% is used as the initial bolus, followed by a 5- to 10-mL/hour continuous infusion of ropivacaine 0.2%. It is essential to allow relatively large patient-controlled boluses of 10 to 15 mL every 60 minutes to recapture unblocked cords in the postoperative period, should this become necessary.

Catheter Removal

The catheter is removed after the patient no longer requires continuous block and full sensation has returned to the limb (see Chapter 12). Any radiating pain during catheter removal may indicate that the catheter is coiled around a nerve or cord, and this situation should be managed with utmost care. Remove the catheter by stabilizing the proximal part and first removing the distal end from the skin bridge. Once this is done, keep the catheter sterile and then remove the remaining catheter.

(See pericoracoid approach for continuous infraclavicular block movie on DVD.)

REFERENCES

1. Raw RM: Brachial plexus blocks below the clavicle. In Boezaart AP (ed): Anesthesia and Orthopaedic Surgery. New York, McGraw-Hill, 2006, pp 311-320.
2. Wilson JL, Brown DL, Wong GY, et al: Infraclavicular brachial plexus block: Parasagittal anatomy important to the coracoid technique. Anesth Analg 1998;87: 870-873.
3. Kilka HG, Geiger P, Mehrkens HH: Infraclavicular vertical brachial plexus blockade: A new method for anesthesia of the upper extremity. An anatomical and clinical study [in German]. Anaesthesist 1995;44:339-344.
4. Klaastad O, Lilleas FG, Rotnes JS, et al: A magnetic resonance imaging study of modifications to the infraclavicular brachial plexus block. Anesth Analg 2000;91:929-933.
5. Klaastad O, Smith HJ, Smedby O, et al: A novel infraclavicular brachial plexus block: The lateral and sagittal technique, developed by magnetic resonance imaging studies. Anesth Analg 2004;98;252-256.
6. Chan VWS: The use of ultrasound for peripheral nerve blocks. In Boezaart AP (ed): Anesthesia and Orthopaedic Surgery. New York, McGraw-Hill, 2006, pp 283-290.
7. Borene S, Edwards JN, Boezaart AP: At the chords, the pinkie towards: Interpreting infraclavicular motor response to neurostimulation. Reg Anesth Pain Med 2004;29:125-129.
8. Candido KD, Winnie AP, Ghaleb AH, et al: Buprenorphine added to the local anesthetic for axillary brachial plexus block prolongs postoperative analgesia. Reg Anesth Pain Med 2002;27:162-167.
9. Ilfeld BM, Morey TE, Enneking FK: Continuous infraclavicular perineural infusion with clonidine and ropivacaine compared with ropivacaine alone: A randomized, double blinded, controlled study. Anesth Analg 2003;97:706-712.
10. Borgeat A, Ekatodramis G, Dumont C: An evaluation of the infraclavicular block via a modified approach of the Raj technique. Anesth Analg 2001;93:436-441.
11. Whiffler K: Coracoid block: A safe and easy technique. Br J Anaesth 1981;53:845-848.

Chapter 7

Nerves in the Axilla: Applied Anatomy

- Radial Nerve in the Axilla
- Median Nerve in the Axilla
- Ulnar Nerve in the Axilla
- Musculocutaneous Nerve in the Axilla

RADIAL NERVE IN THE AXILLA

The radial nerve (see Fig. 1-1, [23]) arises from the posterior cord (see Fig. 1-1, [13]) of the brachial plexus, which in turn receives innervation from all three trunks and the C6, C7, and C8 roots.

Figure 7-1 demonstrates the area that receives sensory innervation from the radial nerve.

In the dissection depicted in Figure 7-2, the medial and lateral cords are retracted and the radial nerve is indicated with an *arrow*. It passes through the triangular space below the lower border of the teres major, between the long head of the triceps muscle and the humerus.

Electrical stimulation of the radial nerve causes extension of the arm at the elbow because of contractions of the triceps. These contractions can be seen clearly in the accompanying recording.

(See radial nerve movie on DVD.)

MEDIAN NERVE IN THE AXILLA

The median nerve (see Fig. 1-1, [24]) arises from the lateral cord (see Fig. 1-1, [12]) and the medial and lateral cords (see Fig. 1-1, [12, 14]). It receives innervation from all the trunks and roots of the brachial plexus. The nerve has no branches in the upper arm.

Figure 7-3 illustrates the areas of sensory innervation of the median nerve.

The *arrow* in Figure 7-4 indicates the median nerve, which is a large nerve in the axilla. It is

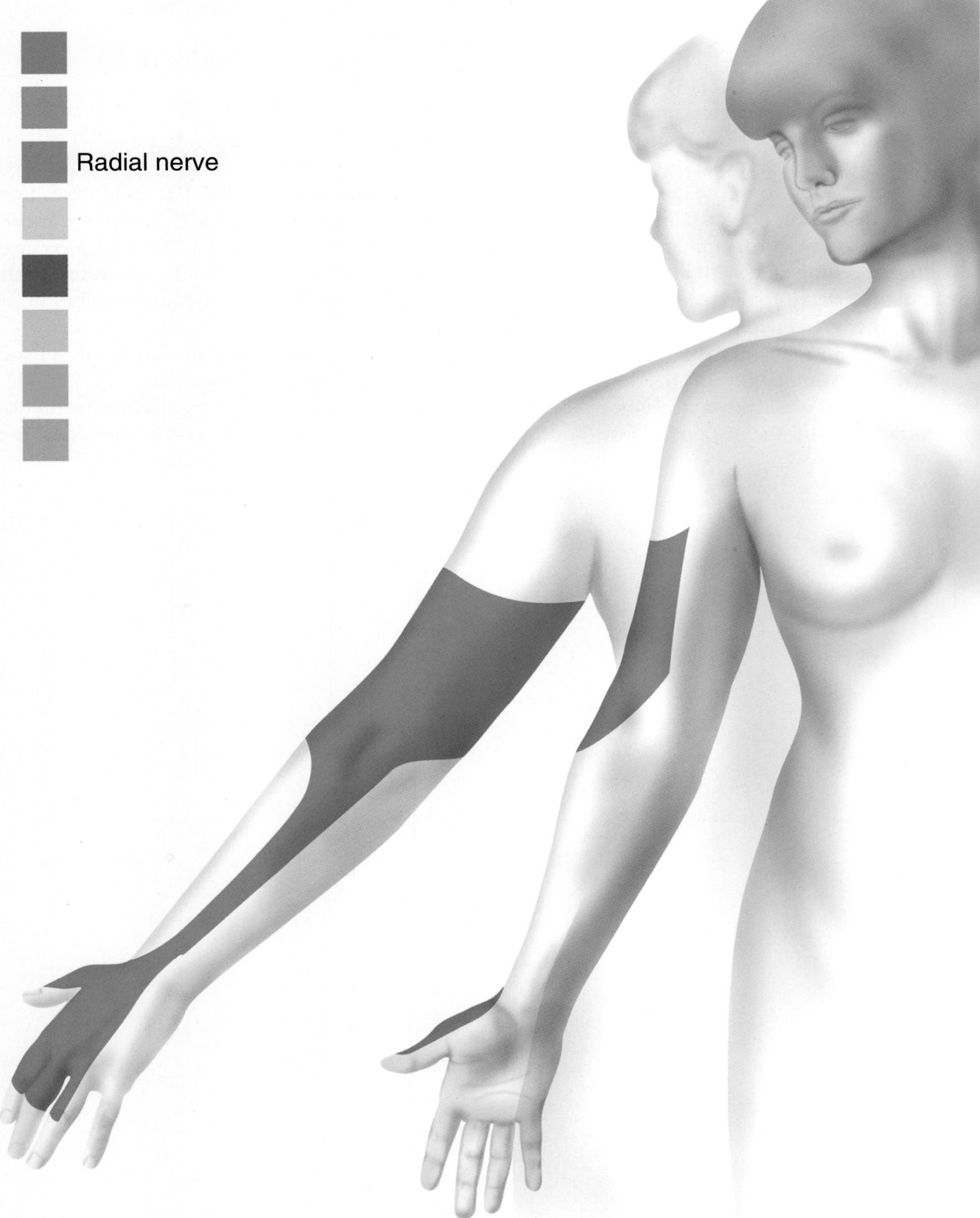

FIGURE 7-1 Sensory neurotome of the radial nerve.

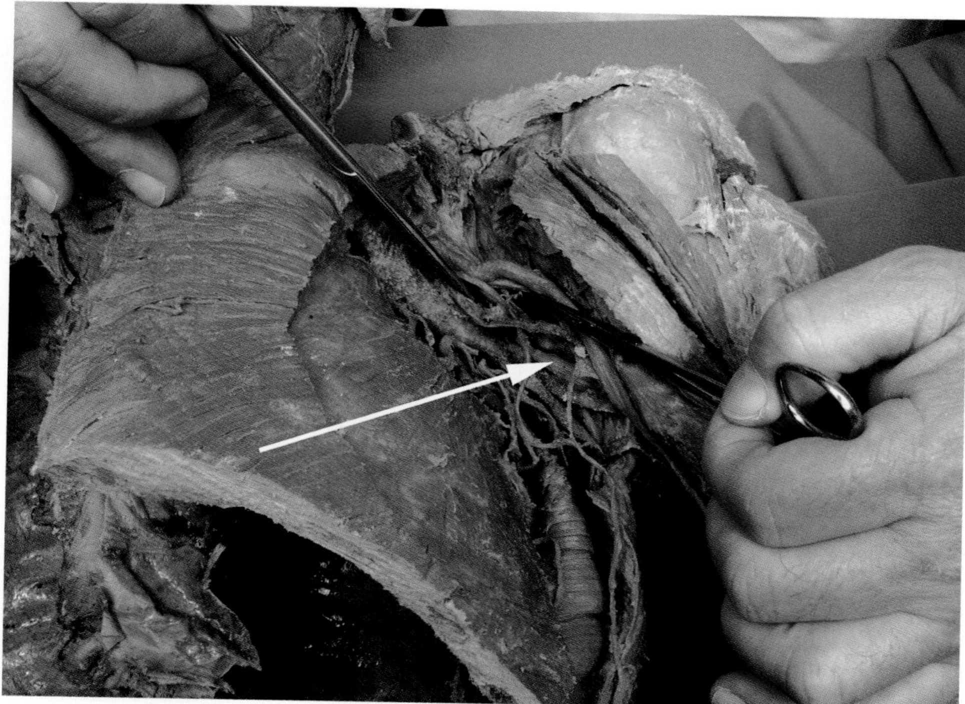

FIGURE 7-2 The *arrow* indicates the radial nerve in the infraclavicular area.

easy to stimulate this nerve electrically in the axilla. Such stimulation leads to pronation of the forearm, flexion of the fingers, and adduction of the thumb.

(See median nerve movie on DVD.)

ULNAR NERVE IN THE AXILLA

The ulnar nerve (see Fig. 1-1, [25]) arises from the medial cord (see Fig. 1-1, [14]) of the brachial plexus, which in turn is derived from the inferior trunk and the C8 and T1 roots.

Figure 7-5 shows the area of sensory innervation of the ulnar nerve.

The ulnar nerve (Fig. 7-6, *arrow*) is smaller than the median nerve, and runs posterior to it.

Stimulation of the ulnar nerve in the axilla causes flexion of the fingers and ulnar deviation at the wrist.

(See ulnar nerve movie on DVD.)

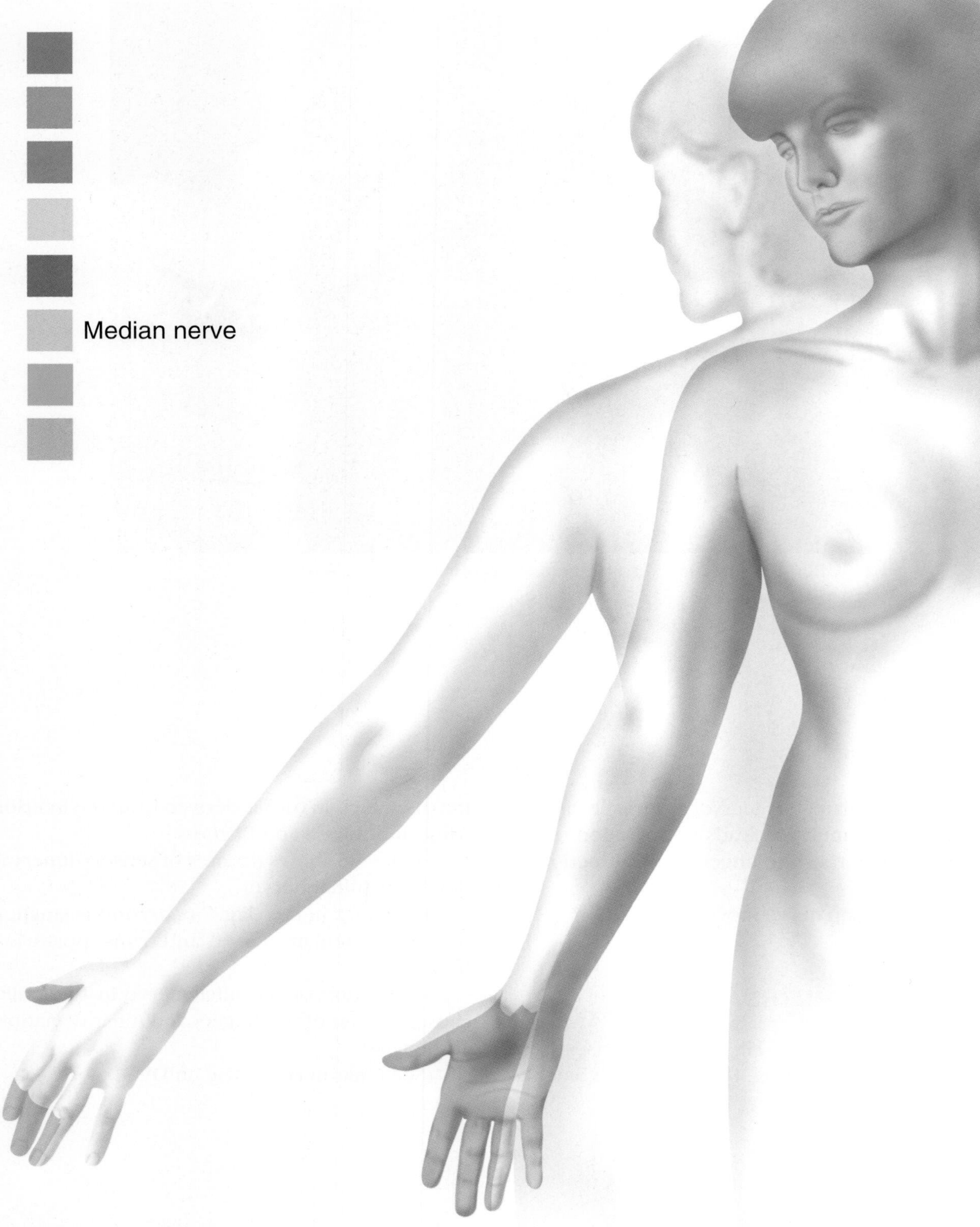

FIGURE 7-3 Sensory neurotome of the median nerve.

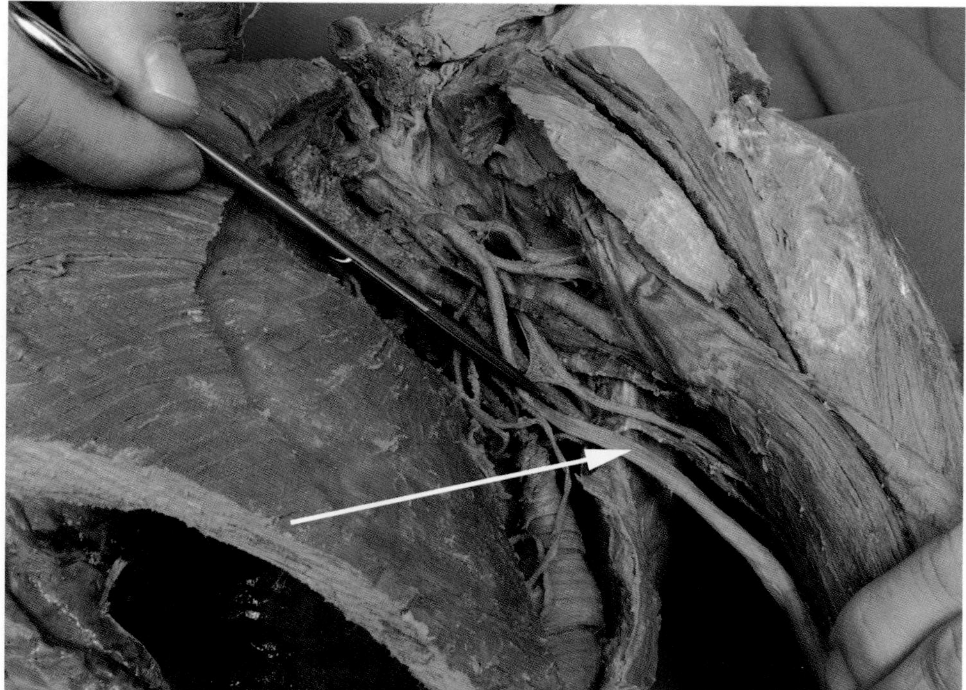

FIGURE 7-4 The *arrow* indicates the median nerve in the subclavian area.

MUSCULOCUTANEOUS NERVE IN THE AXILLA

The musculocutaneous nerve (see Fig. 1-1, [22]) originates as a continuation of the lateral cord (see Fig. 1-1, [12]) of the brachial plexus. It is innervated from the C5, C6, and C7 roots.

Figure 7-7 illustrates the area of sensory innervation of the musculocutaneous nerve.

As can be seen in the dissection illustrated in Figure 7-8, the musculocutaneous nerve (*arrow*) courses around the humerus next to the axillary nerve. It is often damaged here during surgery of the shoulder. The musculocutaneous nerve

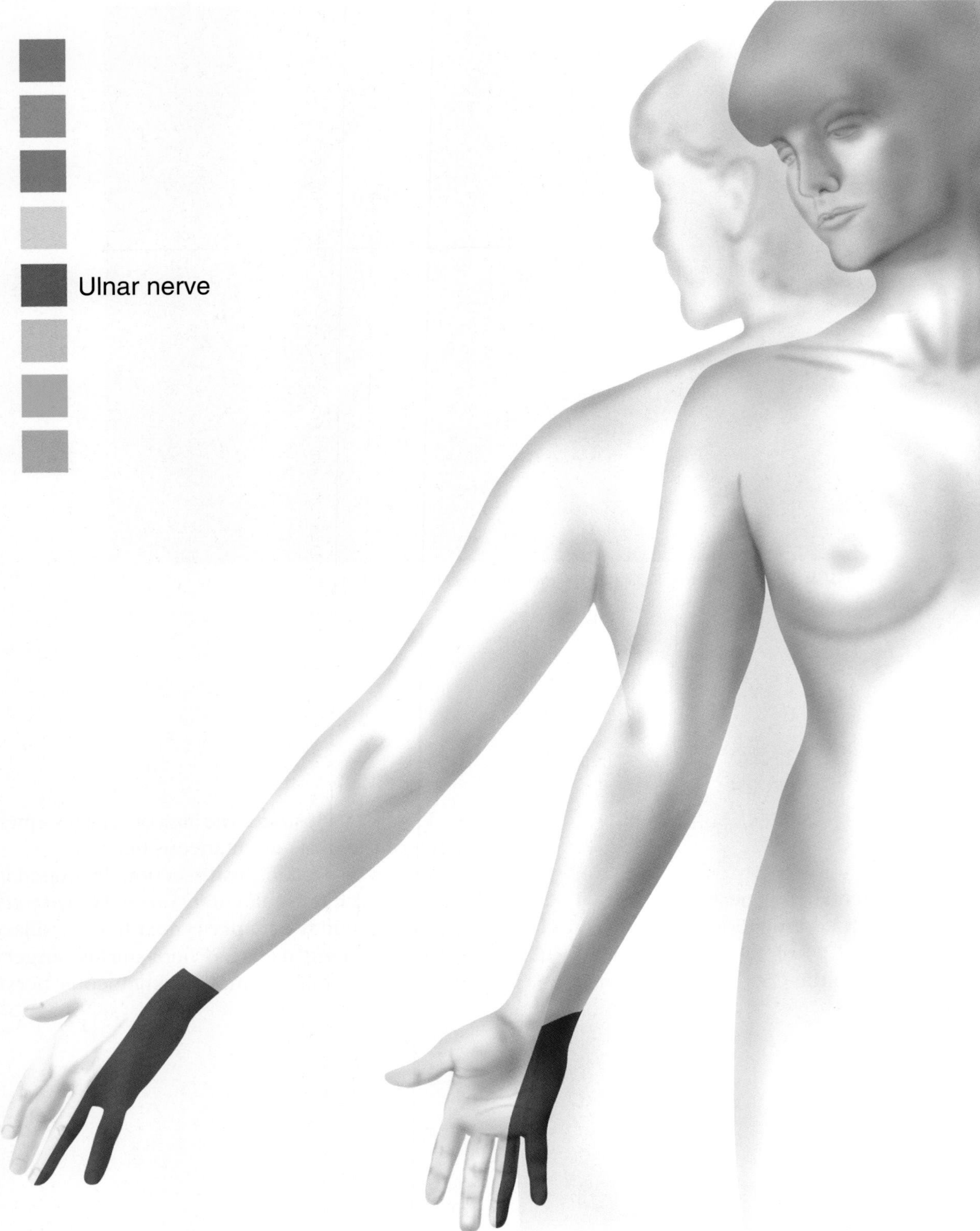

FIGURE 7-5 Sensory neurotome of the ulnar nerve.

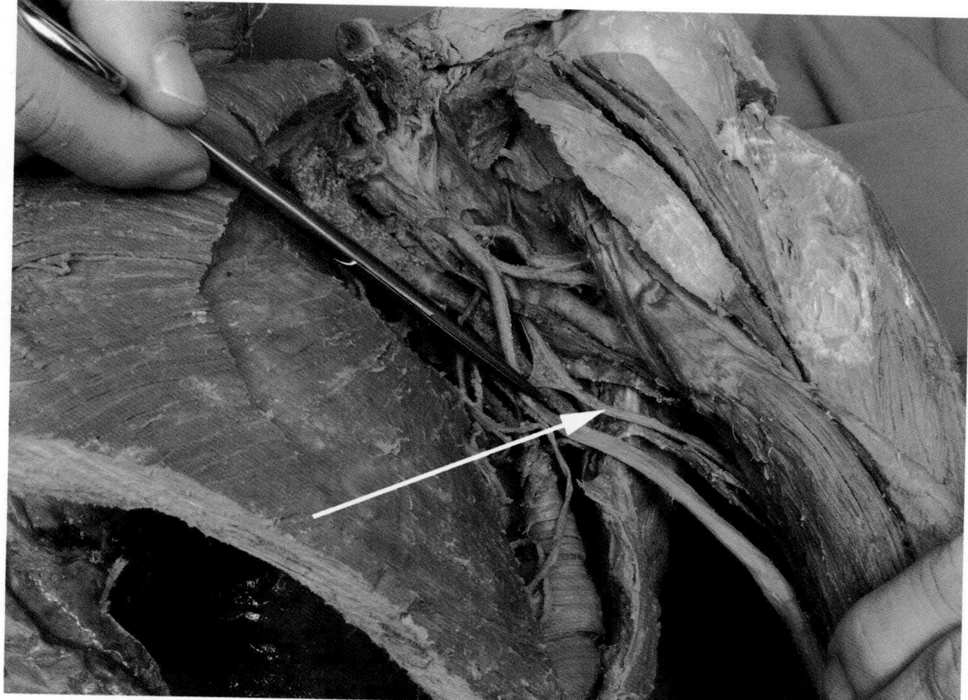

FIGURE 7-6 The *arrow* indicates the ulnar nerve in the subclavian area.

supplies the biceps muscle in the arm and is a pure sensory nerve in the forearm.

Electrical stimulation of the musculocutaneous nerve causes a motor response of the biceps muscle with flexion of the elbow.

(See musculocutaneous nerve movie on DVD.)

Figure 7-9 illustrates the axillary artery (*arrow*).

Figure 7-10 illustrates the axillary nerve (*arrow*) curling around the humerus with the musculocutaneous nerve.

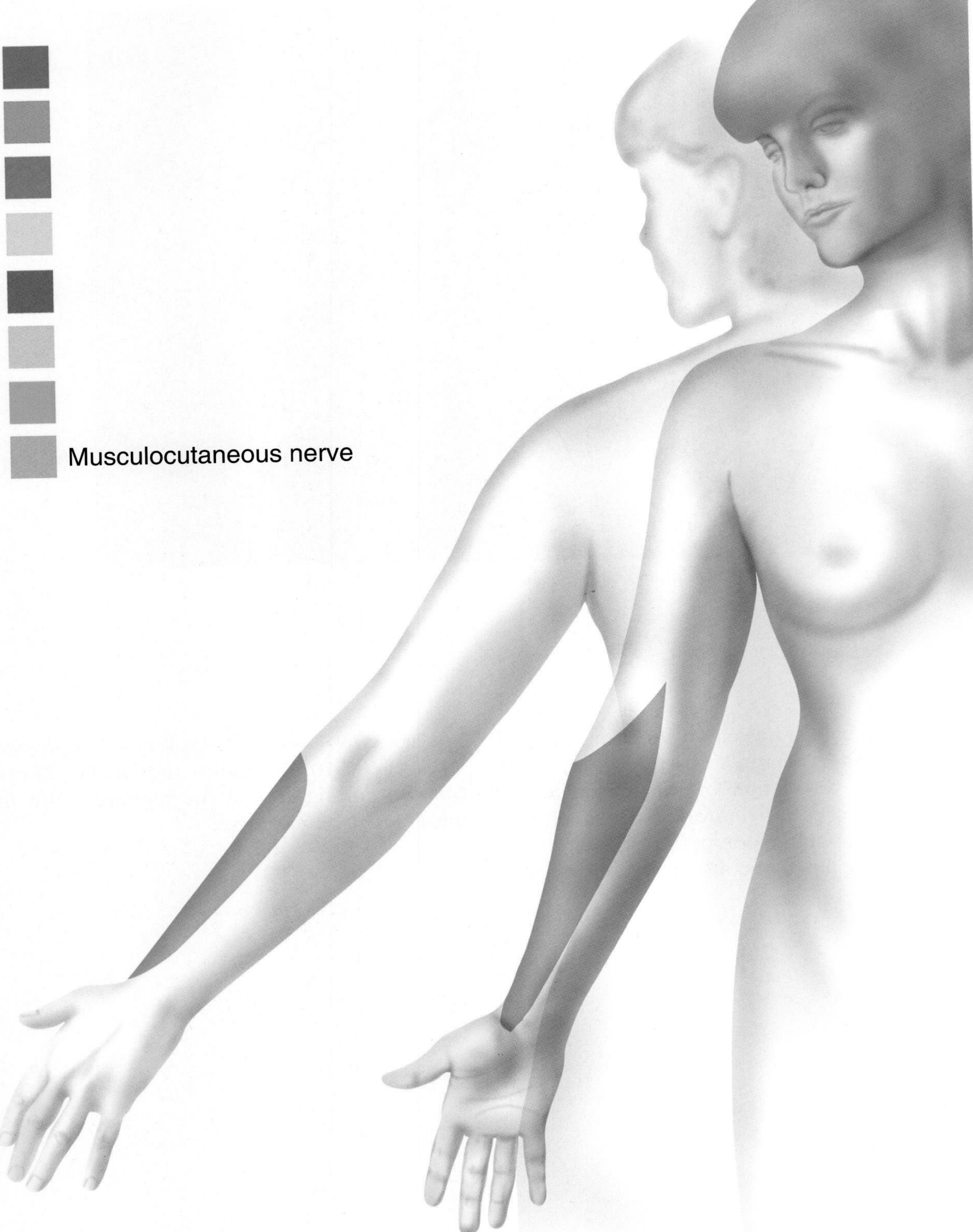

FIGURE 7-7 Sensory neurotome of the musculocutaneous nerve.

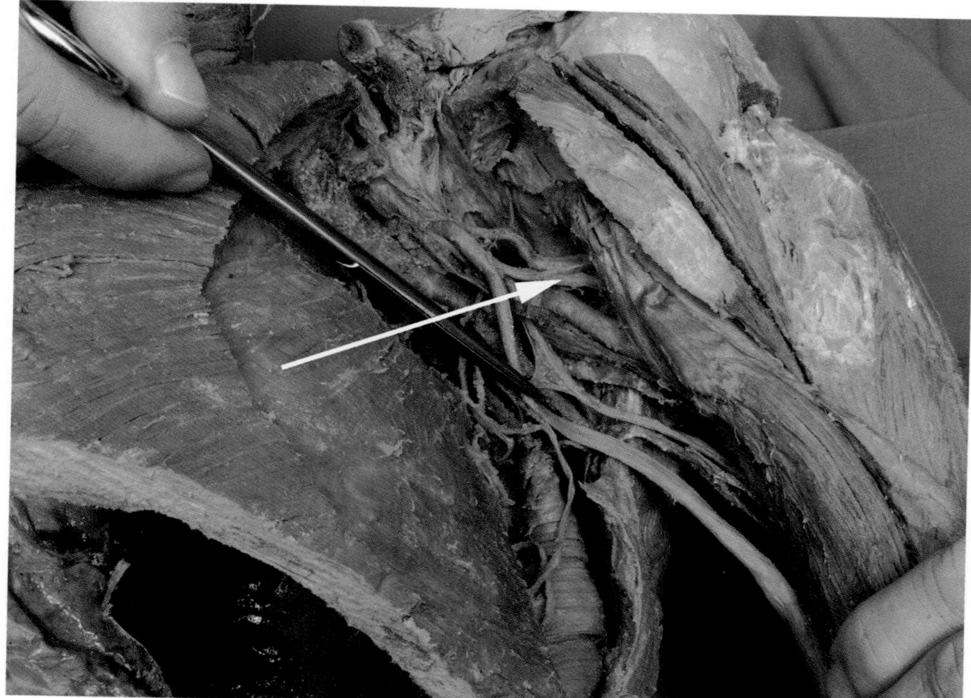

FIGURE 7-8 The *arrow* indicates the musculocutaneous nerve in the subclavian area.

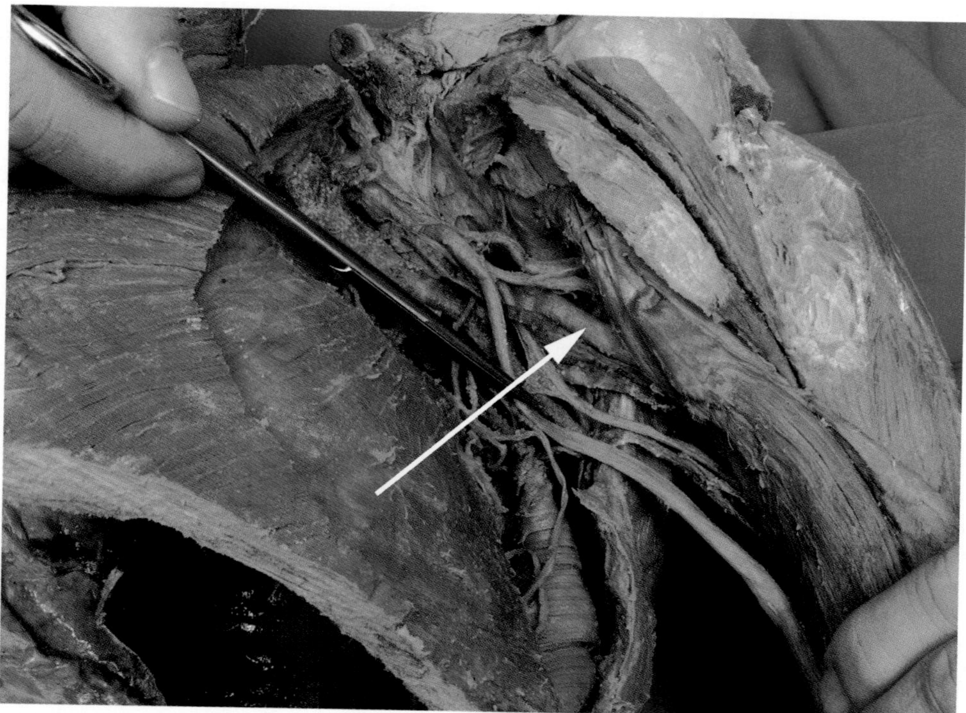

FIGURE 7-9 The *arrow* indicates the axillary artery in the subclavian area.

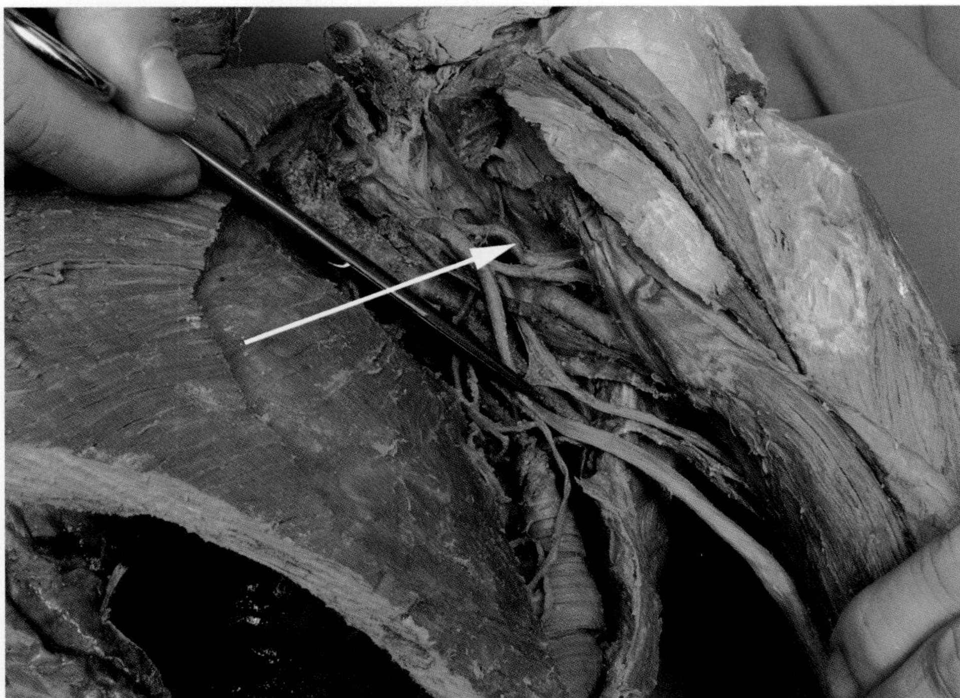

FIGURE 7-10 The *arrow* indicates the axillary nerve in the subclavian area. Note that the axillary and musculocutaneous nerves run together.

SUGGESTED FURTHER READING

1. Gray's Anatomy: The Anatomical Basis of Clinical Practice, 39th ed. Philadelphia, Elsevier, 2005.
2. Netter FH: Atlas of Human Anatomy, 2nd ed. East Hanover, NJ, Novartis, 1997.
3. Abrahams PH, Marks SC Jr, Hutchings RT: McMinn's Color Atlas of Human Anatomy, 5th ed. Philadelphia, Elsevier Mosby, 2003.
4. Boezaart AP: Anesthesia and Orthopaedic Surgery. New York, McGraw-Hill, 2006.
5. Hadzic A, Vloka JD: Peripheral Nerve Blocks: Principles and Practice. New York, McGraw-Hill, 2004.
6. Rathmell JP, Neal JM, Viscomi CM: Regional Anesthesia: The Requisites in Anesthesia. Philadelphia, Elsevier Mosby, 2004.
7. Brown DL: Atlas of Regional Anesthesia, 3rd ed. Philadelphia, Elsevier, 2006.
8. Barret J, Harmon D, Loughnane B, et al: Peripheral Nerve Blocks and Peri-operative Pain Relief. Philadelphia, WB Saunders, 2004.
9. Meier G, Büttner J: Atlas der peripheren Regionalanästhesie. Stuttgart, Georg Thieme Verlag, 2004.
10. Hahn MB, McQuillan PM, Sheplock GJ: Regional Anesthesia: An Atlas of Anatomy and Technique. St. Louis, Mosby, 1996.

Chapter 8

Axillary Blocks

- Single-Injection Axillary Block
- Continuous Axillary Block

SINGLE-INJECTION AXILLARY BLOCK

Introduction

The axillary block is done on the branch level of the brachial plexus (1). Because there are seven branches, of which two are sensory nerves, this block is sometimes difficult to master, and it is often impossible to obtain complete block with a single injection.

Specific Anatomic Considerations

The brachial and antebrachial cutaneous nerves (see Fig. 1-1, [19] and [20]) originate from the medial cord (see Fig. 1-1, [14]). These two nerves and the musculocutaneous nerve in the forearm (see Fig. 1-1, [22]) are sensory nerves. The details of the sheath surrounding the plexus at this level has been described and debated by Thompson and Rorie (2), Winnie and colleagues (3), Partridge and colleagues (4), and Klaastad and associates (5).

Figure 7-1 illustrates the neurotomes of the area that will be blocked if the radial nerve is blocked. This area will likewise be spared if the radial nerve is missed with this block.

Figure 7-3 illustrates the sensory innervation of the median nerve, whereas Figure 7-5 illustrates the area innervated by the ulnar nerve. Figure 7-7 illustrates the area innervated by the musculocutaneous nerve.

The areas supplied by the brachial and antebrachial cutaneous nerves are indicated in Figure 5-7.

Technique

The patient is positioned in the supine position with the shoulder abducted and the elbow flexed. The axillary artery is identified and marked (Fig. 8-1).

The skin and subcutaneous tissue are anesthetized after disinfection of the skin. Care must be taken not to penetrate the nerve sheathes with the needle at this stage.

The stimulating needle, attached to a nerve stimulator set at a current output of 1 to 2 mA, a frequency of 2 Hz, and a pulse width of 100 to 300 μsec, enters the skin angled slightly cephalad next to the artery, and a distinct "pop" can be felt as the brachial plexus sheath is entered (Fig. 8-2).

The needle can now be adjusted to place it close to the most appropriate nerve or nerves for the planned surgery.

The nerve stimulator is turned down to 0.3 to 0.5 mA when the needle is placed on the most appropriate nerve.

While keeping the needle steady and observing the motor response, local anesthetic agent is injected. The motor response stops immediately on injection. This constitutes a positive Raj test, and is an additional indication that the block to this specific nerve will be successful. The other nerves can now be identified and separately blocked. Ultrasound is also very handy for this block (Figure 8.3).

Local Anesthetic Agent Choice

Most local anesthetic agents have been used for this block. Typically, 15 to 40 mL of ropivacaine

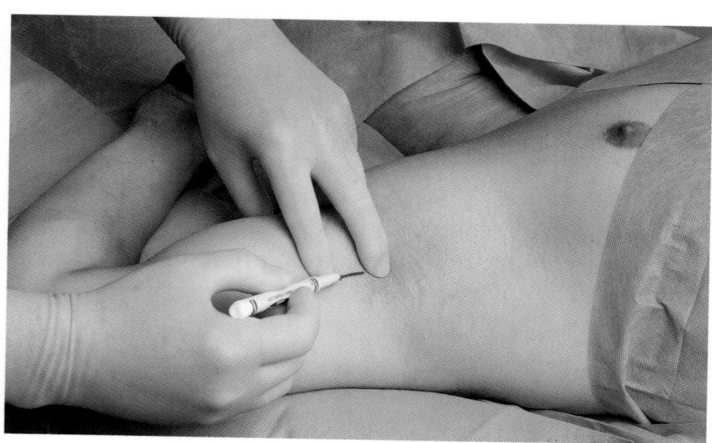

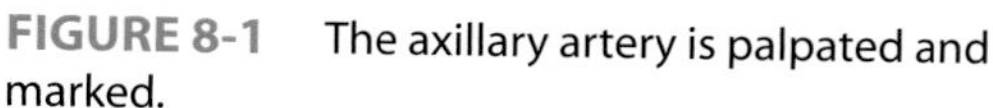

FIGURE 8-1 The axillary artery is palpated and marked.

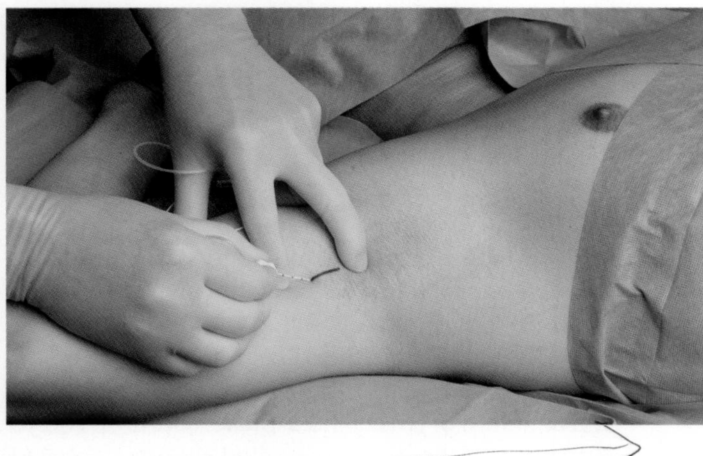

FIGURE 8-2 After a small skin wheal is raised, the needle entry is perpendicular to the axillary artery.

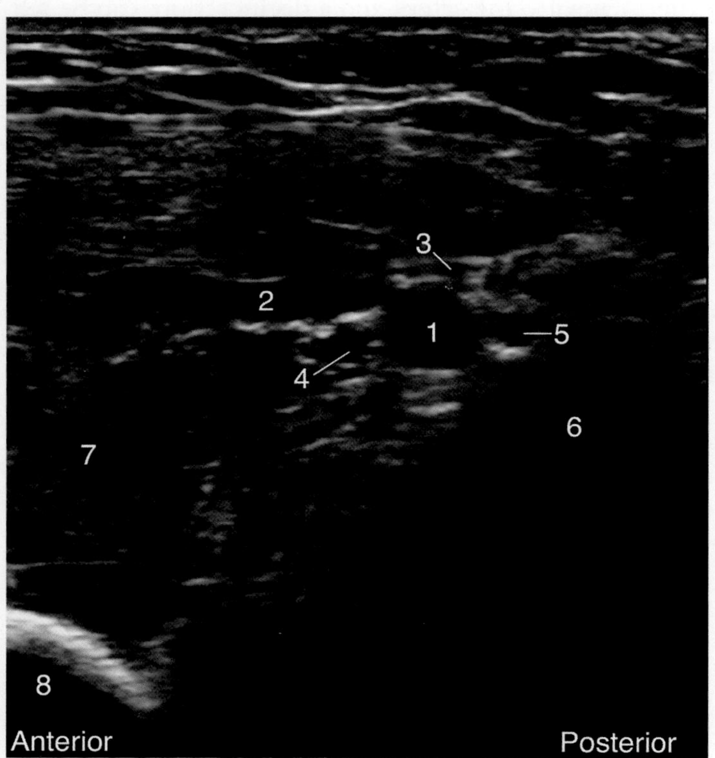

FIGURE 8-3 Ultrasound image of axillary area. 1 = Axillary artery; 2 = Axillary vein; 3 = Ulnar nerve; 4 = Median nerve; 5 = Radial nerve; 6 = Triceps brachii muscle; 7 = Coracobrachialis muscle; 8 = Humerus.

0.5% to 0.75% is used, of which 10 to 25 mL is injected onto the most appropriate nerve and the remainder into at least one of the other nerves. Adding buprenorphine 0.3 mg or dexamethasone 40 mg to the mixture may lengthen the duration of action of the block, but if a long-acting block is required, it is best to place a continuous nerve block.

(See single-injection axillary block movie on DVD.)

CONTINUOUS AXILLARY BLOCK

Introduction

As in the continuous infraclavicular block, the catheter is situated on a specific peripheral nerve for the continuous axillary block (6). This nerve is likely to be the only nerve that will be blocked with the relatively small volumes of local anesthetic agent infused days after surgery,

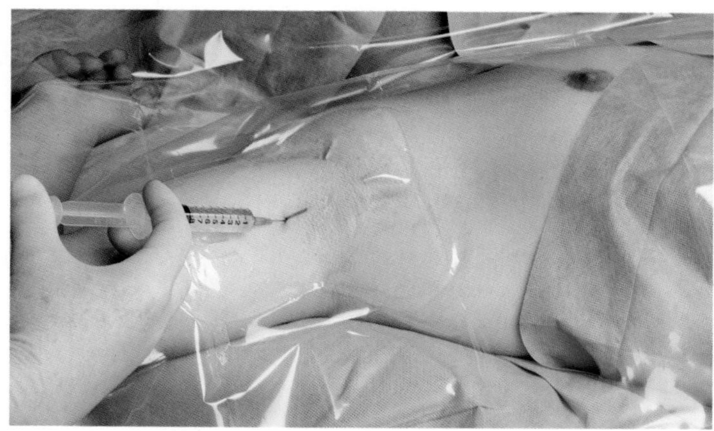

A

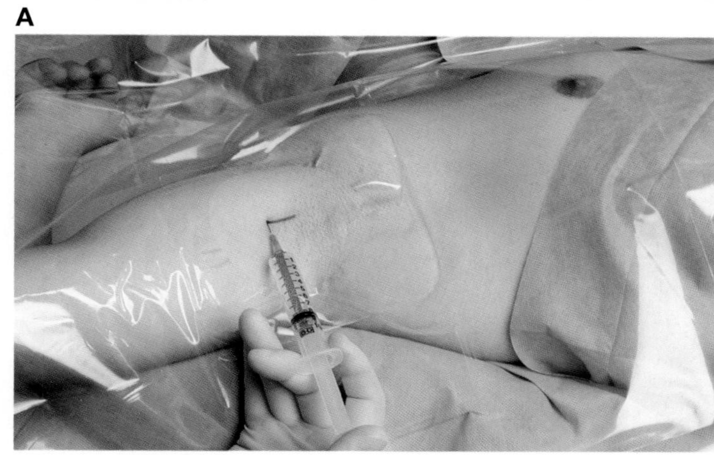

B

FIGURE 8-4 **A,** A small skin wheal is raised. **B,** The area of intended catheter tunneling is also anesthetized.

and this has proved disappointing in clinical practice. All the peripheral nerves to the arm and forearm need to be blocked for elbow and wrist surgery.

Technique

The patient is positioned supine with the shoulder joint abducted and the elbow flexed.The skin and subcutaneous tissue (Fig. 8-4A) and intended path of the tunneling of the catheter (Fig. 8-4B) are anesthetized after the skin has been prepared and the area covered with a sterile, fenestrated, transparent dressing.

An insulated 17- or 18-gauge Tuohy needle, attached to a nerve stimulator set to a current output of 1 to 2 mA, a frequency of 2 Hz, and a pulse width of 100 to 300 μsec, enters the skin next to the axillary artery and is directed medially (Fig. 8-5). The needle is held steady and the stylet removed after the most appropriate nerve has been identified and the nerve stimulator output has been turned down to approximately 0.3 to 0.5 mA. This guarantees accurate needle placement, but not accurate catheter placement.

It is important not to inject any conductive fluids such as local anesthetic agent or normal saline through the needle at this point because this will render stimulating catheter placement impossible. If the anesthesiologist subscribes to the notion of "opening of the space," 5% dextrose and water can be used, which will not abolish the electrical stimulus.

The nerve stimulator is now set to 0.5 to 1 mA and attached to the proximal end of the catheter (Fig. 8-6). Note the special mark on the catheter, which indicates that the catheter tip is now situated at the tip of the needle. The catheter is advanced beyond the needle tip; if the motor response disappears, it means that the catheter tip is moving away from the nerve.

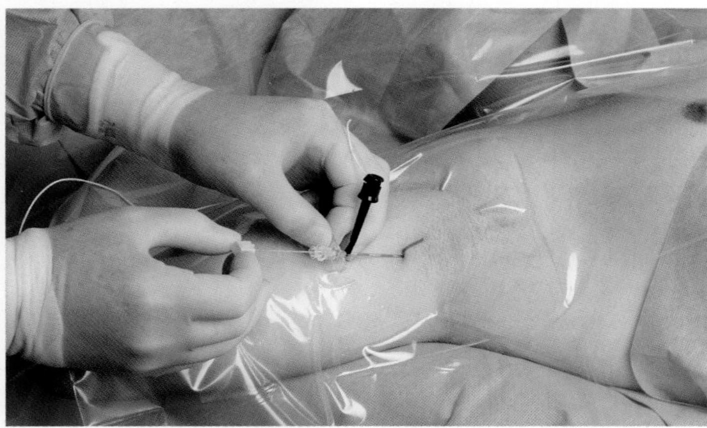

FIGURE 8-5 An insulated Tuohy needle is placed on the appropriate branch of the brachial plexus.

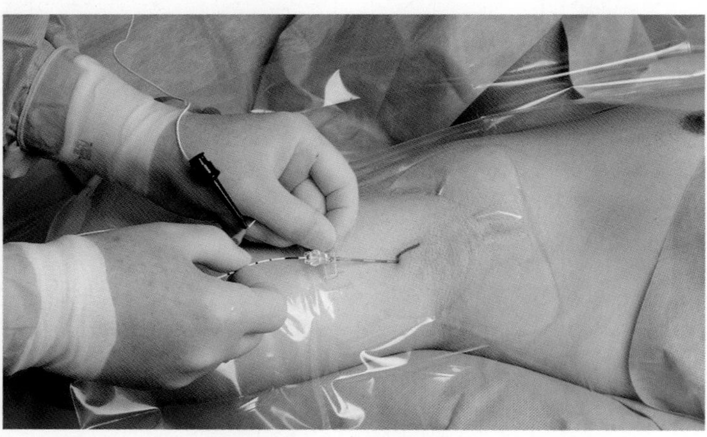

FIGURE 8-6 The nerve stimulator is attached to the proximal end of the stimulating catheter, which is advanced through the needle.

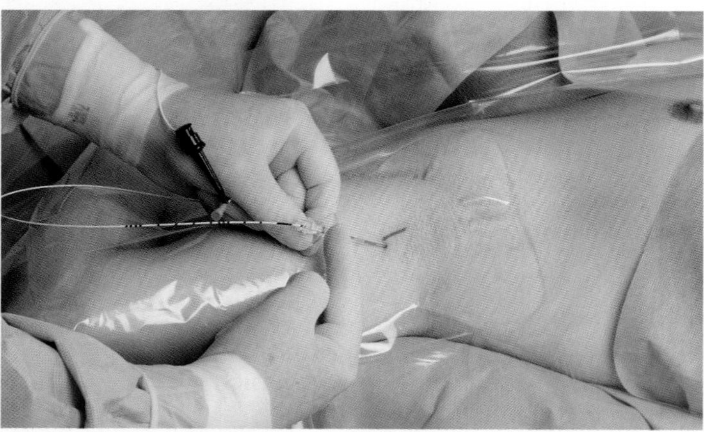

FIGURE 8-7 If the motor response is lost, the needle is rotated counterclockwise after the catheter is withdrawn inside the needle shaft.

Withdraw the catheter tip carefully to inside the needle shaft, make a small adjustment to the needle, such as turning it clockwise or counterclockwise or advancing or withdrawing it slightly (Fig. 8-7). Repeat this maneuver as often as necessary until the motor response remains constant during catheter advancement. Advance the catheter 3 to 5 cm beyond the needle tip, but not more than 5 cm.

The needle is removed without disturbing the catheter position.

A special tunneling device can be used to tunnel the catheter subcutaneously. The Tuohy needle and its stylet can also be used. Tunneling is essential to prevent catheter dislodgement (see Chapter 12). A skin bridge may be important for short- to medium-term catheter use because it facilitates catheter removal. Catheter leakage, however, is common if a skin bridge is used.

The catheter connecting device is attached to the catheter and the nerve stimulator, set to an output of 0 mA, is attached to the fixation device. The nerve stimulator output is slowly turned up until a muscle twitch can just be seen. Local anesthetic agent or any conducting fluids, such as normal saline, can now be injected and the muscle twitches will immediately stop after the injection starts. This constitutes a positive Raj test, which gives further assurance that the secondary block to the particular peripheral nerve will be successful. It does not guarantee complete block to all the nerves, especially not for long-term blocks if low volume infusions are used.

Local Anesthetic Drug and Infusion Choice

All local anesthetic agents have been used for this block. Typically, 15 to 40 mL of ropivacaine 0.5% to 0.75% is used as the initial bolus, followed by a 5- to 10-mL/hour infusion of ropivacaine 0.2%. It is essential to allow for relatively large patient-controlled boluses of 10 to 15 mL every 60 minutes to recapture unblocked peripheral nerves in the postoperative period, should this become necessary.

Catheter Removal

The catheter is removed after the patient no longer requires continuous block and full sensation has returned to the limb (see Chapter 12). Any radiating pain during catheter removal may indicate that the catheter has coiled around a nerve, and this situation should be managed with utmost care. Remove the catheter by stabilizing the proximal part and first removing the distal part of the catheter from the skin bridge. Once this is done, keep the distal part sterile and remove the rest of the catheter.

(See continuous axillary block movie on DVD.)

REFERENCES

1. Steel AC, Harrop-Griffiths W: Nerve blocks in the axilla. In Boezaart AP (ed): Anesthesia and Orthopaedic Surgery. New York, McGraw-Hill, 2006, pp 321-330.
2. Thompson GE, Rorie DL: Functional anatomy of the brachial plexus sheaths. Anesthesiology 1983;59:117-122.
3. Winnie AP, Radonjic R, Akkineni SR, et al: Factors influencing distribution of local anesthetic injected into the brachial plexus sheath. Anesth Analg 1979;58:225-234.
4. Partridge BL, Katz J, Bernischke K: Functional anatomy of the brachial plexus sheath: Implications for anesthesia. Anesthesiology 1987;66:743-747.
5. Klaastad O, Smedby O, Thompson GE, et al: Distribution of local anaesthetic in axillary brachial plexus block: A clinical and magnetic resonance imaging study. Anesthesiology 2002;96:1315-1324.
6. Harrop-Griffiths W: Peripheral nerve catheter techniques. Anaesth Intensive Care Med 2004;4:124.

Chapter 9

Nerves around the Elbow: Applied Anatomy

- **Radial Nerve at the Elbow**
- **Median Nerve at the Elbow**
- **Ulnar Nerve at the Elbow**

RADIAL NERVE AT THE ELBOW

The radial nerve (Fig. 9-1, [23]) runs around the humerus and lies anterior to the lateral epicondyle at the elbow, where it can be electrically stimulated and blocked.

Figure 9-2 illustrates the areas of sensory innervation of the radial nerve. If the block is performed at the elbow, only the areas distal to the block will be affected.

The surface anatomy of the radial nerve (Fig. 9-3, *arrow*) at the elbow is midway between the tendon of the biceps muscle and the lateral epicondyle.

Electrical stimulation of the radial nerve at the elbow causes extension at the wrist.

(See radial nerve movie on DVD.)

MEDIAN NERVE AT THE ELBOW

The median nerve (see Fig. 9-1, [24]) runs anterior to the elbow and medial to the brachial artery.

The palm of the hand on the lateral side and the areas illustrated in Figure 9-4 receive their sensory innervation from the median nerve.

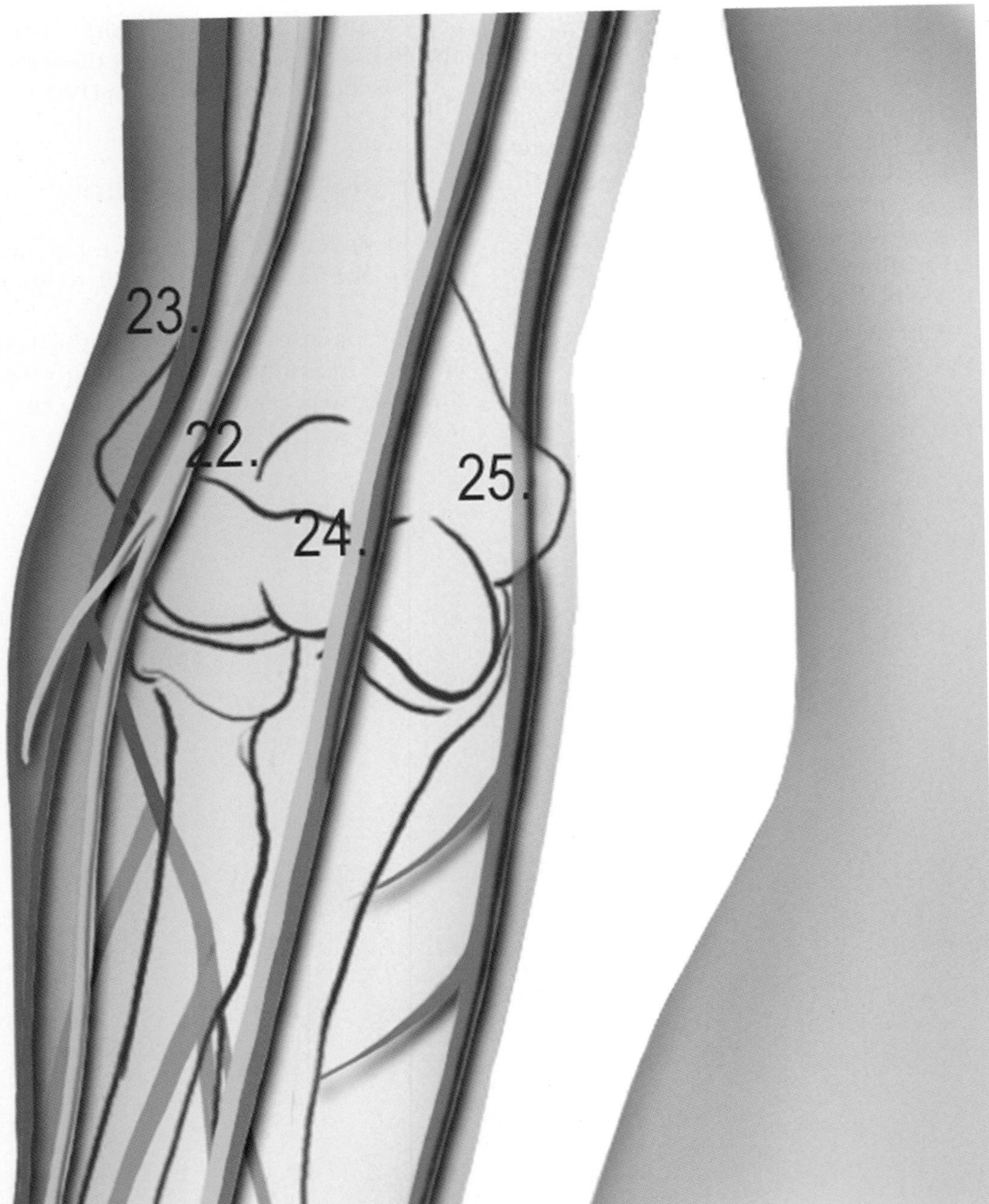

FIGURE 9-1 Schematic representation of the nerves around the elbow. 22, musculocutaneous nerve; 23, radial nerve; 24, median nerve; 25, ulnar nerve.

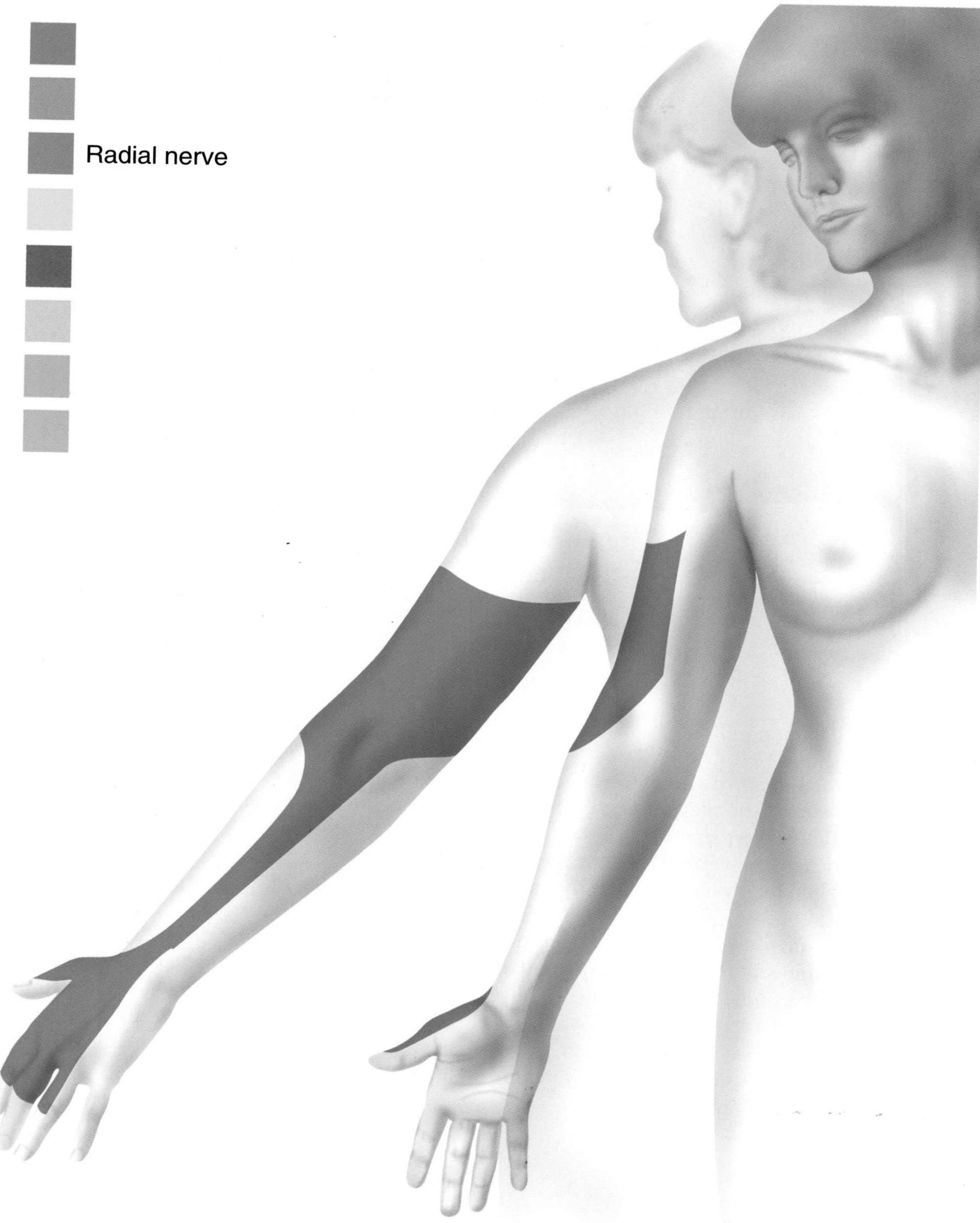

FIGURE 9-2 Sensory distribution of the radial nerve.

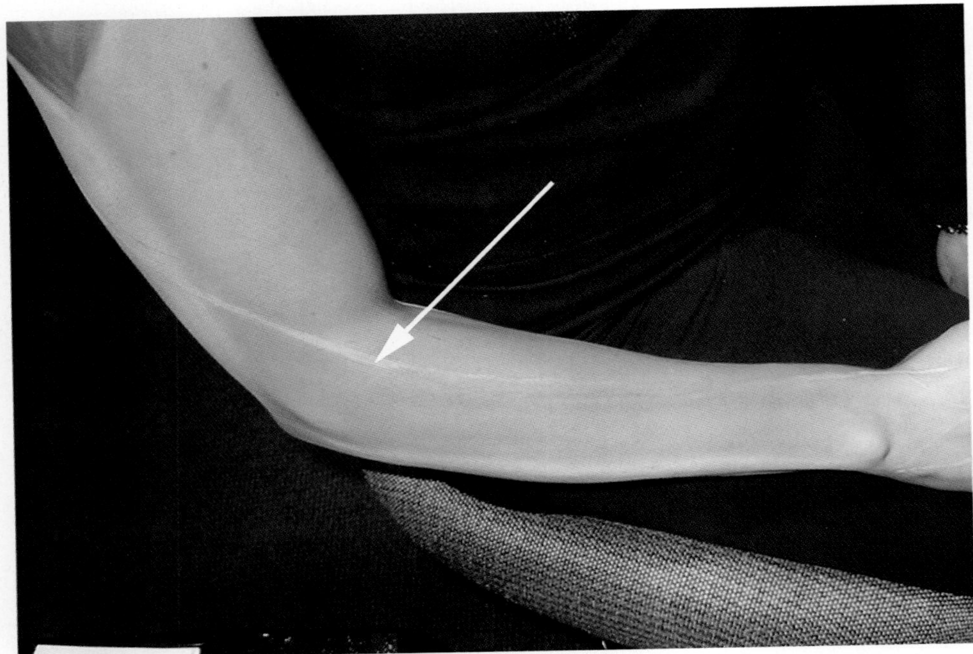

FIGURE 9-3 Surface anatomy of the radial nerve.

In the medial view of the elbow (Fig. 9-5), the dissection shows the median nerve (*arrow*) medial to the brachial artery.

At a slightly higher level (Fig. 9-6), the median nerve (*arrow*) can be seen anterior to the ulnar nerve.

The surface anatomy of the median nerve is approximately midway from the biceps tendon to the medial epicondyle of the humerus, just medial to the brachial artery (Fig. 9-7).

Electrical stimulation of the median nerve at the elbow results in pronation of the forearm, flexion of the fingers, and adduction of the thumb.

(See median nerve movie on DVD.)

ULNAR NERVE AT THE ELBOW

The ulnar nerve (see Fig. 9-1, [25]) passes posterior to the medial epicondyle of the humerus.

Figure 9-8 illustrates the sensory distribution of the ulnar nerve. Note that, like the median nerve, sensory distribution of the ulnar nerve is limited to the hand.

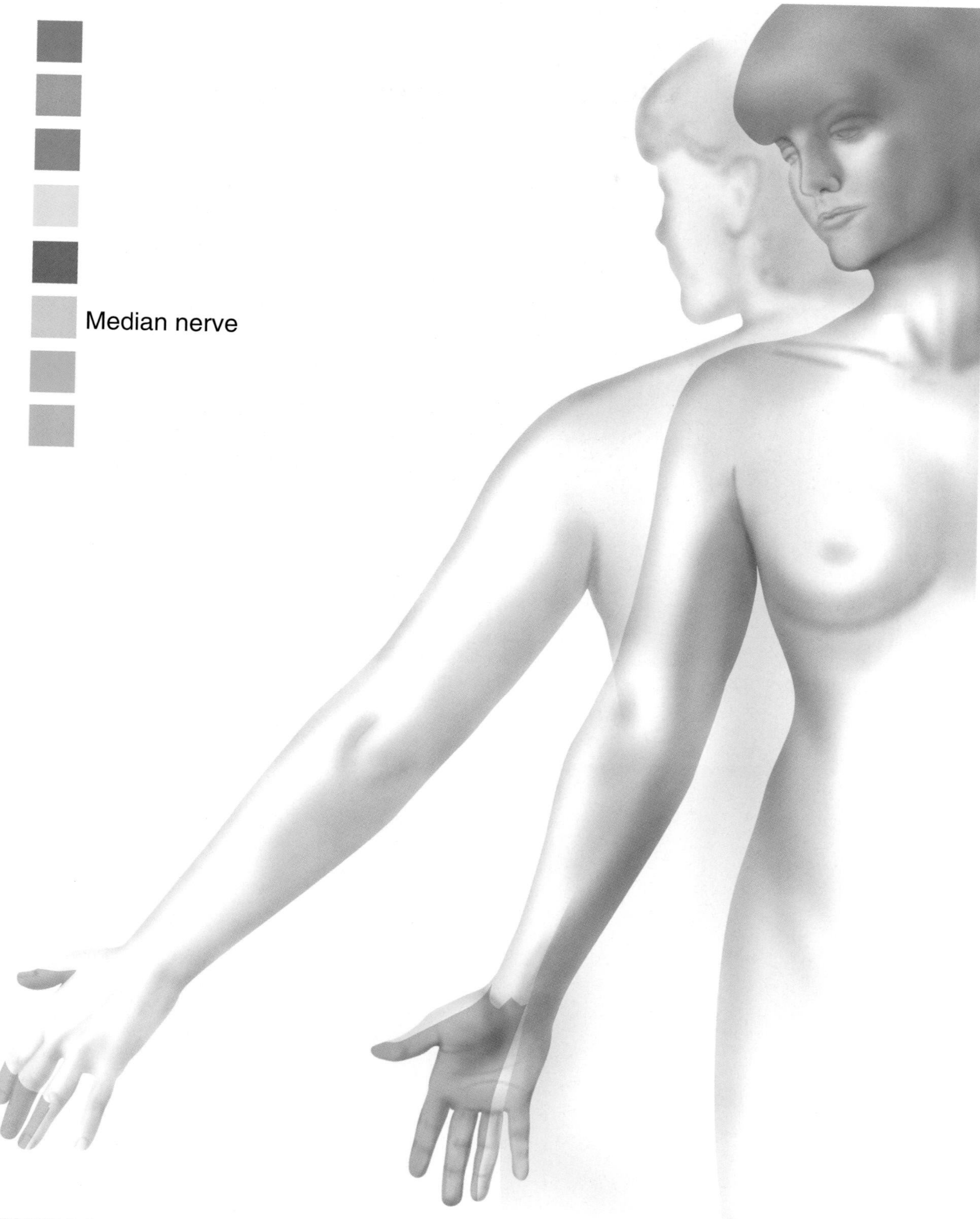

FIGURE 9-4 Sensory distribution of the median nerve.

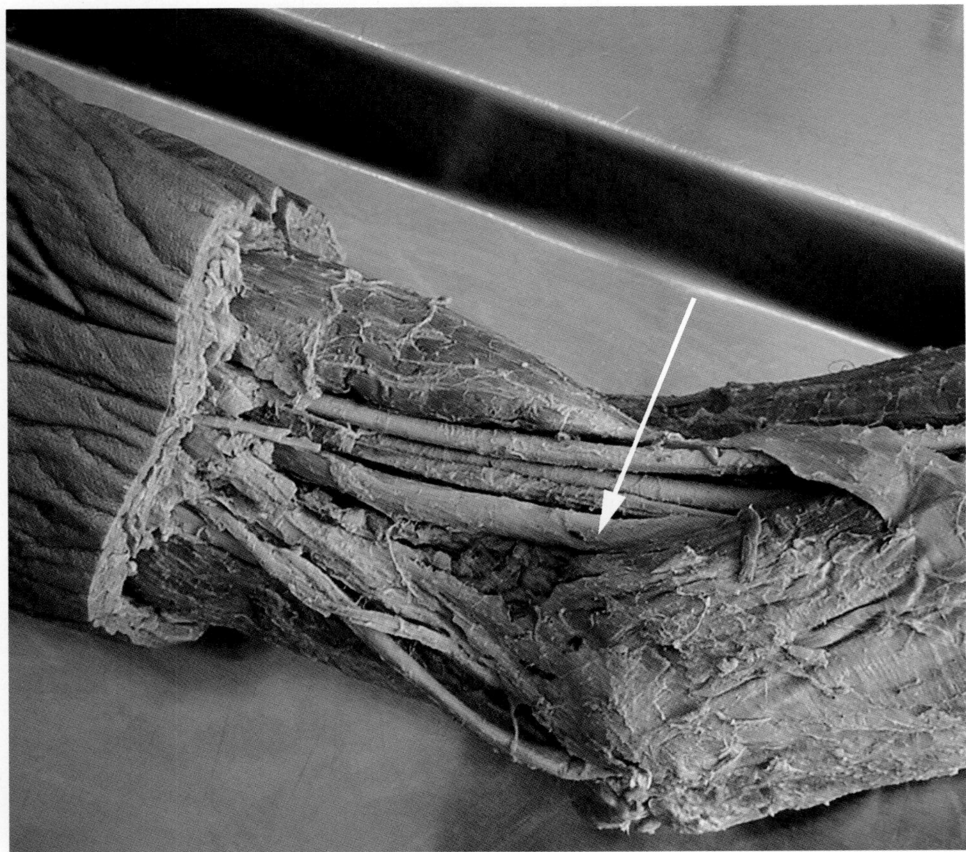

FIGURE 9-5 *Arrow* indicates the median nerve at the elbow.

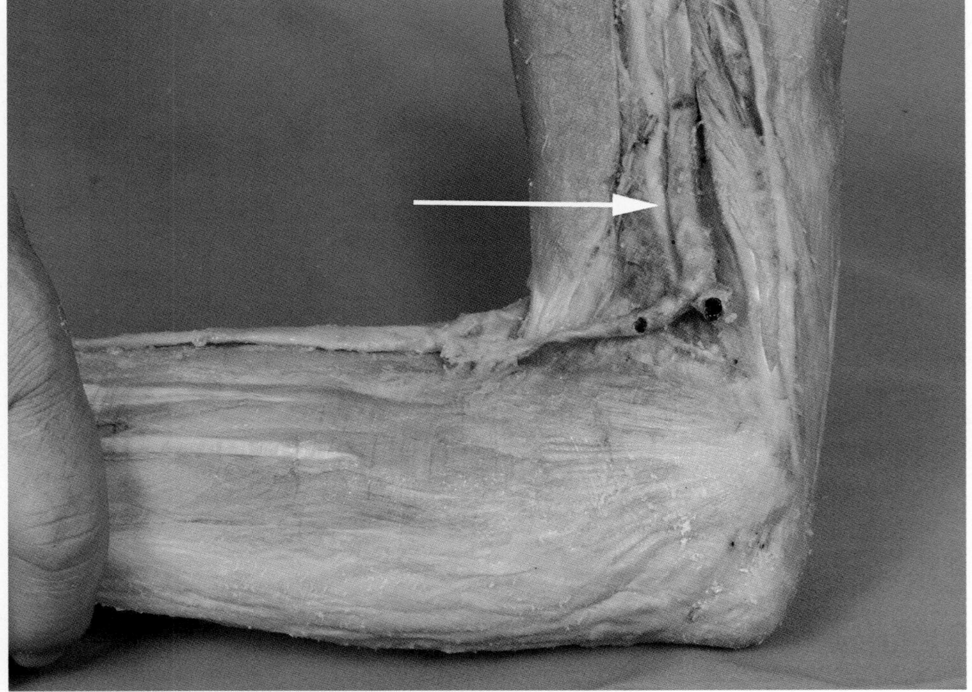

FIGURE 9-6 *Arrow* indicates the median nerve in the upper arm.

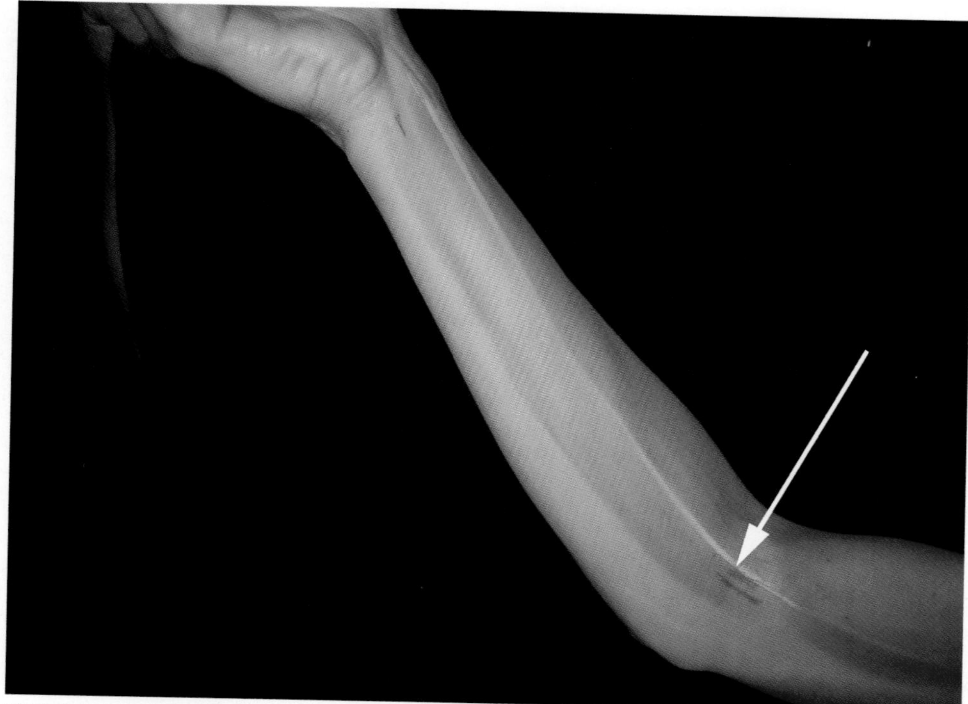

FIGURE 9-7 Surface anatomy of the median nerve at the elbow.

The ulnar nerve (Fig. 9-9, *arrow*) can be seen as it disappears into the sulcus ulnaris, behind the medial epicondyle of the humerus.

Before it reaches the elbow, the ulnar nerve (Fig. 9-10, *arrow*) travels near the upper border of the triceps muscle, where it can easily be electrically stimulated or blocked. It is advisable not to attempt an ulnar nerve block at the sulcus ulnaris level.

Electrical stimulation of the ulnar nerve at the level of the elbow results in flexion of the fingers and ulnar deviation of the wrist.

(See ulnar nerve movie on DVD.)

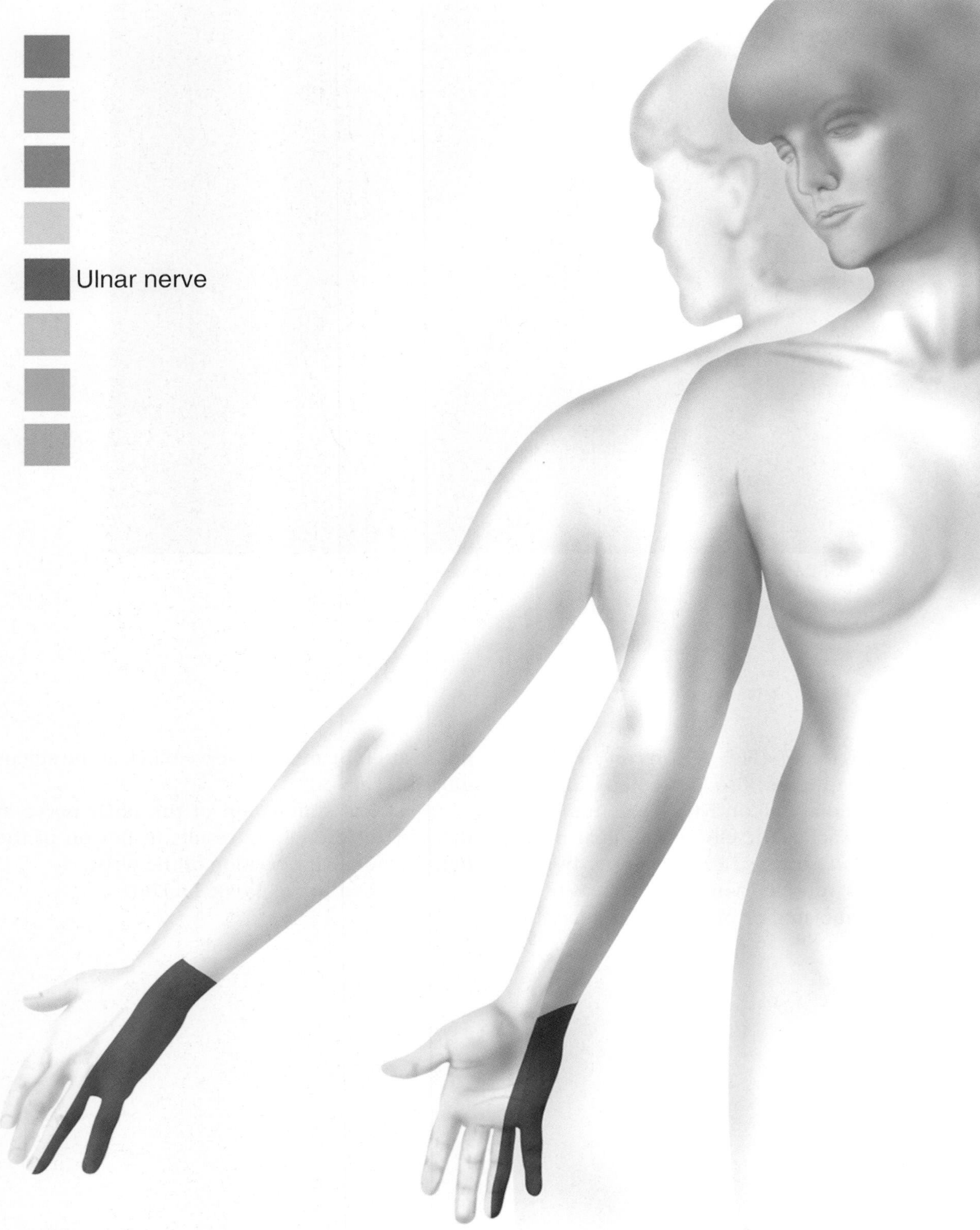

FIGURE 9-8 Sensory distribution of the ulnar nerve.

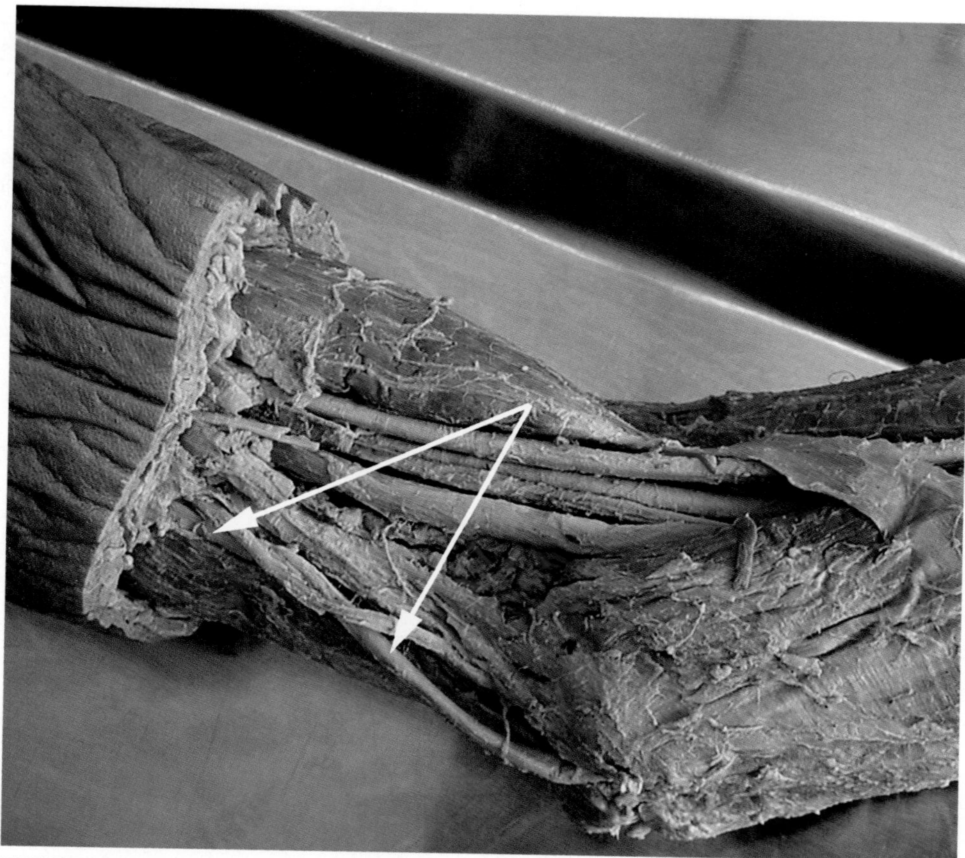

FIGURE 9-9 *Arrows* indicate the ulnar nerve at the elbow.

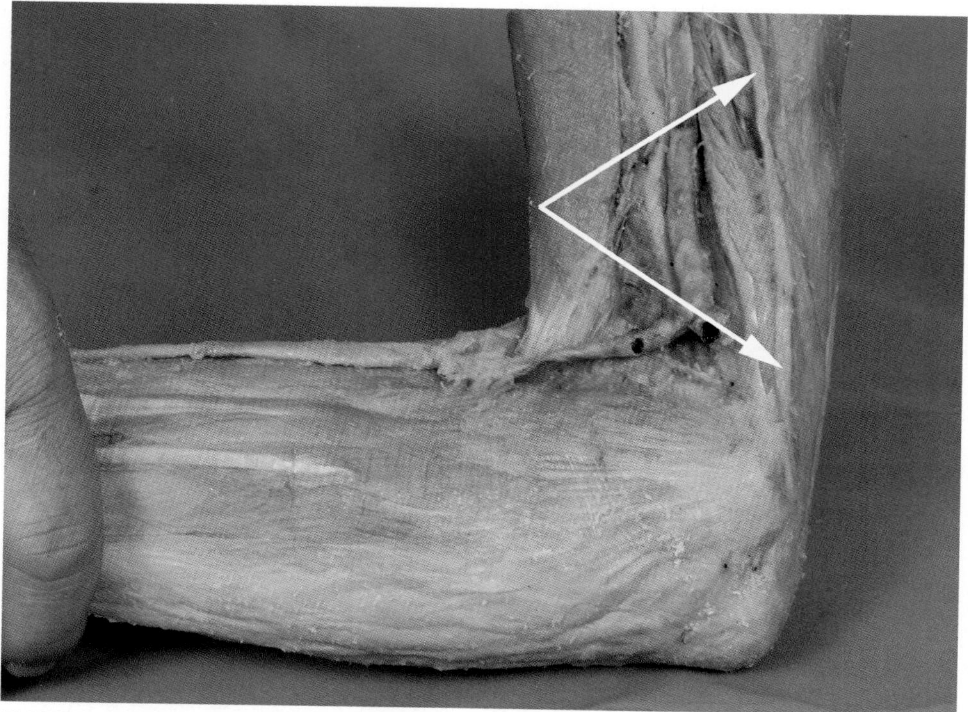

FIGURE 9-10 *Arrows* indicate the ulnar nerve in the upper arm.

SUGGESTED FURTHER READING

1. Gray's Anatomy: The Anatomical Basis of Clinical Practice, 39th ed. Philadelphia, Elsevier, 2005.
2. Netter FH: Atlas of Human Anatomy, 2nd ed. East Hanover, NJ, Novartis, 1997.
3. Abrahams PH, Marks SC Jr, Hutchings RT: McMinn's Color Atlas of Human Anatomy, 5th ed. Philadelphia, Elsevier Mosby, 2003.
4. Boezaart AP: Anesthesia and Orthopaedic Surgery. New York, McGraw-Hill, 2006.
5. Hadzic A, Vloka JD: Peripheral Nerve Blocks: Principles and Practice. New York, McGraw-Hill, 2004.
6. Rathmell JP, Neal JM, Viscomi CM: Regional Anesthesia: The Requisites in Anesthesia. Philadelphia, Elsevier Mosby, 2004.
7. Brown DL: Atlas of Regional Anesthesia, 3rd ed. Philadelphia, Elsevier, 2006.
8. Barret J, Harmon D, Loughnane B, et al: Peripheral Nerve Blocks and Peri-operative Pain Relief. Philadelphia, WB Saunders, 2004.
9. Meier G, Büttner J: Atlas der peripheren Regionalanästhesie. Stuttgart, Georg Thieme Verlag, 2004.
10. Hahn MB, McQuillan PM, Sheplock GJ: Regional Anesthesia: An Atlas of Anatomy and Technique. St. Louis, Mosby, 1996.

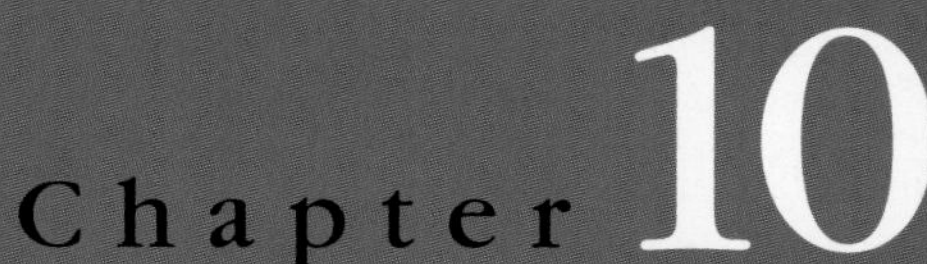

Chapter 10

Blocks around the Elbow

- Musculocutaneous Nerve Block at the Elbow
- Radial Nerve Block at the Elbow
- Median Nerve Block at the Elbow
- Ulnar Nerve Block at the Elbow

These blocks are typically used as "rescue" blocks or if longer-acting blocks are required for postoperative pain relief. For example, if an infraclavicular, axillary, or supraclavicular block has been done and a specific peripheral nerve has been missed, the nerve can be blocked at the elbow. Similarly, if a short-acting drug such as mepivacaine has been used and a longer action of the block in a specific area of the distal arm is required, that specific nerve can be blocked at the elbow using a longer-acting drug. The use of an elbow block for total surgical anesthesia of the distal arm has proved disappointing because the antebrachial cutaneous nerve and cutaneous part of the musculocutaneous nerve are sensory nerves. These sensory nerves are difficult to block reliably, although the use of ultrasonography may facilitate this aspect of the procedure.

MUSCULOCUTANEOUS NERVE BLOCK AT THE ELBOW

Technique

The nerve is situated between the biceps brachii and brachialis muscles on the lateral side of the arm, just proximal to the elbow. Placing two fingers of the nonoperative hand into the groove between these two muscles to separate them and injecting approximately 10 mL of local anesthetic agent between these muscles will block the musculocutaneous nerve (Fig. 10-1). At this level, the nerve is a sensory nerve.

The musculocutaneous nerve can also be blocked at the elbow by subcutaneous infiltration, as illustrated in Figure 10-2, but blockade of the musculocutaneous nerve in the axilla, where it is still a mixed motor and sensory nerve, is probably

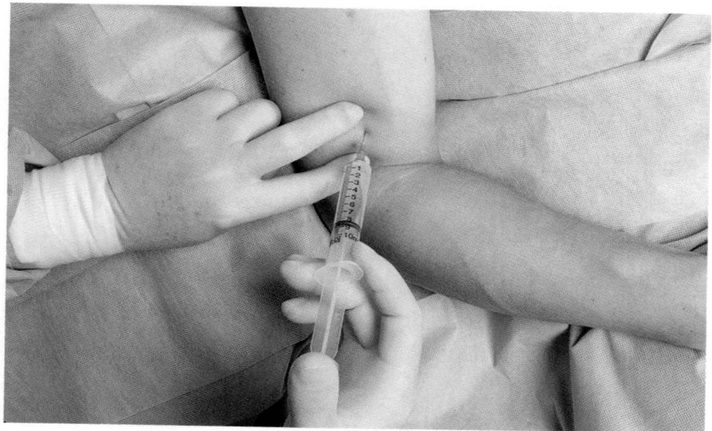

FIGURE 10-1 Injection of the musculocutaneous nerve at the elbow.

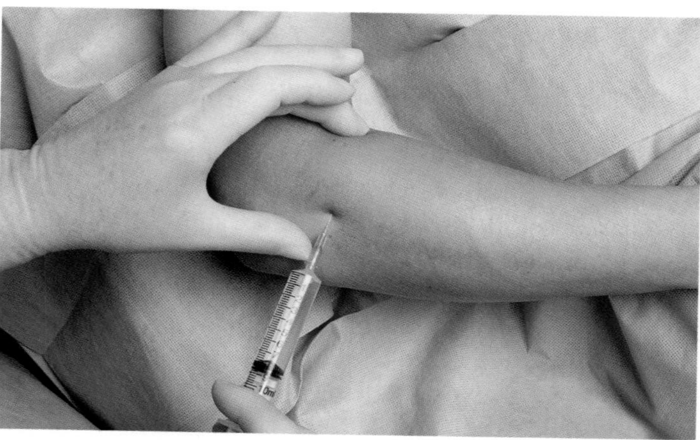

FIGURE 10-2 Injection of the musculocutaneous nerve below the elbow.

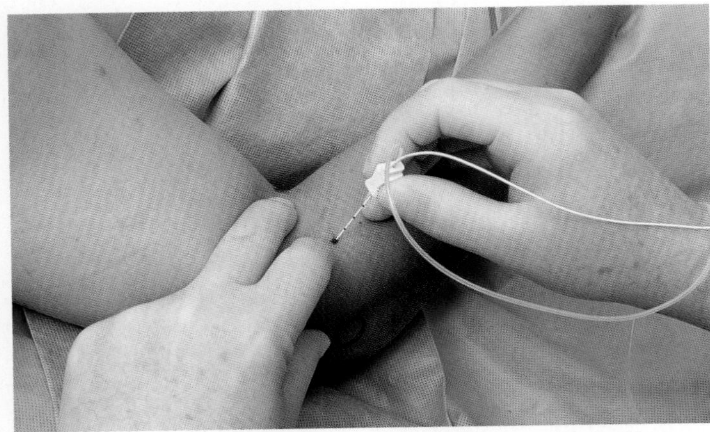

FIGURE 10-3 Injection of the radial nerve at the elbow.

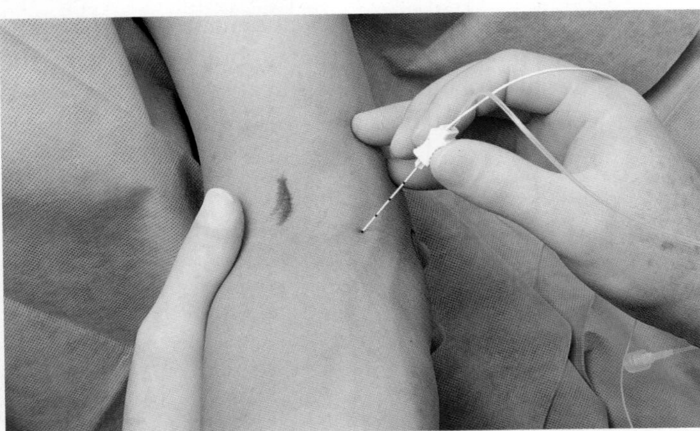

FIGURE 10-4 Injection of the median nerve at the elbow.

more reliable. The musculocutaneous nerve innervates the biceps brachii and brachialis muscles, and stimulation of the nerve causes elbow flexion.

RADIAL NERVE AT THE ELBOW

Technique

The point of needle entry is halfway from the biceps brachii tendon to the lateral epicondyle of the elbow joint, as demonstrated in Figure 10-3. After a skin wheal is raised, a 22-gauge, 50-mm stimulating needle, attached to a nerve stimulator set at a current output of 1 to 2 mA, a frequency of 2 Hz, and pulse length of 100 to 300 μsec, enters the skin perpendicularly. A distinct "pop" can be felt as the needle penetrates the extensor muscle, and this is immediately followed by an extensor motor response at the wrist joint.

The nerve stimulator is now turned down and the needle adjusted such that a brisk motor response is still detectable at the wrist at a stimulator output of 0.3 to 0.5 mA. This indicates correct needle placement, and 5 to 10 mL of local anesthetic agent can be injected.

MEDIAN NERVE BLOCK AT THE ELBOW

Technique

The point of needle entry is halfway from the biceps brachii tendon to the medial epicondyle of the elbow joint, as demonstrated in Figure 10-4. The blue mark in Figure 10-4 indicates the biceps tendon, whereas the median artery can usually be palpated, and the nerve is situated just lateral of this artery. After a skin wheal is raised, a 22-gauge, 50-mm stimulating needle,

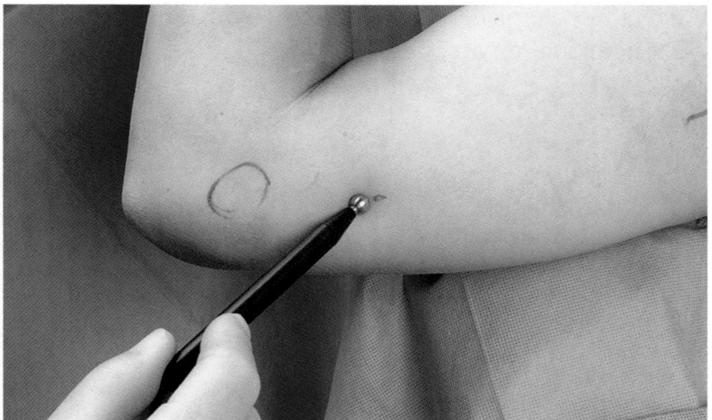

FIGURE 10-5 Transcutaneous stimulation of the ulnar nerve proximal to the elbow.

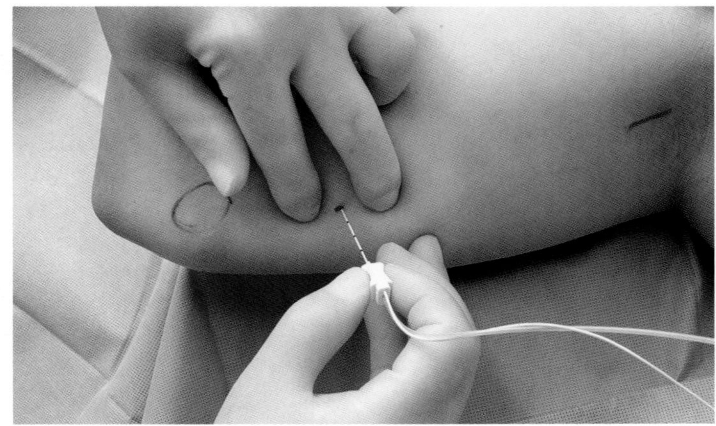

FIGURE 10-6 Injection of the ulnar nerve proximal to the elbow.

attached to a nerve stimulator set at a current output of 1 to 2 mA, a frequency of 2 Hz, and pulse length of 100 to 300 μsec, enters the skin perpendicularly. A flexion and pronation motor response at the wrist joint indicates that the median nerve is stimulated.

The nerve stimulator is now turned down and the needle adjusted such that a brisk motor response is still detectable at the wrist at a stimulator output of 0.3 to 0.5 mA. This indicates correct needle placement, and 5 to 10 mL of local anesthetic agent can be injected.

ULNAR NERVE BLOCK AT THE ELBOW

Technique

It is important to avoid the ulnar nerve in the sulcus ulnaris area because injection here inevitably causes ischemic nerve injury.

The ulnar nerve is situated just anterior to the triceps muscle in the medial aspect of the arm, as demonstrated in Figure 9-10.

The ulnar nerve can be stimulated transcutaneously by using a specially designed transcutaneous probe (Fig. 10-5), or it can be palpated anterior to the triceps muscle by following it proximally from the sulcus ulnaris.

The point of needle entry is approximately 5 cm proximal to the elbow joint (Fig. 10-6). After a skin wheal is raised, a 22-gauge, 50-mm stimulating needle, attached to a nerve stimulator set at a current output of 1 to 2 mA, a frequency of 2 Hz, and pulse length of 100 to 300 μsec, enters the skin perpendicularly. Flexor and ulnar deviation at the wrist joint indicates ulnar nerve stimulation.

The nerve stimulator is now turned down and the needle adjusted such that a brisk motor response is still detectable at the wrist at a stimulator output of 0.3 to 0.5 mA. This indicates correct needle placement, and 5 to 10 mL of local anesthetic agent can be injected.

REFERENCES

1. Abrahams PH, Marks SC Jr, Hutchings RT: McMinn's Color Atlas of Human Anatomy, 5th ed. Philadelphia, Elsevier Mosby, 2003.
2. Boezaart AP: Anesthesia and Orthopaedic Surgery. New York, McGraw-Hill, 2006.
3. Hadzic A, Vloka JD: Peripheral Nerve Blocks: Principles and Practice. New York, McGraw-Hill, 2004.
4. Rathmell JP, Neal JM, Viscomi CM: Regional Anesthesia: The Requisites in Anesthesia. Philadelphia, Elsevier Mosby, 2004.
5. Brown DL: Atlas of Regional Anesthesia, 3rd ed. Philadelphia, Elsevier, 2006.
6. Barret J, Harmon D, Loughnane B, et al: Peripheral Nerve Blocks and Peri-operative Pain Relief. Philadelphia, WB Saunders, 2004.
7. Meier G, Büttner J: Atlas der peripheren Regionalanästhesie. Stuttgart, Georg Thieme Verlag, 2004.
8. Hahn MB, McQuillan PM, Sheplock GJ: Regional Anesthesia: An Atlas of Anatomy and Technique. St. Louis, Mosby, 1996.

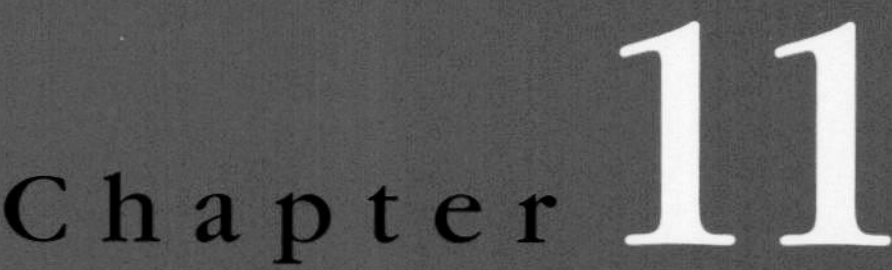

Lumbar Plexus: Applied Anatomy

- **Anterior Lumbar Plexus**

ANTERIOR LUMBAR PLEXUS

Femoral Nerve

The femoral nerve (Fig. 11-1, [1]) arises from the posterior divisions of the anterior primary rami of the second, third, and fourth lumbar roots of the lumbar plexus, the same segments as the obturator nerve. But the obturator nerve, which innervates the adductor muscles of the leg, is derived from the anterior divisions of the nerves.

Figure 11-2 illustrates the sensory innervation of the femoral nerve and its branch, the saphenous nerve.

Note that the medial portion of the upper leg, proximal to the knee, is not supplied by the femoral nerve, but is instead supplied by the obturator nerve. Also, the femoral nerve does not innervate the anterolateral portion of the upper leg, which is supplied by the lateral cutaneous nerve of the thigh.

Obturator Nerve

Figure 11-3 shows the sensory distribution of the obturator nerve, which, after leaving the obturator foramen, splits into anterior and posterior branches that run in the anterior and posterior aspect of the adductor brevis muscle.

Lateral Cutaneous Nerve of the Thigh

Figure 11-4 shows the sensory innervation of the lateral cutaneous nerve of the thigh. This nerve shares some common roots with the femoral nerve (L2, L3).

The femoral nerve (Fig. 11-5, *arrow*) lies deep to the fascia iliaca, deep to the inguinal ligament, and at the lateral edge of the femoral sheath, which separates it from the femoral artery and vein. On Figure 11-5, the anterior obturator nerve is marked 1 and the lateral cutaneous nerve of the thigh, 2.

Nerve to the Sartorius Muscle

The sartorius muscle implants on the anterior superior iliac spine and the medial tibia, and therefore crosses two major joints, the hip and the knee. The nerve supply to the sartorius is the nerve to the sartorius, which is an anterior branch of the femoral nerve (Fig. 11-6, *arrow*). This nerve, the nerve to the pectineus, and two cutaneous branches are the superficial branches of the femoral nerve.

Note the sartorius muscle crossing the quadriceps muscles in this illustration. The saphenous nerve (see Fig. 11-5, [4]) tracks distally on the medial border of the sartorius muscle.

The femoral nerve emerges approximately at the midpoint of the inguinal ligament. The

Text continued on page 133

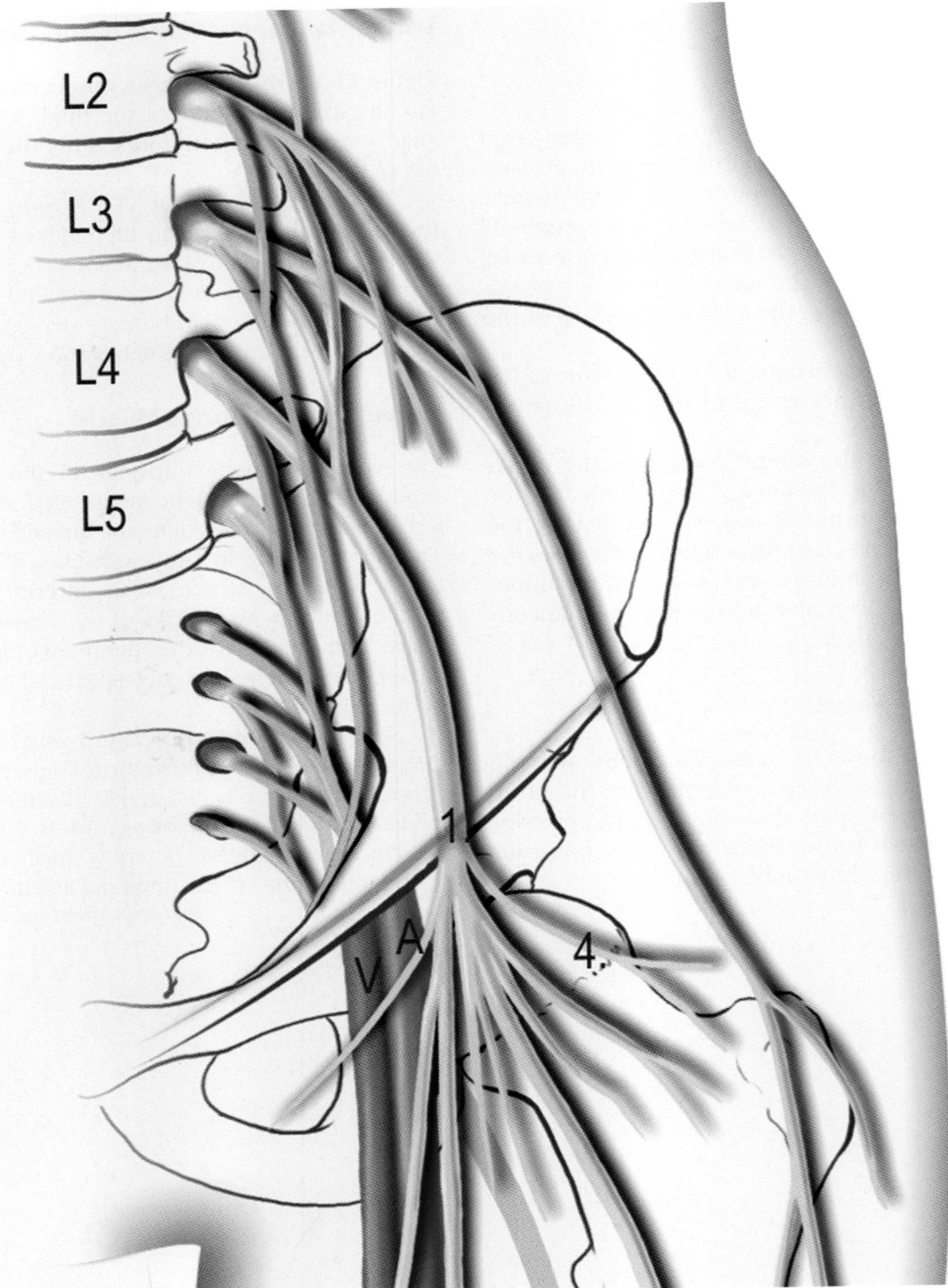

FIGURE 11-1 Schematic representation of the femoral nerve in the groin area. V, femoral vein; A, femoral artery.

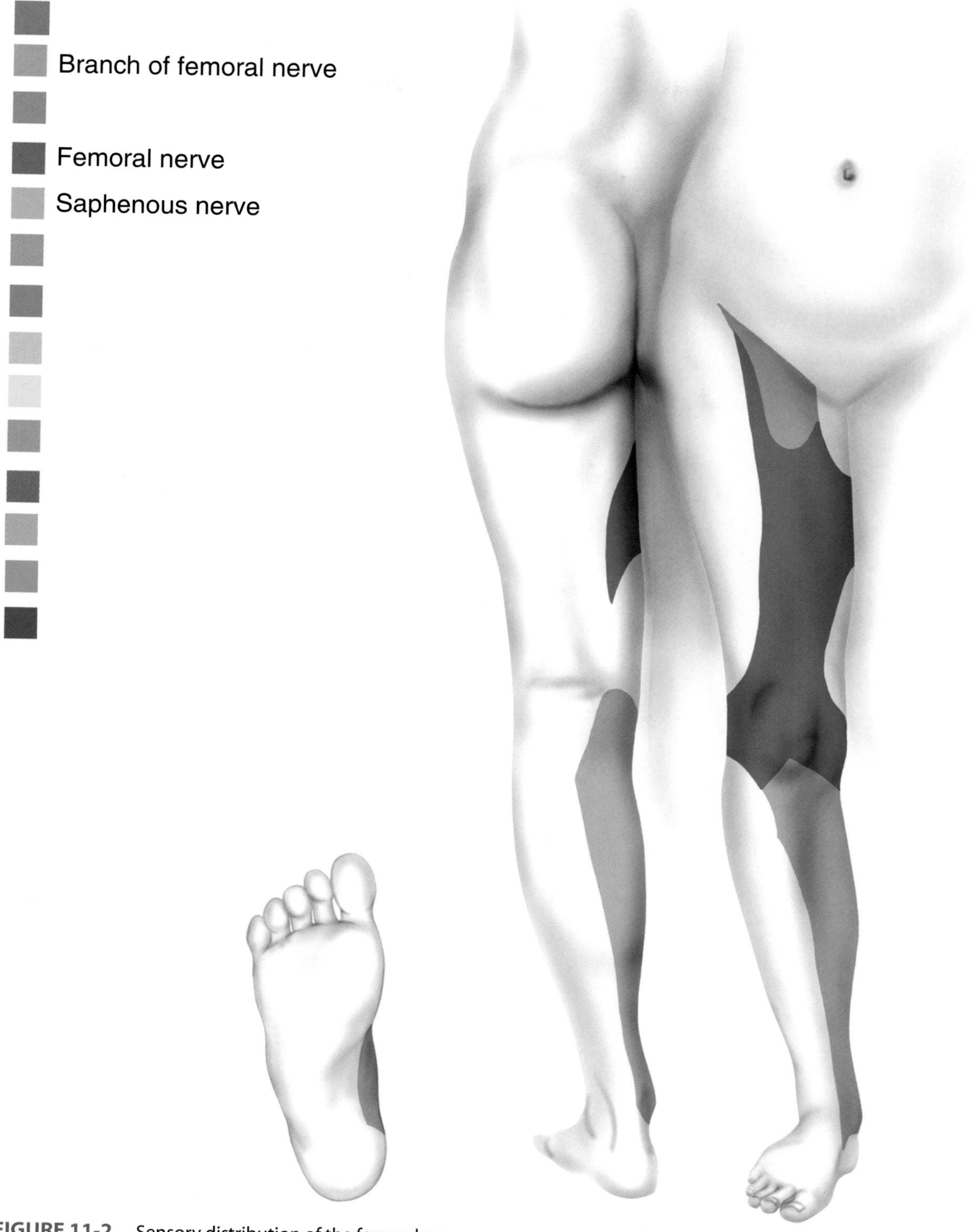

FIGURE 11-2 Sensory distribution of the femoral nerve.

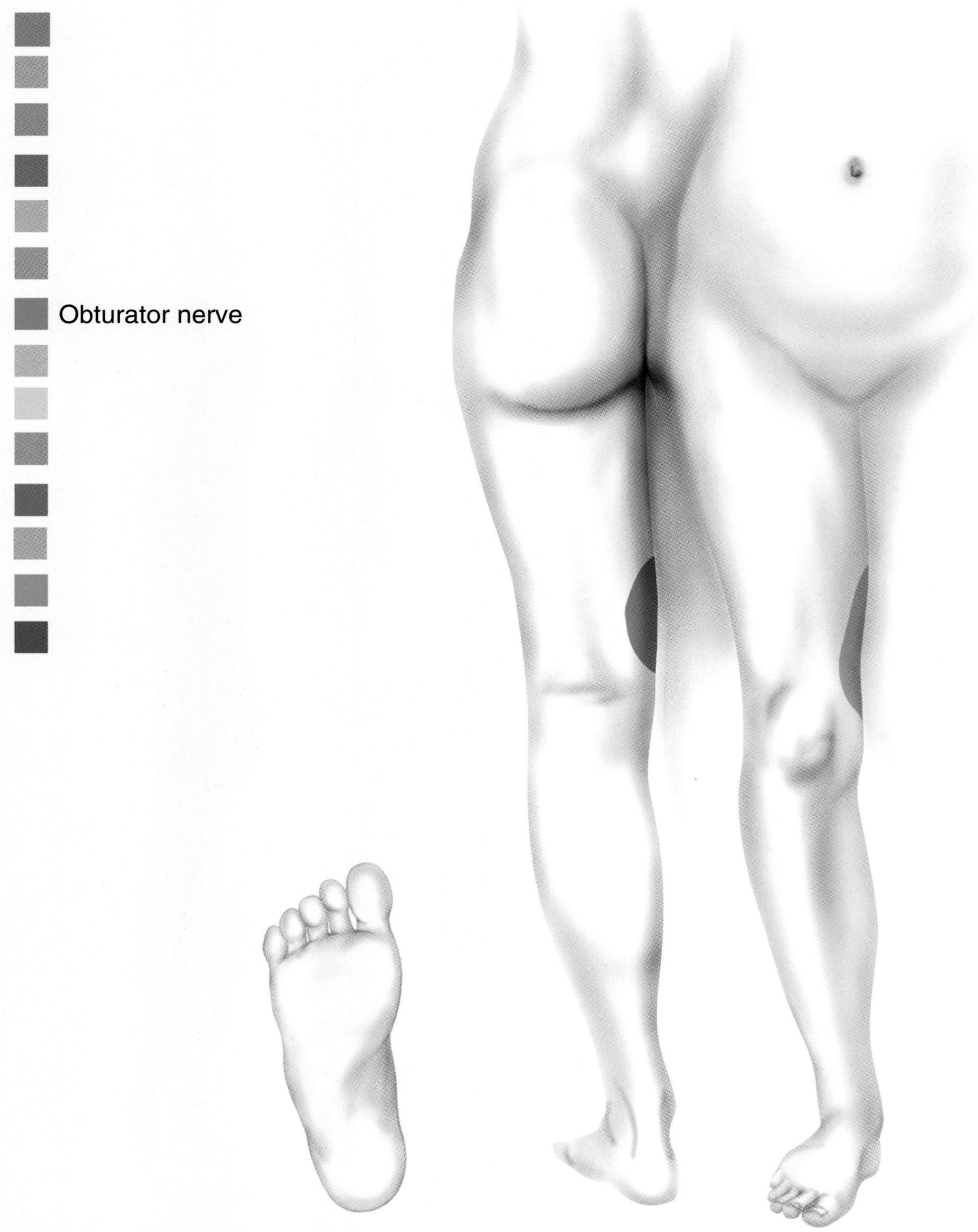

FIGURE 11-3 Sensory distribution of the obturator nerve.

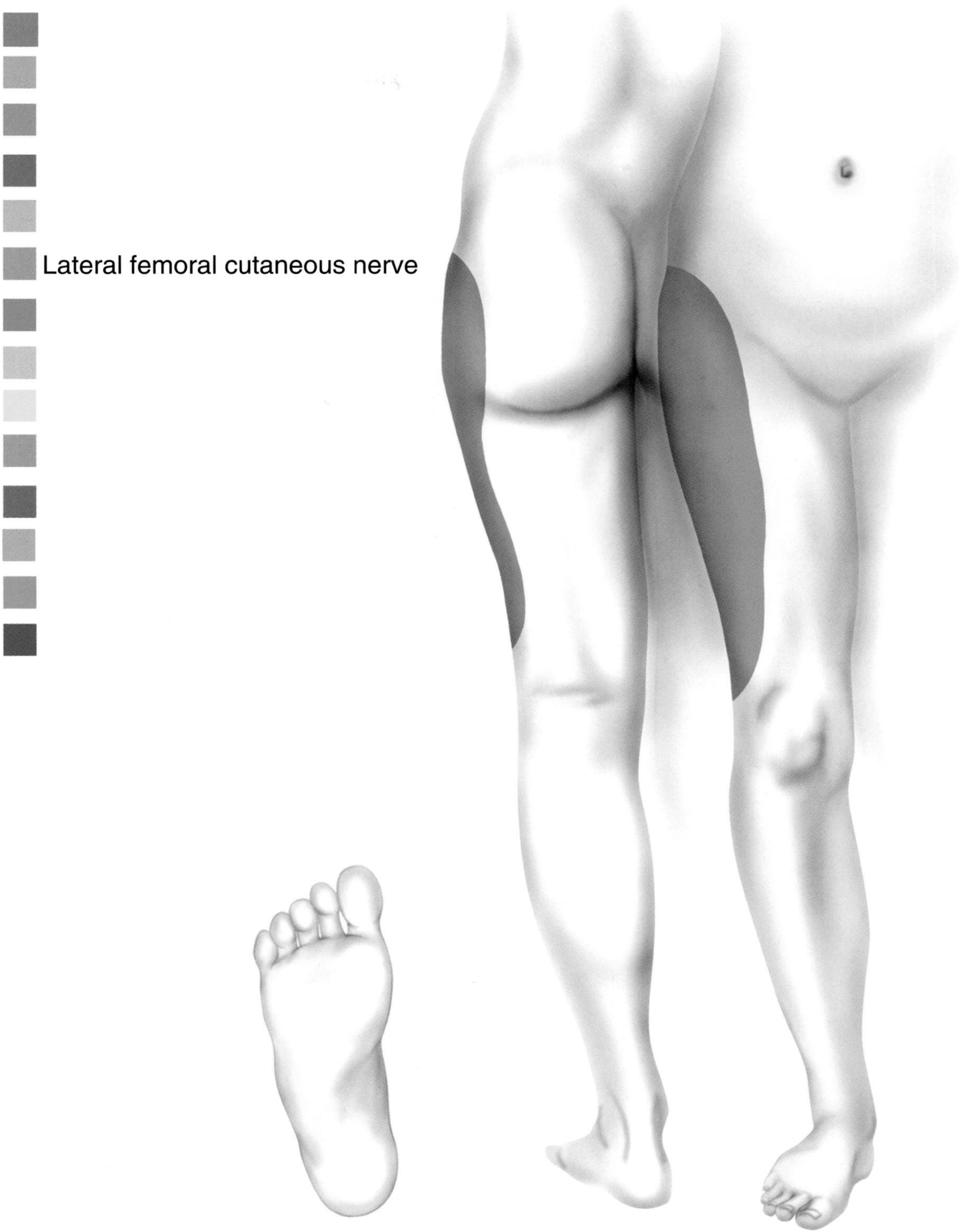

FIGURE 11-4 Sensory distribution of the lateral cutaneous nerve of the thigh.

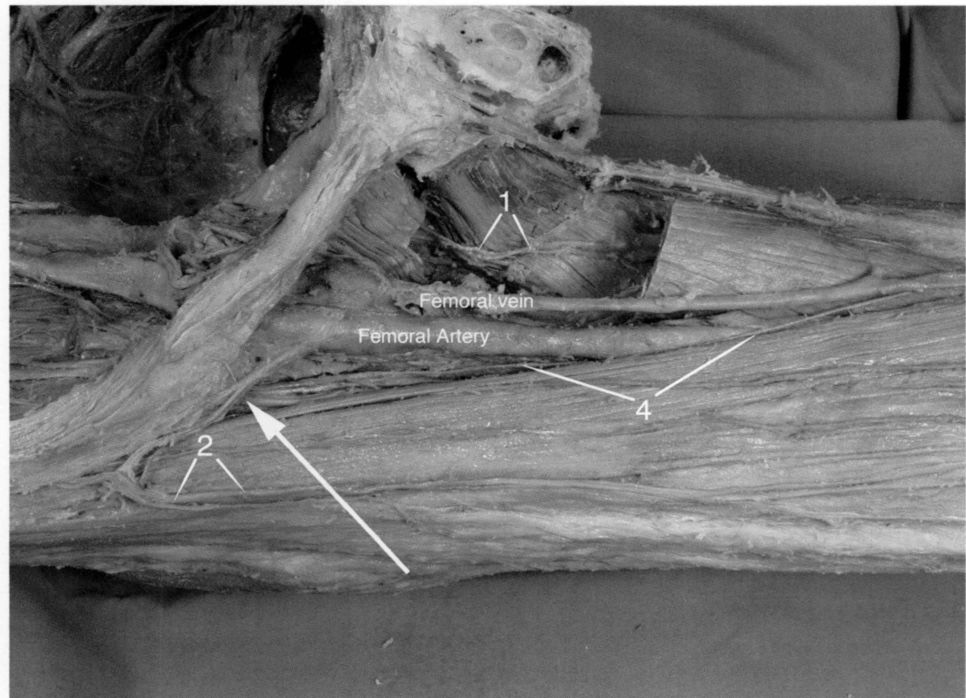

FIGURE 11-5 *Large arrow* indicates the femoral nerve. 1, Obturator nerve; 2, lateral cutaneous nerve of the thigh; 4, saphenous nerve.

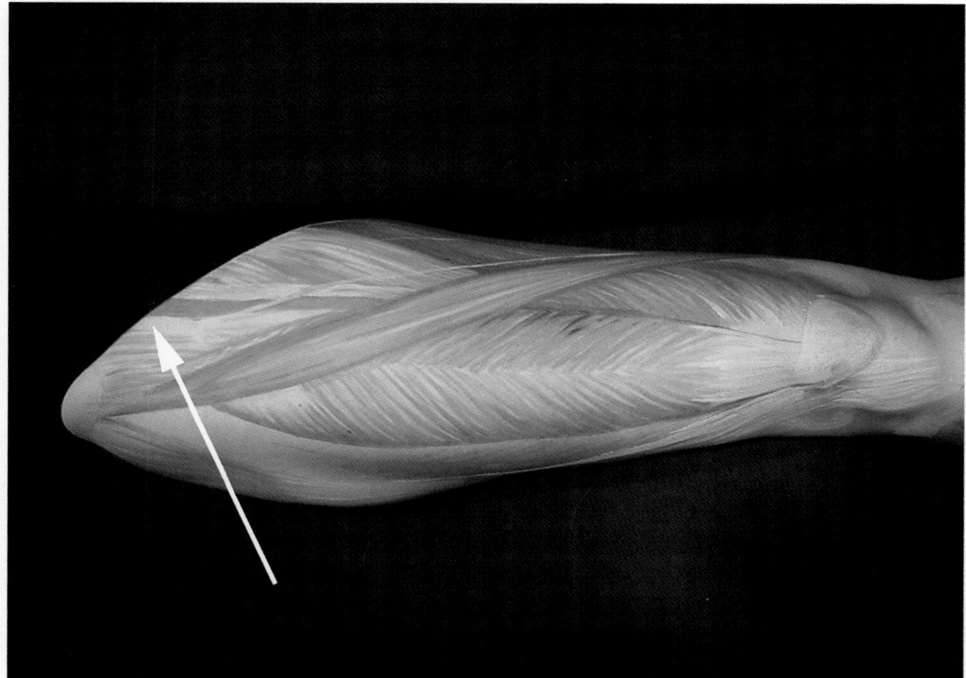

FIGURE 11-6 Surface anatomy of the femoral nerve.

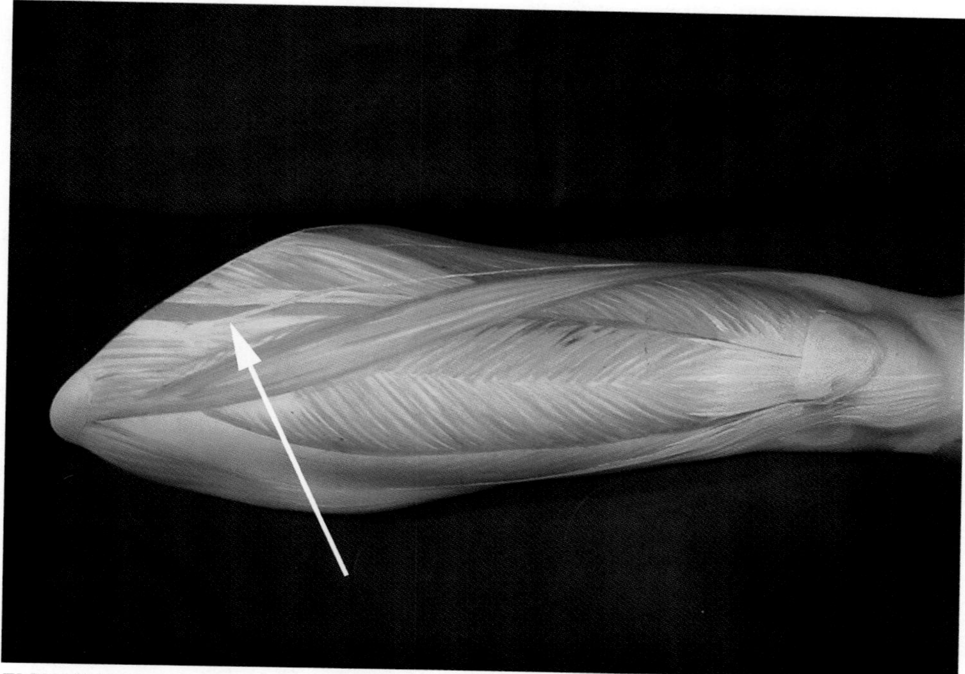

FIGURE 11-7 Surface anatomy of the nerve to the sartorius muscle.

nerve to the sartorius is often encountered during femoral nerve block, and it can be lateral or medial to the femoral nerve, but it is usually more superficial.

Electrical stimulation of the femoral nerve causes contractions of all four of the quadriceps muscles, with subsequent elevation of the patella. This should not be confused with contractions of the sartorius muscle.

The surface landmarks of the nerve to the sartorius (Fig. 11-7, *arrow*) are identical to those of the femoral nerve.

Electrical stimulation of the nerve to the sartorius causes contractions of the sartorius muscle, which are frequently confused with quadriceps muscle contractions but do not cause the patella to move. Note the saphenous nerve medial to the sartorius.

Figure 11-8 illustrates the osteotomes of the lower limb.

Figure 11-9 illustrates the dermatomes of the lower limb.

Figure 11-10 illustrates the neurotomes of the lower limb.

(See percutaneous femoral nerve and nerve sartorius muscle stimulation movie on DVD.)

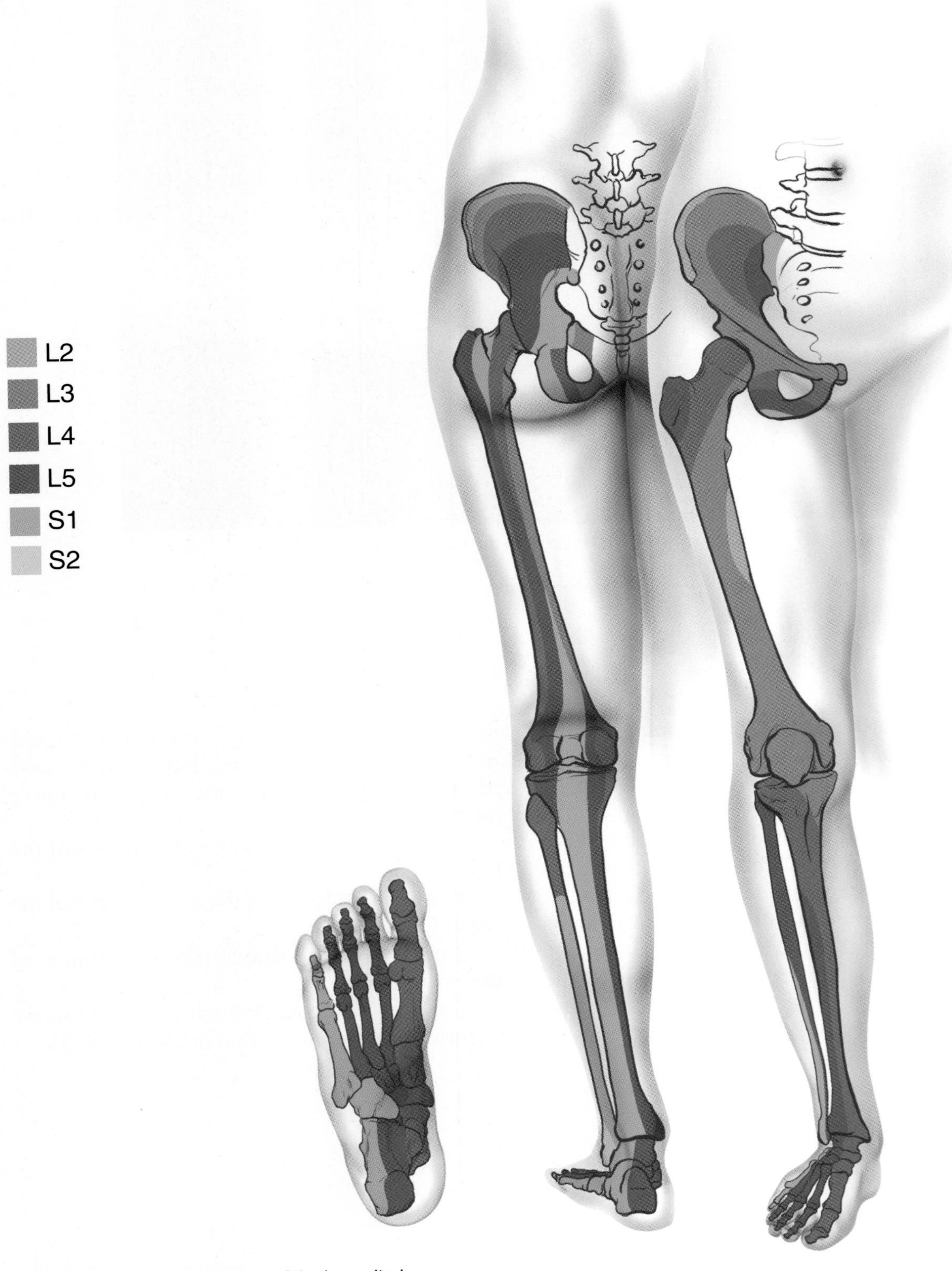

FIGURE 11-8 Osteotomes of the lower limb.

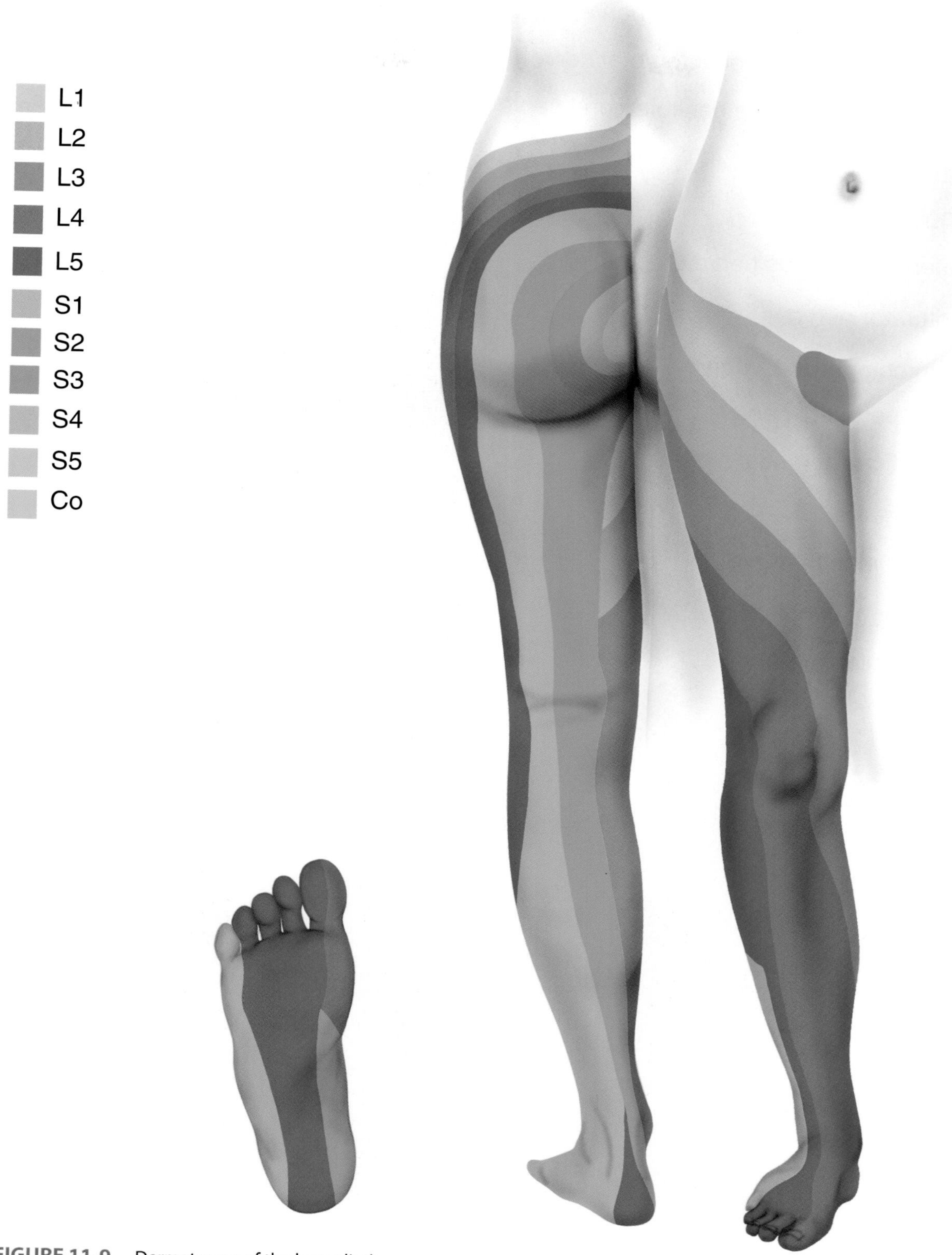

FIGURE 11-9 Dermatomes of the lower limb.

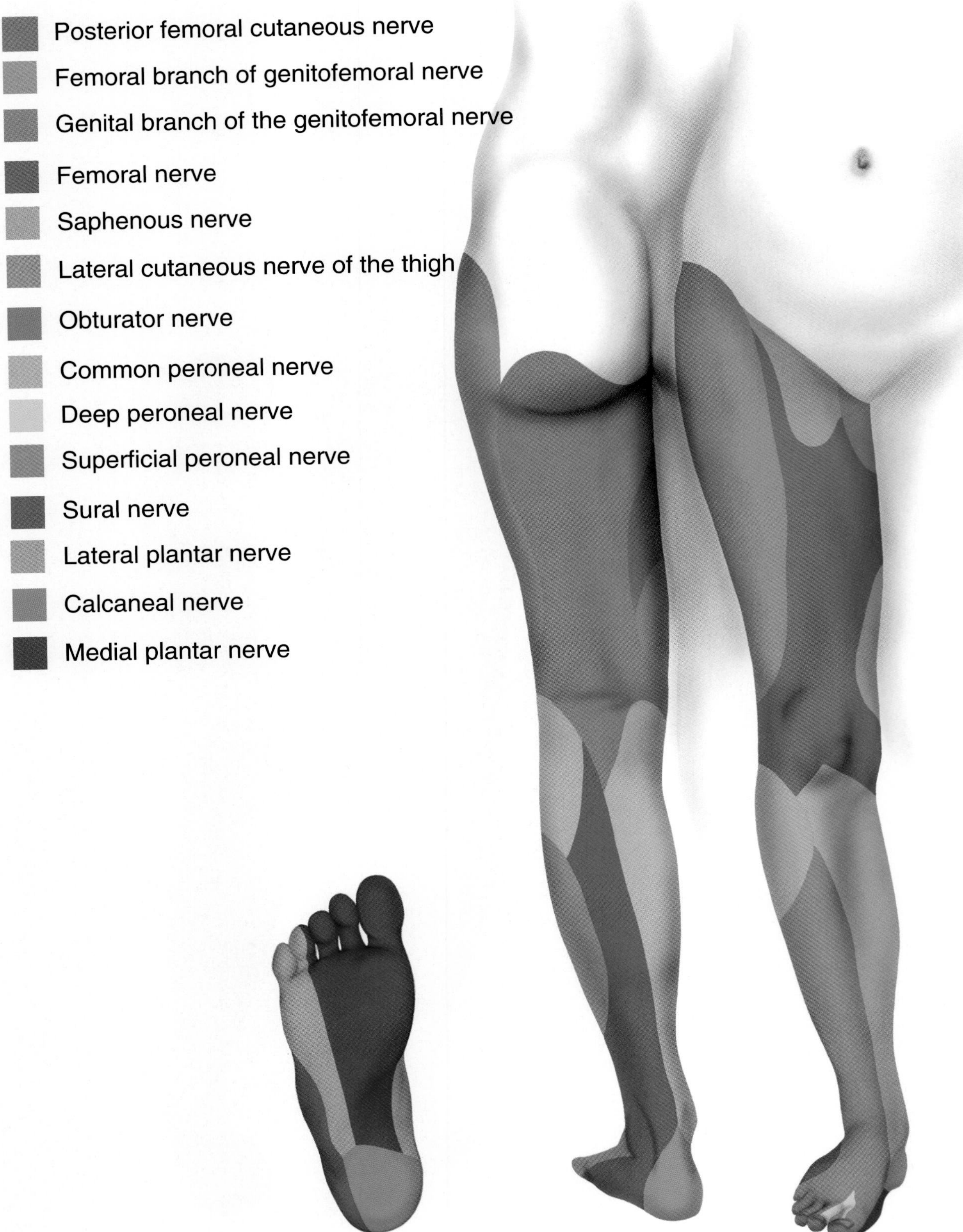

FIGURE 11-10 Neurotomes of the lower limb.

SUGGESTED FURTHER READING

1. Gray's Anatomy: The Anatomical Basis of Clinical Practice, 39th ed. Philadelphia, Elsevier, 2005.
2. Netter FH: Atlas of Human Anatomy, 2nd ed. East Hanover, NJ, Novartis, 1997.
3. Abrahams PH, Marks SC Jr, Hutchings RT: McMinn's Color Atlas of Human Anatomy, 5th ed. Philadelphia, Elsevier Mosby, 2003.
4. Boezaart AP: Anesthesia and Orthopaedic Surgery. New York, McGraw-Hill, 2006.
5. Hadzic A, Vloka JD: Peripheral Nerve Blocks: Principles and Practice. New York, McGraw-Hill, 2004.
6. Rathmell JP, Neal JM, Viscomi CM: Regional Anesthesia: The Requisites in Anesthesia. Philadelphia, Elsevier Mosby, 2004.
7. Brown DL: Atlas of Regional Anesthesia, 3rd ed. Philadelphia, Elsevier, 2006.
8. Barret J, Harmon D, Loughnane B, et al: Peripheral Nerve Blocks and Peri-operative Pain Relief. Philadelphia, WB Saunders, 2004.
9. Meier G, Büttner J: Atlas der peripheren Regionalanästhesie. Stuttgart, Georg Thieme Verlag, 2004.
10. Hahn MB, McQuillan PM, Sheplock GJ: Regional Anesthesia: An Atlas of Anatomy and Technique. St. Louis, Mosby, 1996.
11. Salinas FV: Femoral nerve block. In Boezaart AP (ed): Anesthesia and Orthopaedic Surgery. New York, McGraw-Hill, 2006, pp 331-341.
12. Capdevila X, Nadeau M-J: Lumbar paravertebral (psoas compartment) block. In Boezaart AP (ed): Anesthesia and Orthopaedic Surgery. New York, McGraw-Hill, 2006, pp 358-370.

Chapter 12

Anterior Lumbar Plexus Blocks

- Single-Injection Femoral Nerve Block
- Continuous Femoral Nerve Block
- Single-Injection Obturator Nerve Block
- Single-Injection Lateral Cutaneous Nerve of the Thigh Block

SINGLE-INJECTION FEMORAL NERVE BLOCK

Introduction

The single-injection femoral nerve block is indicated for surgery to the knee, femur, medial tibia, first toe, and medial side of the foot (1). It is essential to study the osteotomes (see Fig. 11-8), dermatomes (see Fig. 11-9), and neurotomes (see Fig. 11-10) of the lower limb to understand the extent of this block.

Specific Anatomic Considerations

The femoral nerve originates from the second, third, and fourth lumbar roots (see Fig. 13-1), and the bones of the L2, L3, and L4 osteotomes are covered by this block (see Fig. 11-8) (2). Note that this area starts with the femur and continues down to the medial aspect of the tibia and medial side of the foot.

Included in this block are the skin areas supplied by the L2, L3, and L4 dermatomes (see Fig. 11-9). Note again that coverage will extend all the way down to the big toe and the medial aspect of the foot.

The single-injection femoral nerve block usually does not involve the area innervated by the lateral cutaneous nerve of the thigh on the side of the thigh (see Fig. 11-4), nor does it commonly involve the medial area of the thigh innervated by the obturator nerve (see Fig. 11-3). The obturator nerve originates from the anterior rami of L2, L3, and L4 (see Fig. 13-1) and gives off branches to the hip joint and the posterior aspects of the knee joint capsule (2).

A pure femoral nerve block usually involves the areas shown in Figure 11-2, which include the anterior aspect of the thigh, as well as the medial aspect of the lower leg and the medial aspect of the foot by way of the saphenous nerve.

The single-injection femoral nerve block is therefore almost always combined with a sciatic nerve block for knee, ankle, and foot surgery. It is best suited for situations in which pain is expected to be of relatively short duration. For pain of longer duration, such as after anterior cruciate ligament repair or total knee replacement, a continuous nerve block is optimal.

Technique

The patient is positioned supine and the femoral artery is palpated and marked (Fig. 12-1). Figure 12-2 illustrates the sono-anatomy for ultrasound-assisted femoral nerve block.

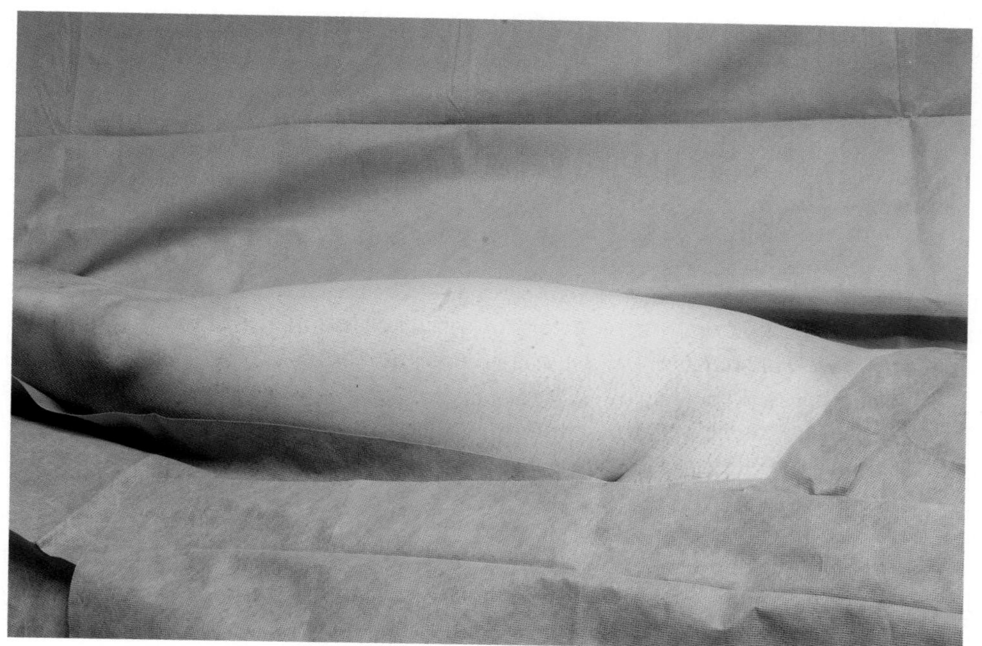

FIGURE 12-1 The patient is positioned in the supine position with the foot neutral, neither externally nor internally rotated.

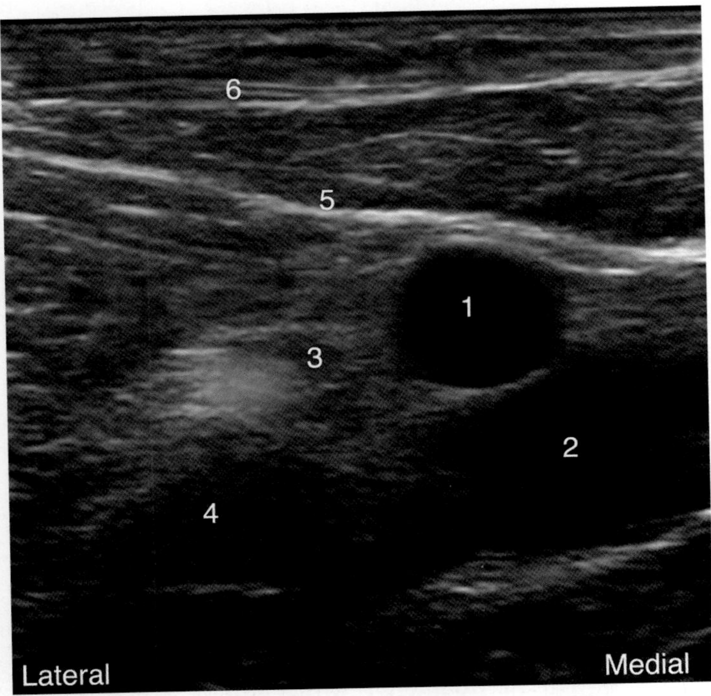

FIGURE 12-2 Transverse sonogram of femoral nerve area. 1 = Femoral artery; 2 = Femoral vein; 3 = Femoral nerve; 4 = iliacus muscle; 5 = Fascia iliaca; 6 = Fascia lata.

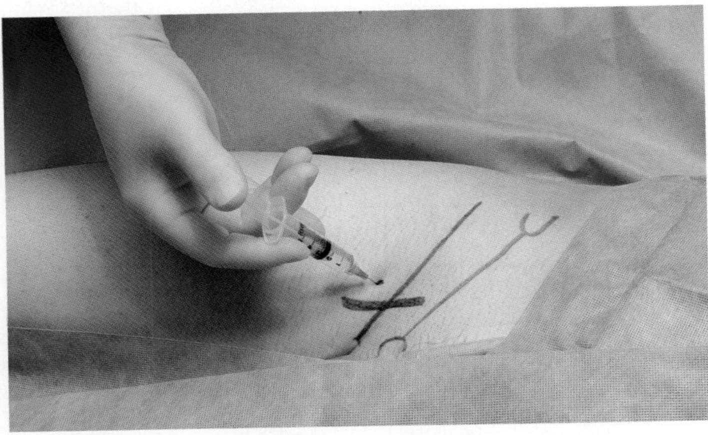

FIGURE 12-3 The *solid vertical line* indicates the position of the femoral artery, and the *horizontal line* the inguinal groove. The *line joining the two semicircles* indicates the position of the inguinal ligament. The skin and subcutaneous tissue are anesthetized.

The point of needle entry (Fig. 12-3, *single dot*) is approximately 1 to 1.5 cm lateral to the artery (see Fig. 12-2, *broad blue vertical line*) and 1 cm caudal to the inguinal crease (see Fig. 12-2, *thin blue horizontal line*). The *semicircles* in Figure 12-2 represent the anterior superior iliac spine and the pubic tubercle. Some anesthesiologists prefer needle entry inside the inguinal crease, whereas others prefer entry above the inguinal crease. Personal preference and the clinical situation should dictate the choice. Above the crease, however, the nerve is closer to the artery and sometimes deep to the artery.

After disinfecting the skin with an appropriate solution, the skin and subcutaneous tissue are anesthetized (Fig. 12-3).

The stimulating needle enters the skin at a slightly cephalic angle and two clear "pops" can usually be felt as the fascia lata and fascia iliaca are penetrated (Fig. 12-4). The nerve stimulator is now typically set at an output of 1 to 2 mA, a frequency of 2 Hz, and a pulse width of 100 to 300 µsec.

The nerve to the sartorius muscle is often encountered, and this should not be confused with femoral nerve stimulation.

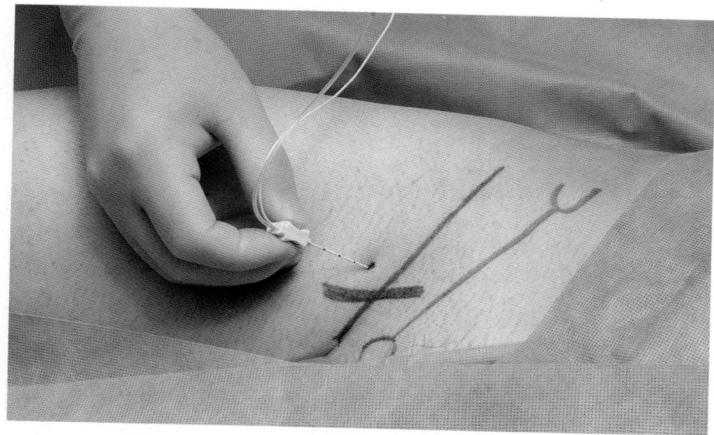

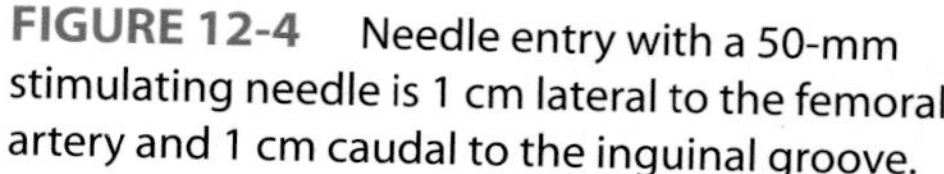

FIGURE 12-4 Needle entry with a 50-mm stimulating needle is 1 cm lateral to the femoral artery and 1 cm caudal to the inguinal groove.

Slight adjustment to the needle, first by advancing it slightly, then by moving it laterally, and finally by moving it medially, will bring it in contact with the femoral nerve with resulting clear cephalad movements of the patella owing to quadriceps muscle contractions. The nerve stimulator is now turned down to 0.3 to 0.5 mA.

Injection of local anesthetic agent or any other conducting fluid, such as normal saline, will cause the muscle twitches to stop immediately. This is a positive Raj test, which gives further assurance that the block will be successful.

Local Anesthetic Agent Choice

Almost all local anesthetics agents in various volumes, concentrations, and combinations have been used for this block. The author prefers to use 15 to 40 mL of ropivacaine 0.5% to 0.75%, or bupivacaine 0.5%. Ropivacaine 0.5% or bupivacaine 0.5% plus 0.3 mg of buprenorphine or 40 mg of dexamethasone may make this block last up to three times longer, but if a long-acting block is required, it is better to place a continuous femoral nerve block. It is, however, essential to place the needle deep to both the fascia lata and fascia iliaca for a successful femoral nerve block.

(See single-injection femoral nerve block movie on DVD.)

CONTINUOUS FEMORAL NERVE BLOCK

Introduction

The main indication for continuous femoral nerve block is anterior knee surgery such as anterior cruciate ligament repair or total knee replacement (3,4,5). It is essential to realize that there is an area behind the knee supplied by the sciatic or obturator nerves that may still be painful in approximately 20% to 80% of patients after major knee surgery. This pain, however, is usually short lived; if it bothers the patient, a single-injection sciatic nerve block may be performed after confirmation of an intact sciatic nerve in the postoperative period. If this is not successful in treating the pain, an obturator nerve block may be required.

If the tendon for anterior cruciate ligament repair is harvested from the hamstrings, a single-injection sciatic nerve block may also be needed. Continuous femoral nerve block is further indicated for painful surgery to the ankle joint (e.g., ankle arthroplasty and triple arthrodesis) in combination with a continuous sciatic nerve block.

If the catheter is placed on the femoral nerve deep to the fascia iliaca, the block will almost always incorporate the lateral cutaneous nerve of the thigh and the obturator nerve (6). Figure 12-5 indicates the spread of 3 mL (Fig. 12-5A), 5 mL (Fig. 12-5B), and 20 mL (Fig. 12-5C) of local anesthetic agent after a continuous femoral nerve block. Notice that 20 mL spreads all the way to the lumbar plexus. This probably makes the continuous femoral nerve block a more appropriate option than a continuous lumbar plexus block if a careful risk-benefit ratio is calculated (7).

Specific Anatomic Considerations

The femoral nerve originates from the second, third, and fourth lumbar roots, and the bones

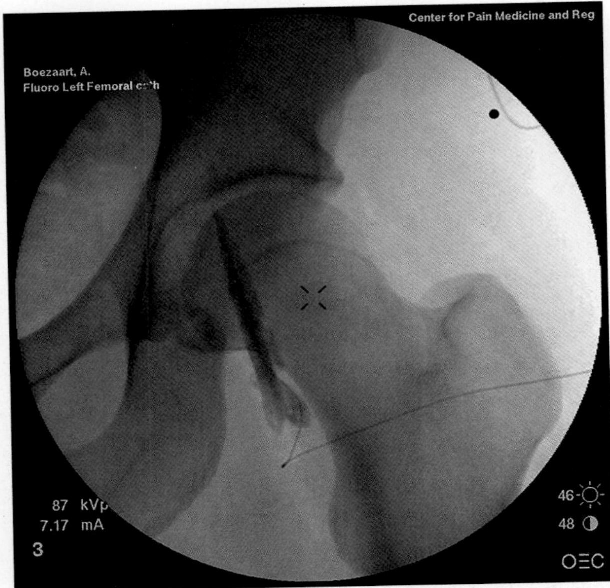

A

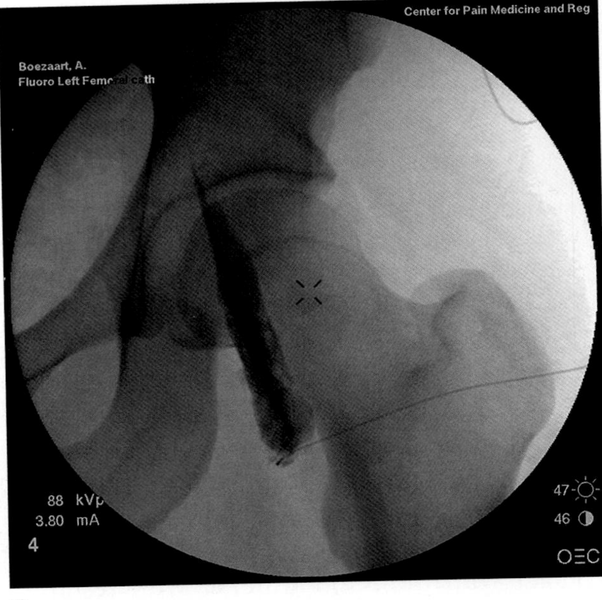

B

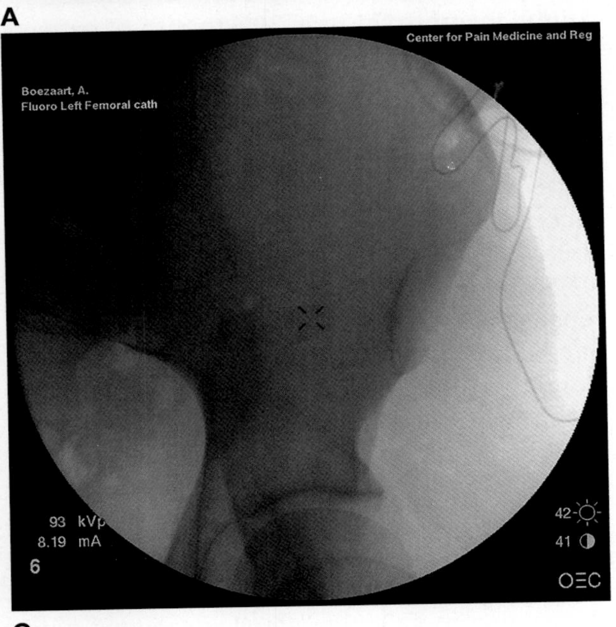

C

FIGURE 12-5 **A,** Injection of 3 mL of contrast medium through a femoral catheter. **B,** Injection of 5 mL of contrast medium through a femoral catheter. **C,** Injection of 20 mL of contrast medium through a femoral catheter.

of the L2, L3, and L4 osteotomes are covered by this block (see Fig. 11-8). Note that this includes almost the entire femur and continues down to the medial aspect of the tibia and medial aspect of the foot.

The skin area of the leg supplied by the L2, L3, and L4 dermatomes is covered by the continuous femoral nerve block (see Fig. 11-9). Note again that this area extends to the big toe.

The continuous femoral nerve block almost always involves the lateral cutaneous nerve of the thigh, the obturator nerve, and femoral nerve if the catheter is advanced under nerve stimulator control next to the nerve (see Figs. 11-2 to 11-4).

In young, fit, healthy patients, there is no or very little brown fat surrounding the femoral nerve, which makes catheter placement in these patients more challenging than in older patients and patients with more adipose tissue. Patience is required for accurate catheter placement in such patients. It is, however, preferable to place a stimulating catheter on the femoral nerve to achieve a successful secondary block.

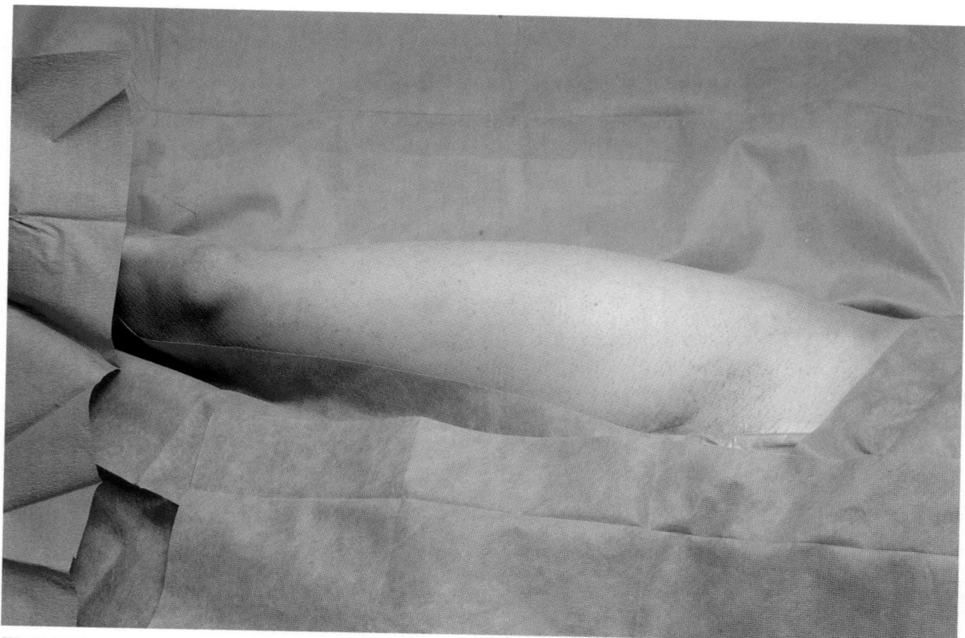

FIGURE 12-6 The patient is positioned supine with the foot in the neutral position.

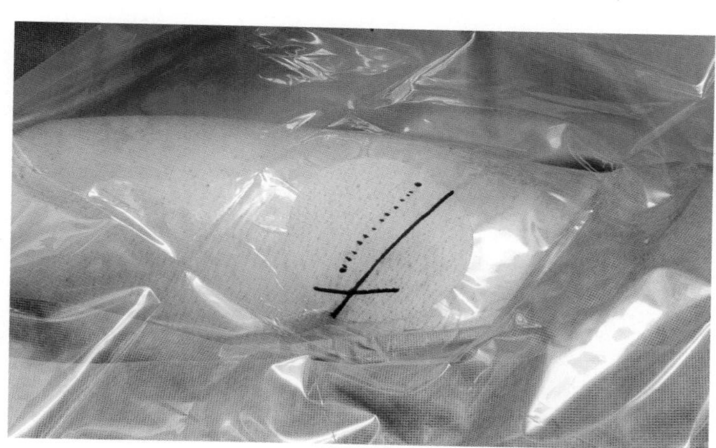

FIGURE 12-7 The *horizontal dotted line* indicates the intended path for tunneling the catheter. The *vertical solid line* indicates the position of the femoral artery, and the *horizontal solid line* the inguinal groove.

Technique

The patient is positioned supine with the foot neutral, neither externally nor internally rotated (Fig. 12-6).

After palpating and marking the femoral artery and inguinal crease, and disinfecting the skin, the area is covered with a sterile, fenestrated, transparent plastic drape (Fig. 12-7).

The skin, subcutaneous tissue (Fig. 12-8A), and the intended path for tunneling of the catheter (Fig. 12-8B) is anesthetized with lidocaine and 1:200,000 epinephrine.

An insulated 17- or 18-gauge Tuohy needle is attached to the nerve stimulator, which is set to an output of 1 to 1.5 mA, a frequency of 2 Hz, and a pulse width of 100 to 300 μsec, and enters the skin 1 to 1.5 cm lateral of the femoral artery and 1 cm caudal of the inguinal crease (Fig. 12-9). The bevel of the needle points upward and the needle enters at a cephalic angle of approximately 45 degrees. The needle can also be placed by ultrasound-assistance (Fig. 12-2).

Some anesthesiologists prefer needle entry inside the inguinal crease, whereas others prefer entry above the inguinal crease. Personal

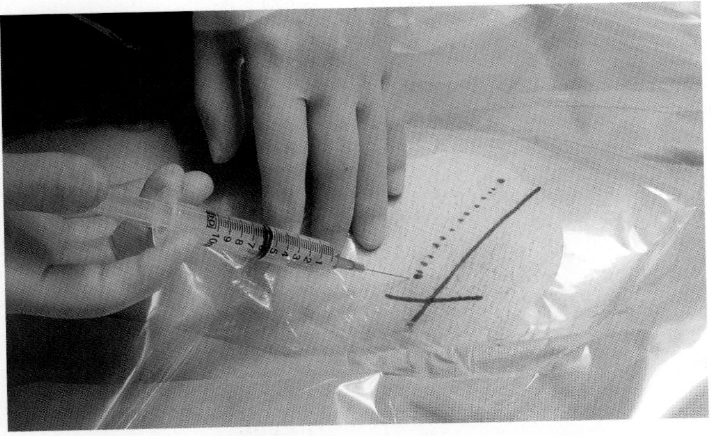

A

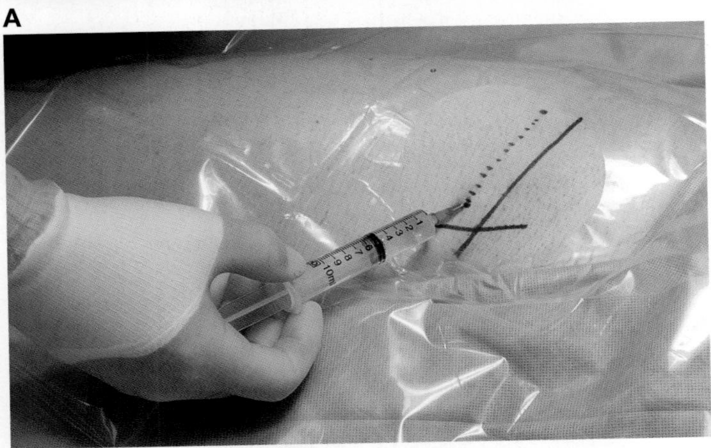

B

FIGURE 12-8 **A,** The skin and subcutaneous tissues are anesthetized. **B,** The intended path for tunneling the catheter is anesthetized.

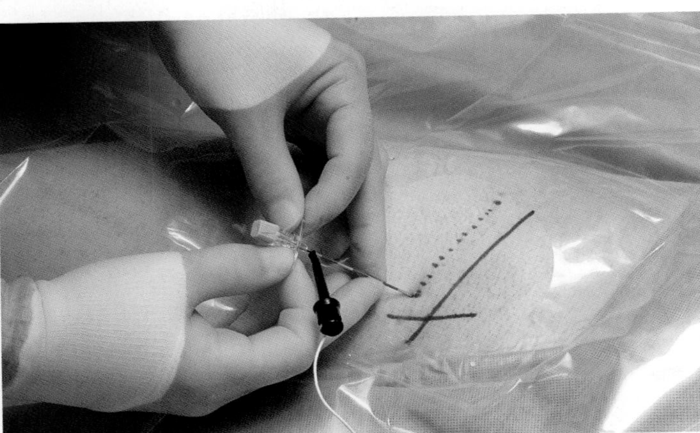

FIGURE 12-9 An insulated 18-gauge Tuohy needle, attached to a nerve stimulator, enters 1 cm lateral to the artery and 1 cm caudal to the inguinal groove.

preference and the clinical situation should dictate the choice. Above the crease, however, the nerve is closer to the artery and sometimes deep to the artery.

There are usually two distinct "pops" as the fascia lata and fascia iliaca are penetrated. Cephalad movement of the patella is clearly observed as the femoral nerve is stimulated.

After identifying the femoral nerve with the needle, the nerve stimulator output is turned down to between 0.3 and 0.5 mA and a brisk motor response of the quadriceps muscle should

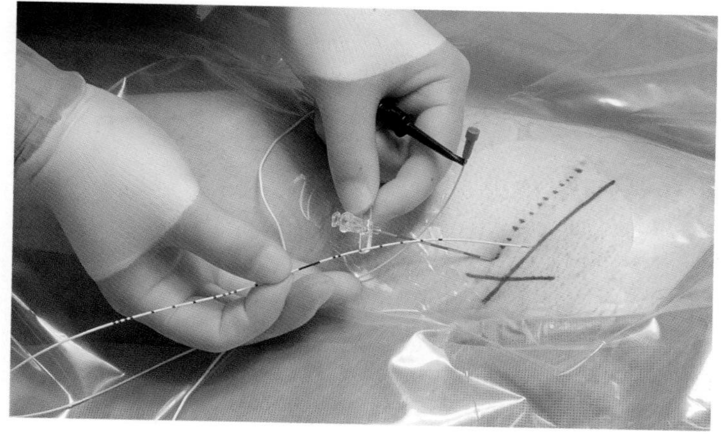

FIGURE 12-10 Once the nerve has been located with the needle, the nerve stimulator is attached to the proximal end of the catheter, and the distal end of the catheter is inserted into the needle shaft.

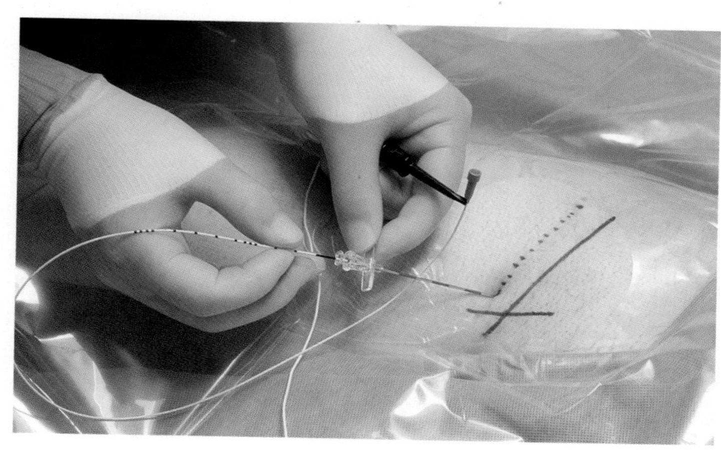

FIGURE 12-11 The special mark on the catheter indicates that the catheter tip is now situated at the needle tip.

still be present. This ensures correct needle placement deep to the fascia iliaca, but it does not ensure accurate catheter placement. It is essential not to inject any local anesthetic agent or other electrically conductive fluid such as normal saline through the needle at this point because this will render stimulating catheter placement impossible. The notion of using normal saline to "open up the space" in which to advance the catheter is not based on scientific fact because in live tissue it only infiltrates the tissue, making it edematous and rendering further nerve stimulation impossible or very difficult. If the anesthesiologist does subscribe to the notion of "opening up the space," he or she should use 5% dextrose in water because it will not abolish the motor response and will allow stimulating catheter placement.

The nerve stimulator is now attached to the proximal end of the stimulating catheter, which is placed in the palm of the operator's left hand, and the catheter is held with the right hand at the area of the special mark, which is 10 cm from the catheter tip (Fig. 12-10).

The catheter tip is inserted into the shaft of the needle. The motor response will immediately resume, and the special mark on the catheter indicates that the catheter tip is situated at the tip of the needle, but it is not yet protruding from the needle tip. The needle should not be manipulated if this broad black mark is not completely visible (Fig. 12-11).

If the twitches disappear on advancement of the catheter, the catheter is carefully withdrawn into the needle shaft such that the entire special mark is visible once again. A small adjustment to the needle is made by rotating it one-fourth turn clockwise or counterclockwise or by withdrawing or advancing the needle slightly, and the catheter is advanced again (Fig. 12-12). This maneuver is repeated as often as necessary to ensure correct and accurate catheter placement

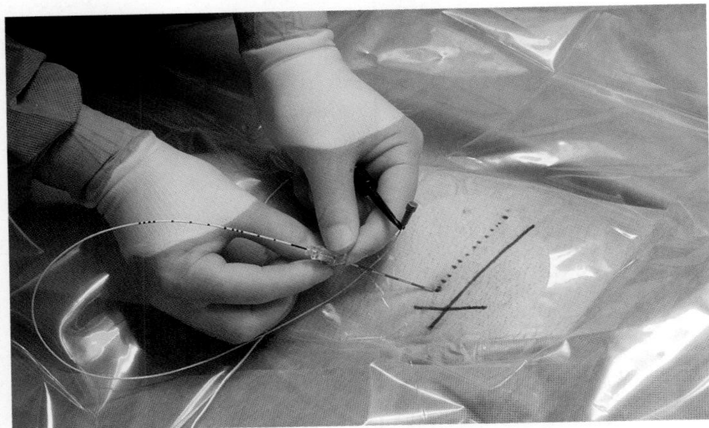

FIGURE 12-12 If the motor response is lost during catheter advancement, the catheter is withdrawn to inside the needle shaft and the needle manipulated—in this case, it is turned a quarter turn clockwise.

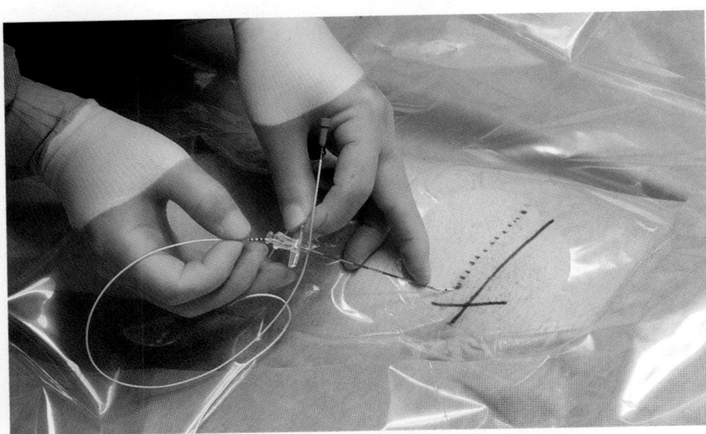

FIGURE 12-13 The catheter is advanced again and after correct catheter placement, the needle is removed without disturbing the catheter.

and successful secondary block. In young, fit adults, it may be necessary to repeat these maneuvers many times, and patience is required. If the catheter is placed without quadriceps stimulation during catheter advancement, it simply means that the catheter is not on or near the nerve and the block cannot be expected to be successful. If required, the catheter can be advanced until adduction of the thigh due to obturator nerve stimulation is observed, but this maneuver is usually unnecessary because the local anesthetic agent will spread along the femoral nerve if the catheter is properly placed (see Fig. 12-5C).

Remove the needle without disturbing the catheter (Fig. 12-13).

Catheter Tunneling with a Skin Bridge

The catheter is tunneled by first inserting the inner stylet of the needle 1 to 2 mm from the catheter exit site if a skin bridge is required (Fig. 12-14A), and advancing it subcutaneously to a point approximately 8 to 10 cm lateral if this is appropriate for the surgery (Fig. 12-14B). This area has previously been anesthetized. The skin bridge tends to make catheter removal easier, but this is offset by a higher frequency of leakage.

The needle is "railroaded" retrogradely over the stylet (Fig. 12-14C, D).

The stylet is removed, the catheter is fed through the needle, and the needle is removed (Fig. 12-14E, F).

The piece of silicone tubing that protected the catheter tip while packaged is handy for placing in the loop made by the catheter to protect the skin under the skin bridge (Fig. 12-14G).

Catheter Tunneling without a Skin Bridge

Figure 12-15 explains the steps involved in catheter tunneling without a skin bridge.

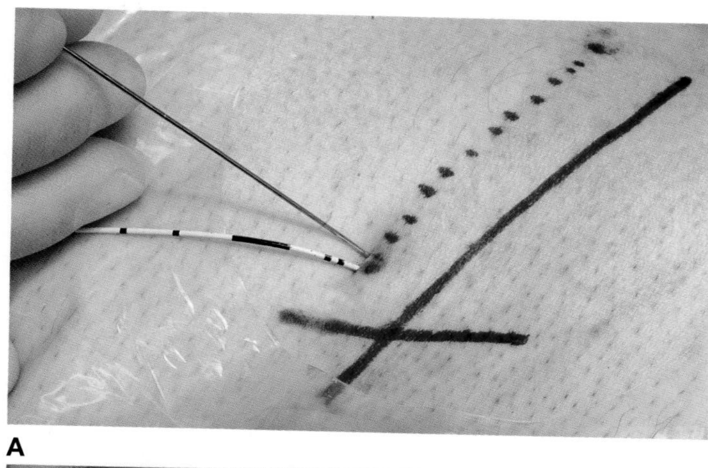
A

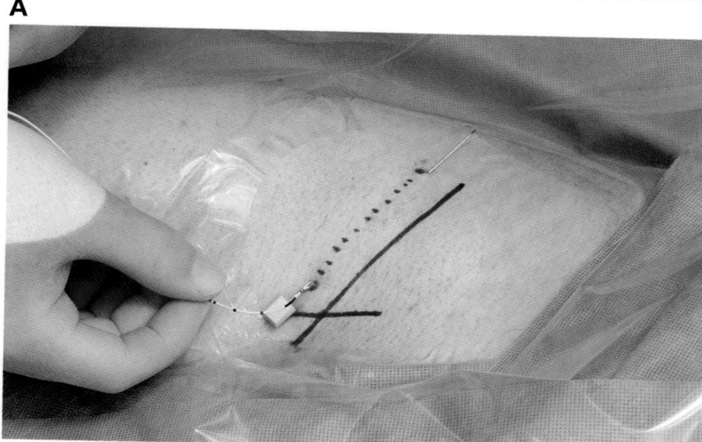
B

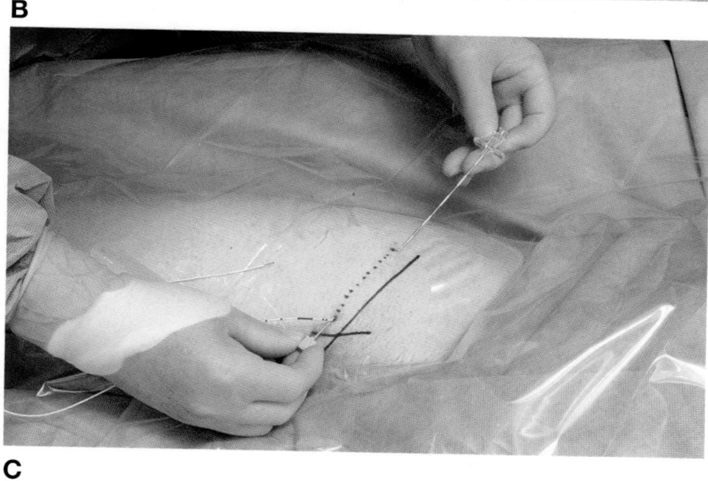
C

FIGURE 12-14 Tunneling with a skin bridge. **A,** The needle stylet enters the skin 1 to 2 mm lateral to the exit site of the catheter. **B,** The inner stylet of the needle is advanced 8 to 10 cm laterally. **C,** The needle is "railroaded" over the stylet.

Raj Test

The Luer lock connecting device is attached to the proximal end of the catheter, the nerve stimulator is clipped to the connecting device, and the nerve stimulation is set to an output of 0 mA.

The nerve stimulator output is turned up slowly until a quadriceps muscle twitch can just be seen. Local anesthetic agent or normal saline is injected and the motor response immediately stops. This constitutes a positive Raj test, which is a further indication that the secondary block will be successful.

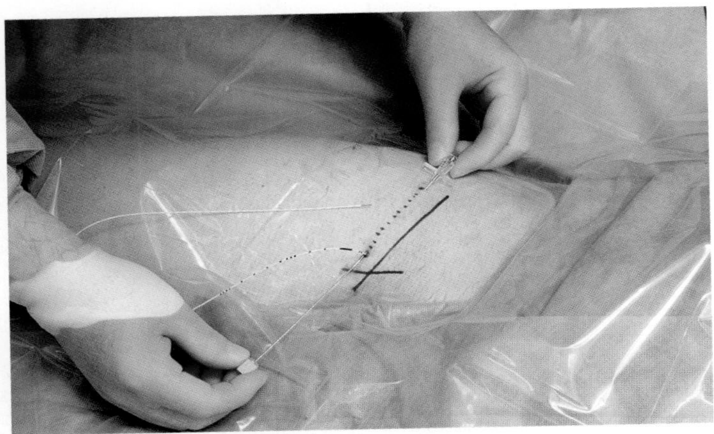

D

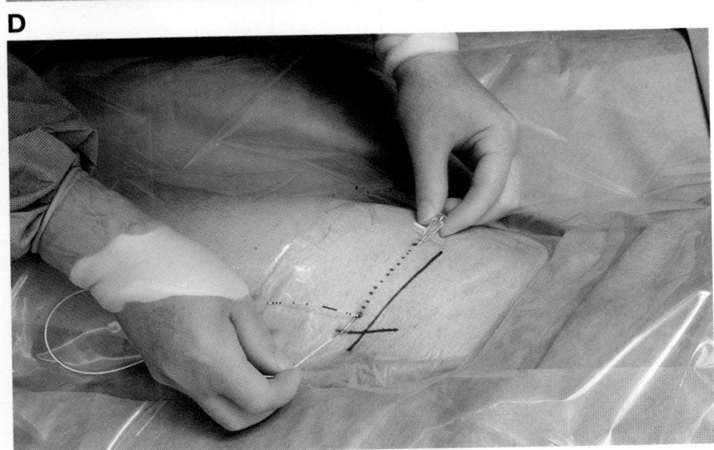

E

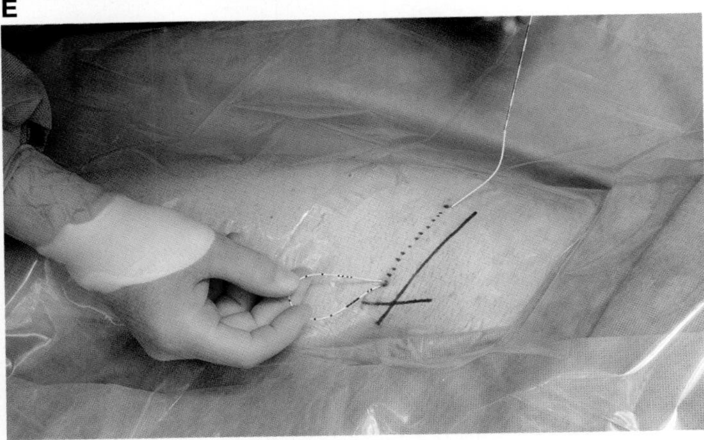

F

FIGURE 12-14 *(continued)* **D,** The stylet is removed. **E,** The catheter is advanced retrogradely through the needle. **F,** The needle is removed.

The catheter and connecting device is placed in the fixation device, which is placed in a convenient position, usually on the patient's abdomen.

Catheter Removal

Catheter removal is a sterile procedure done after the patient no longer requires the continuous nerve block and full sensation has returned to the leg. A common strategy is to discontinue the infusion for 3 to 6 hours when it is anticipated that the patient will not need the block any longer. This gives the patient and health care providers an opportunity to judge the efficacy of the other analgesics. If the patient experiences severe pain again, a bolus is activated through the

FIGURE 12-14 ***(continued)*** **G,** Silicone tubing is placed to protect the skin.

G

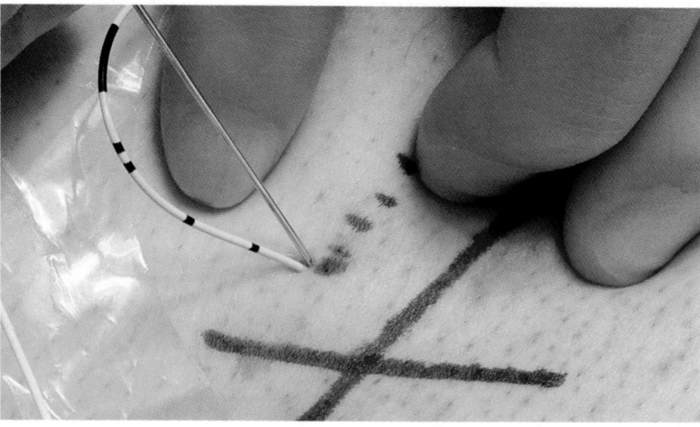

A

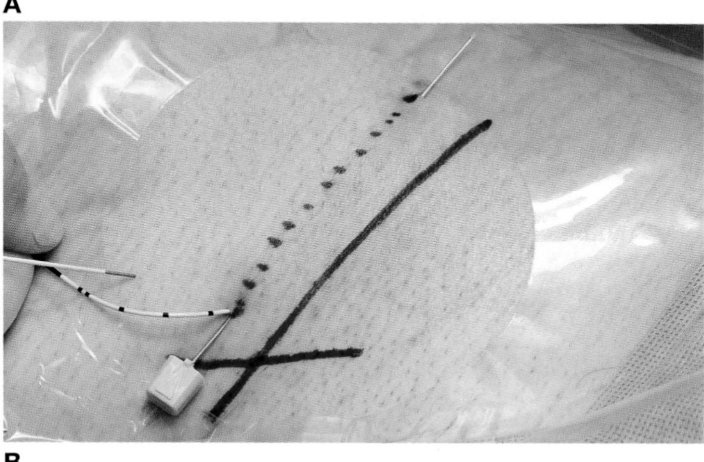

B

FIGURE 12-15 Catheter tunneling without a skin bridge. **A,** The needle stylet enters the exit wound of the catheter. **B,** The needle stylet is advanced 8 to 10 cm laterally.

catheter and the infusion restarted at its previous settings. If the alternative analgesic agents seem to be effective, the catheter can be removed.

The proximal end of the catheter is held with the left hand and the distal end is removed from the skin bridge. This part of the catheter is kept sterile and the rest of the catheter is removed (Fig. 12-16).

Local Anesthetic Agent Choice

Almost all local anesthetic agents and combinations of agents have been used for this block, but the

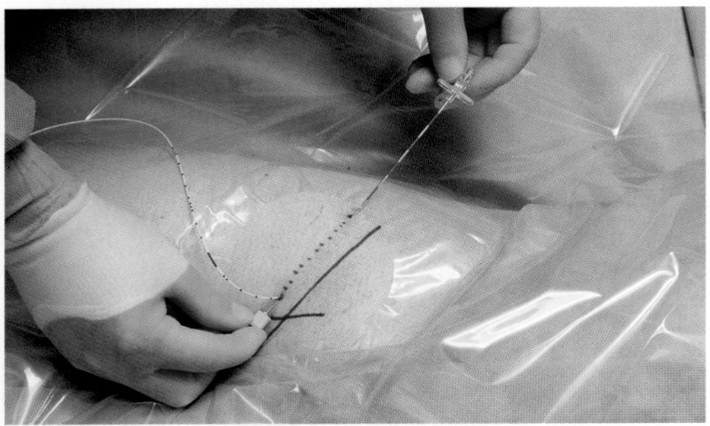

C

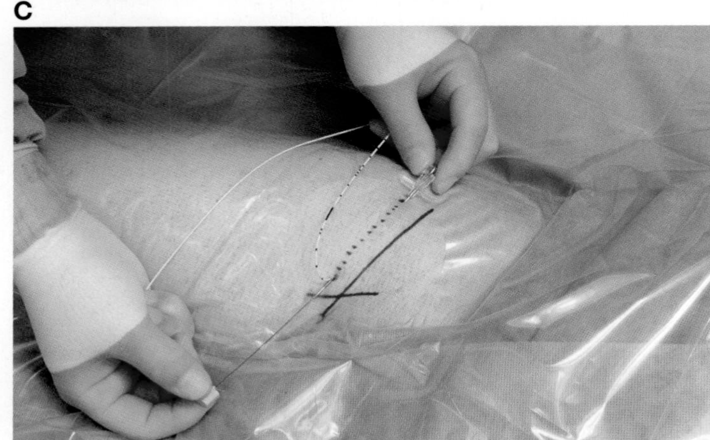

D

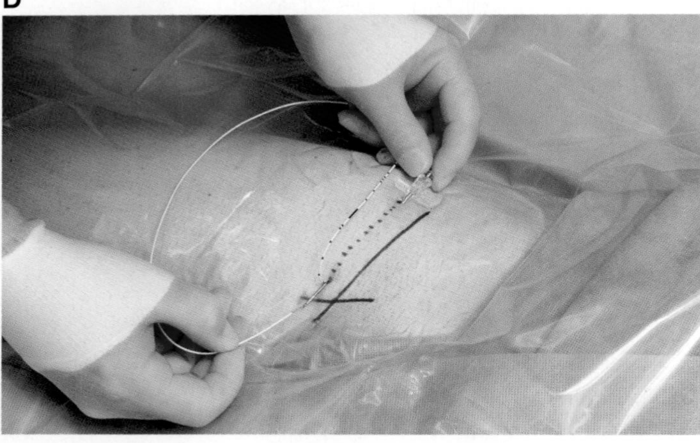

E

FIGURE 12-15 ***(continued)*** **C,** The needle is "railroaded" over the stylet. **D,** The catheter is advanced retrogradely through the needle. **E,** Catheter advancement through the needle.

author prefers to use 15 to 40 mL of ropivacaine 0.5% to 0.75% as the initial bolus for intraoperative analgesia, followed with a 2- to 10-mL/hour continuous infusion of ropivacaine 0.1% to 0.2%. Patient-controlled boluses of 5 to 10 mL every hour are usually sufficient to control breakthrough pain.

This block can jeopardize quadriceps function and some authorities believe that quadriceps function may be essential for knee rehabilitation. Although the importance of quadriceps function for knee rehabilitation has not yet been verified by research, it is advisable to use a dilute concentration of ropivacaine (i.e., 0.1% or 0.05%) to preserve quadriceps function during the postoperative period. Research is ongoing to evaluate buprenorphine in this role.

(See continuous femoral nerve block movie on DVD.)

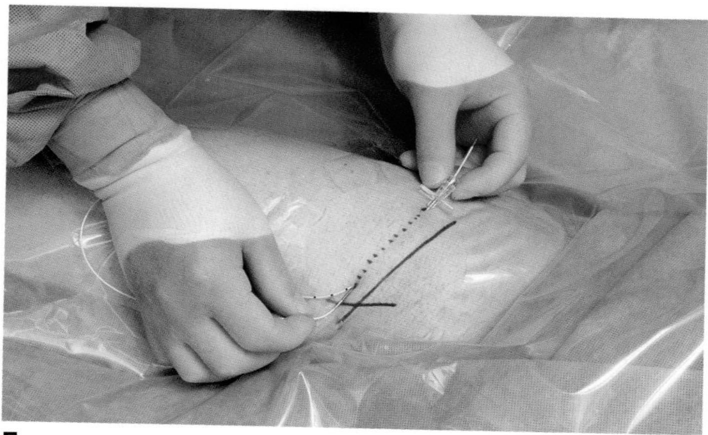

F

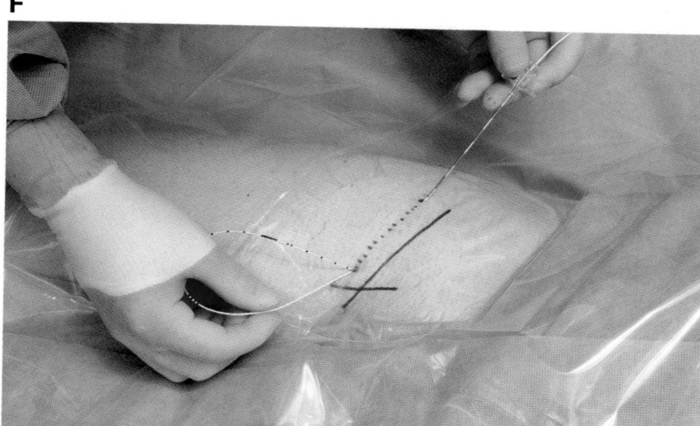

G

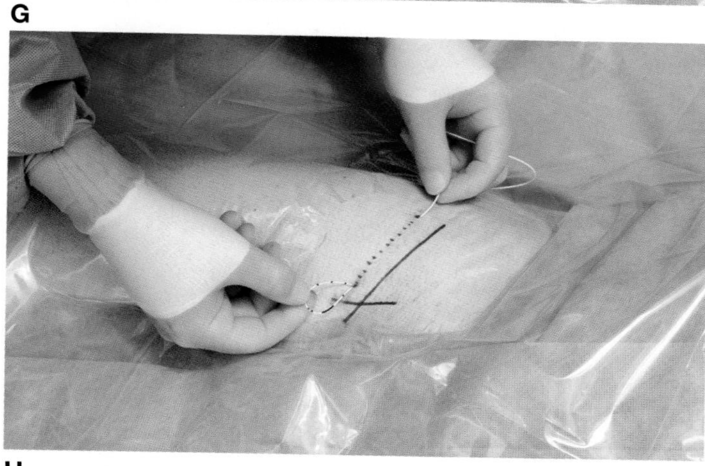

H

FIGURE 12-15 ***(continued)*** **F,** The needle is removed. **G,** The loop in the catheter is reduced. **H,** The loop in the catheter disappears under the skin.

SINGLE-INJECTION OBTURATOR NERVE BLOCK

Introduction

The obturator nerve block is seldom indicated, but after knee surgery and incomplete lumbar plexus block by the anterior approach (femoral nerve block), the patient may experience posterior or medial knee pain. A single-injection sciatic nerve block usually alleviates posterior pain, but an obturator nerve block may be indicated. The anterior division of the obturator nerve supplies the skin over the medial aspect of the lower thigh and does not contribute to the innervation of the

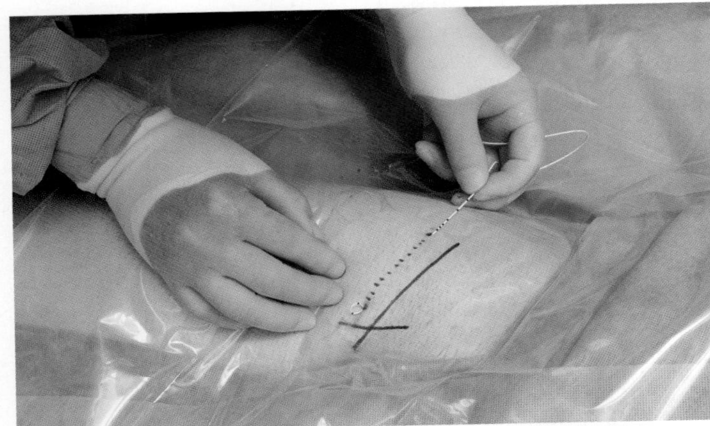

I

FIGURE 12-15 ***(continued)*** **I,** Finished.

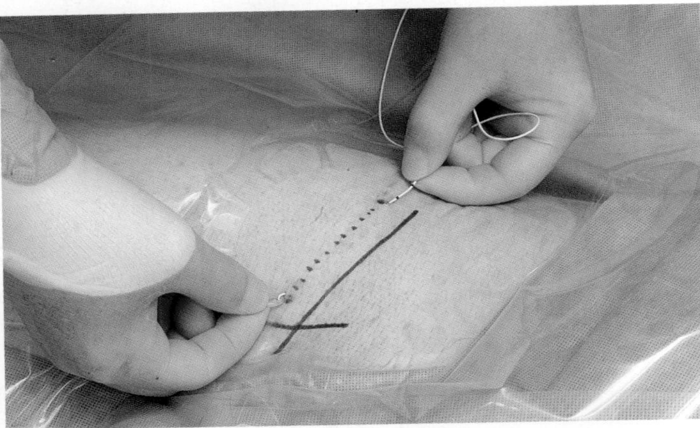

A

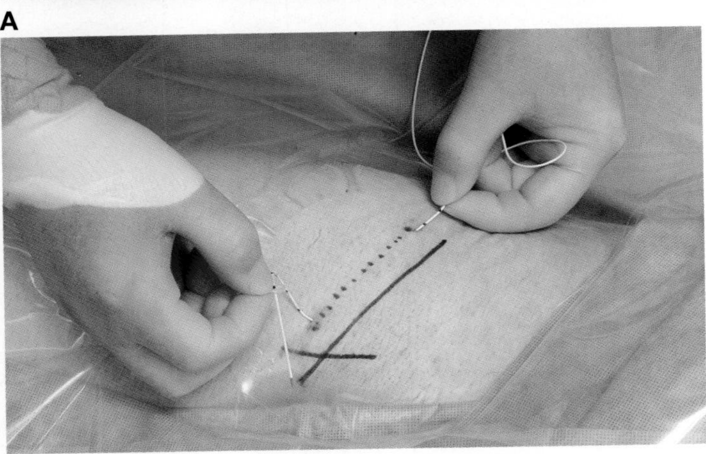

B

FIGURE 12-16 Catheter removal. **A,** The proximal end of the catheter is fixed with one hand and the silicone tubing held in the other hand. **B,** The distal end of the catheter is removed while keeping it sterile.

knee joint itself, whereas the posterior division innervates the posterior knee capsule. There are few indications for either a single-injection or a continuous obturator nerve block.

Specific Anatomic Considerations

The obturator nerve is a branch of the lumbar plexus formed from the anterior rami of the second, third, and fourth lumbar nerves (see

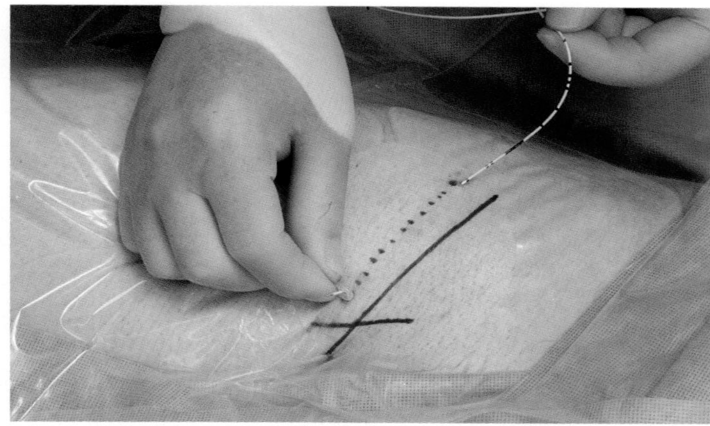

C

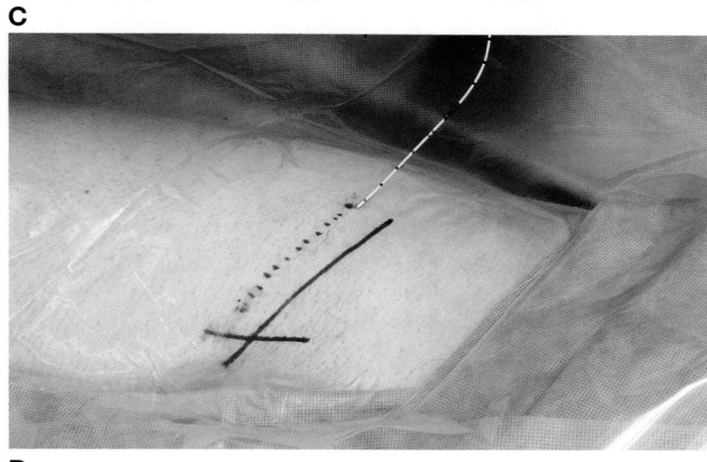

D

FIGURE 12-16 *(continued)* **C,** Traction is applied to the proximal end while still keeping the distal end sterile. **D,** The entire catheter is removed.

Fig. 13-1) (8). It passes on the brim of the pelvis (Fig. 12-17) to leave the pelvis through the obturator foramen. After exiting the foramen, it divides into an anterior and a posterior division. The anterior division passes above the external obturator muscle, whereas the posterior division passes through the upper border of this muscle.

Obeying Hilton's law that a nerve supplying a muscle that moves a joint also innervates that joint (see Chapter 19), the anterior division of the obturator nerve gives off a branch that provides sensory innervation to the hip. It then descends in the inner thigh behind the adductor longus muscle, which it supplies. It continues on the anterior surface of the adductor brevis muscle, supplying it and the gracilis muscle, finally joining up with the subsartorial plexus, the branches of which supply the skin over the medial aspect of the thigh. The obturator nerve often gives off direct branches to the skin of the medial aspect of the thigh before joining the subsartorial plexus.

The posterior division of the obturator nerve passes downward on the adductor magnus muscle deep to the other adductor muscles. It supplies this muscle and terminates in a fine branch that joins the femoral artery and then joins the middle geniculate artery to supply the posterior capsule of the knee joint. The adductor brevis muscle separates the anterior and posterior divisions of the obturator nerve (8).

Technique

The patient is positioned supine, exposing the pubic area (9). The pubic tubercle is palpated and the needle entry point is 2 cm lateral and 2 cm caudal to the tubercle (Fig. 12-18).

After numbing the skin with a small amount of local anesthetic agent by fine

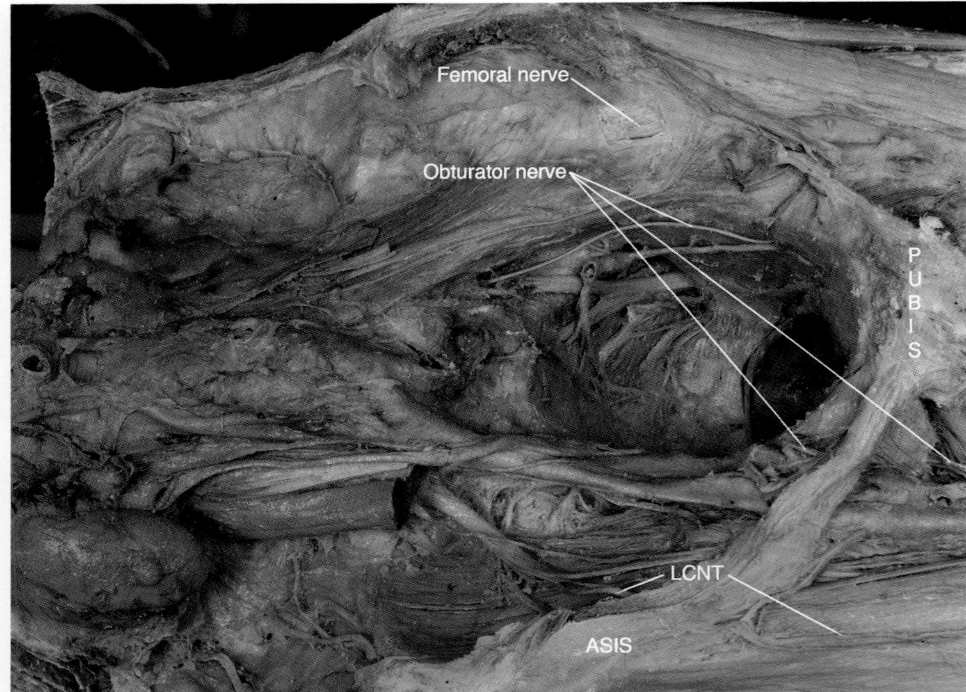

FIGURE 12-17 Dissection showing femoral nerve, obturator nerve, and lateral cutaneous nerve of the thigh. ASIS, anterior superior iliac spine; LCNT, lateral cutaneous nerve of the thigh.

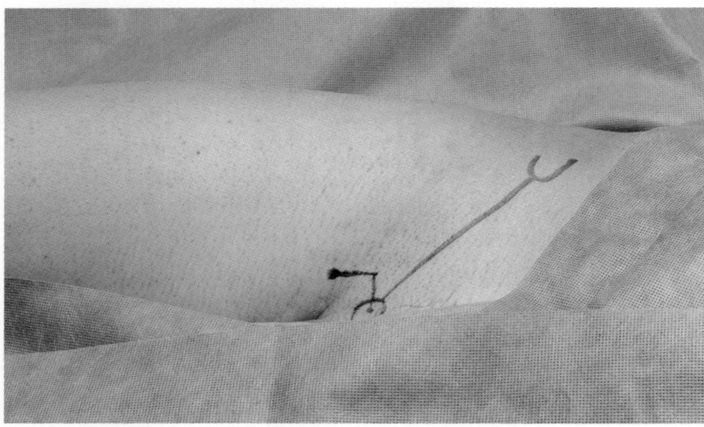

FIGURE 12-18 The pubic tubercle is identified and needle entry is 2 cm lateral and 2 cm caudal to the pubic tubercle.

needle, a 22-gauge stimulating needle, attached to a nerve stimulator set to an output of 1 mA, a frequency of 2 Hz, and a pulse width of 100 to 300 µsec, enters perpendicular to the skin until adductor motor responses are encountered (Fig. 12-19). If the needle is aimed too cephalad, the ramus of the pubis may be encountered. The needle tip is then "walked" posteriorly until the obturator membrane is encountered. The obturator nerve is usually encountered simultaneously, but care must be taken not to penetrate this membrane.

The nerve stimulator output is now turned down to 0.3 to 0.5 mA, while brisk adductor muscle twitches are still present. A small amount of normal saline injection stops the motor response (i.e., a positive Raj test), and the main local anesthetic dose can be injected.

Local Anesthetic Agent Choice

Most local anesthetic agents have been used for this block. It is usually not necessary to have a long-lasting block because the pain originating from the

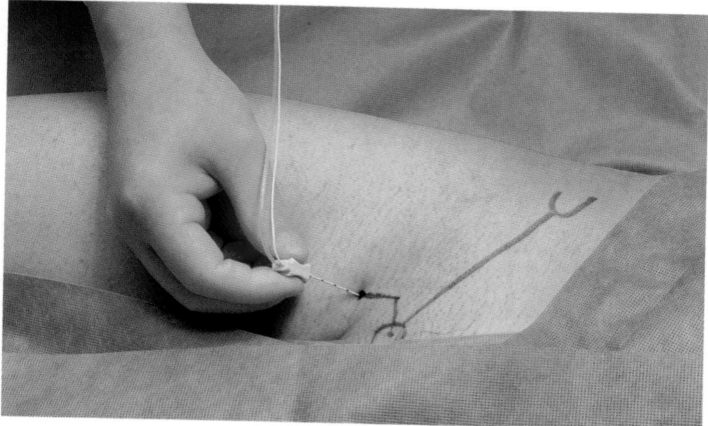

FIGURE 12-19 A 50-mm stimulating needle enters the skin until an adductor motor response is evoked.

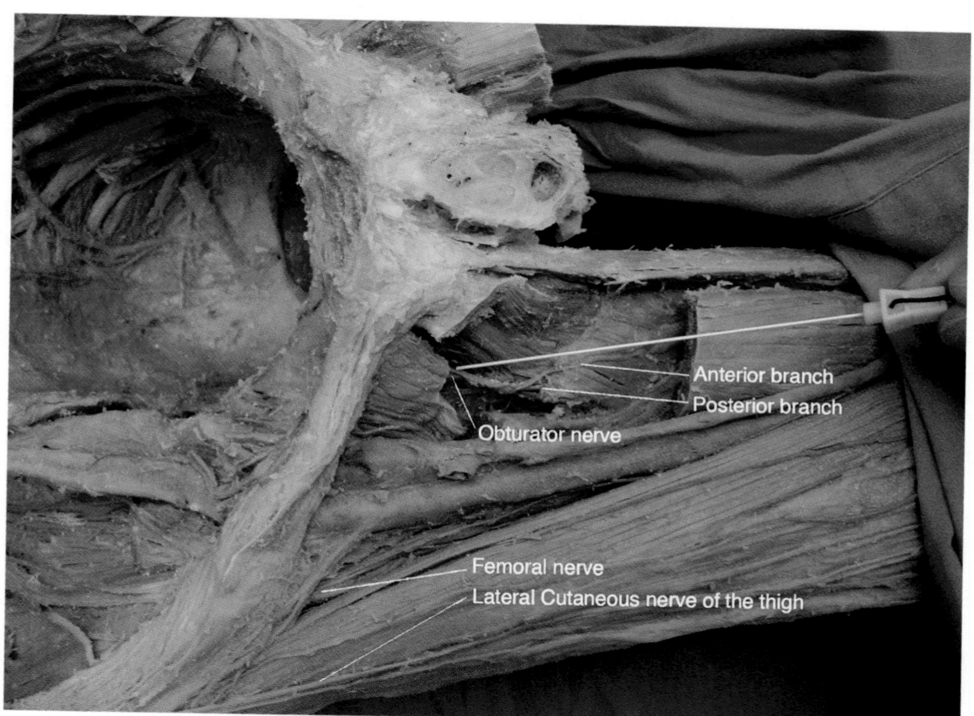

FIGURE 12-20 Dissection showing the anterior and posterior branches of the obturator nerve separated by the adductor brevis muscle.

posterior knee capsule is not long lived—usually 6 to 8 hours. Twenty milliliters of ropivacaine 0.5% is typically all that is required for this block.

Doing the block more distally, as advocated by some authors, may result in only one of the divisions being blocked, leaving the skin on the medial aspect of the thigh (anterior division) or posterior knee capsule (posterior division) unblocked (Fig. 12-20). Ultrasonography has effectively removed this potential problem, however. Because this block is almost always used to supplement another block, typically a femoral nerve block, attention must be given to the possibility of toxic doses of local anesthetic agents, and smaller volumes can be used.

SINGLE-INJECTION LATERAL CUTANEOUS NERVE OF THE THIGH BLOCK

Introduction

Like the obturator nerve block, the lateral cutaneous nerve of the thigh (LCNT) block is usually

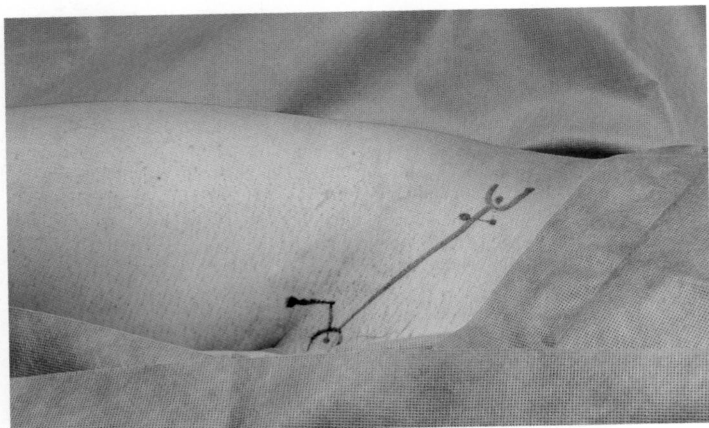

FIGURE 12-21 The *lateral semicircle* indicates the anterior superior iliac spine.

used to supplement an incomplete femoral nerve block. It is seldom indicated on its own, and continuous LCNT block is seldom indicated. Pain originating from the area supplied by this nerve, the lateral skin of the thigh, is seldom long lasting and usually only single-injection blocks are indicated (10).

Specific Anatomic Considerations

The LCNT is derived from the L2 and L3 roots of the lumbar plexus (8). It passes from the lateral border of the psoas muscle across the iliac fossa and lies behind the fascia iliaca at first (see "LCNT" in Fig. 12-17). Further down, it is incorporated within the substance of the fascia iliaca, which is a thick, tough membrane in the fossa iliaca. The nerve passes deep to the inguinal ligament, where it lies free in a fibrous tunnel 1 cm to the medial side of the anterior superior iliac spine (ASIS; see Fig. 12-17). (Meralgia paraesthetica may be due to irritation or compression of the nerve in this fibrous canal.)

The LCNT enters the thigh deep to the fascia lata and divides into anterior and posterior branches that pierce the fascia lata separately 2 to 5 cm below the ASIS (see Fig. 12-20). The anterior branch contains L3 fibers and is distributed along the anterolateral surface of the thigh. Its terminal branch joins the prepatellar plexus, whereas the posterior division, which contains only L3 fibers, passes down the thigh along the posterolateral aspect of the iliotibial tract (8).

Technique

The patient is positioned supine with the ASIS exposed (Fig. 12-21). The ASIS is palpated and marked, and the needle entry point is 2 cm medial and 2 cm caudal to the ASIS (the lateral semicircle in Fig. 12-21).

After raising a small skin wheal with a small volume of local anesthetic agent, the block needle with a B-beveled tip is inserted until a distinct "pop" is felt as the fascia lata is penetrated (Fig. 12-22). Local anesthetic agent is injected at this point, with the anesthesiologist "fanning" it somewhat to ensure that the nerve is blocked.

Local Anesthetic Agent Choice

Most local anesthetic agents have been used for this block, but because the LCNT supplies only the skin over the lateral aspect of the thigh, and pain originating from this area is not long lasting, single-injection blocks with long-acting drugs are not indicated. Because the nerve provides no muscle innervation, long-lasting agents such as 5 to 10 mL of 0.5% bupivacaine can comfortably be used. Other drugs (e.g., ropivacaine, levobupivacaine) can also be used depending on the anesthesiologist's preferences. Because this block is almost always done to supplement an incomplete femoral nerve block or psoas compartment block, attention must be given to the possibility of drug toxicity. The block is also sometimes indicated for meralgia paraesthetica

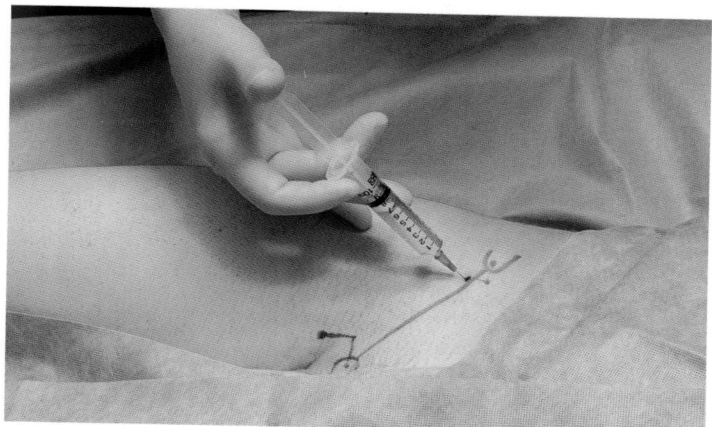

FIGURE 12-22 Needle entry is 2 cm medial and 2 cm caudal to the anterior superior iliac spine.

before surgery is considered, and 5 to 10 mL of 0.5% to 0.75% ropivacaine typically is used for this. Steroid injection is sometimes helpful in this condition.

REFERENCES

1. Parkinson SK, Mueller JB, Little WL, et al: Extent of blockade with various approaches to the lumbar plexus. Anesth Analg 1989;68:243-248.
2. Salinas FV: Femoral nerve block. In Boezaart AP (ed): Anesthesia and Orthopaedic Surgery. New York, McGraw-Hill, 2006, pp 331-341.
3. Capdevila X, Biboulet P, Rubenovitch J, et al: Comparison of the three-in-one and fascia iliaca compartment blocks in adults: Clinical and radiographic analysis. Anesth Analg 1998;86:1039-1044.
4. Capdevila X, Barthelet Y, Biboulet P, et al: Effects of perioperative analgesic technique on the surgical outcome and duration of rehabilitation after major knee surgery. Anesthesiology 1999;91:8-15.
5. Singelyn FJ, Deyaert M, Joris D, et al: Effects of intravenous patient-controlled analgesia with morphine, continuous epidural analgesia, and continuous three-in-one block on postoperative pain and knee rehabilitation after total knee arthroplasty. Anesth Analg 1998;87:88-92.
6. Salinas FV, Neal JM, Sueda LA, et al: Prospective comparison of continuous femoral nerve block with nonstimulating catheter placement versus stimulating catheter-guided perineural placement in volunteers. Reg Anesth Pain Med 2004;29:212-220.
7. Capdevila X, Macaire P, Dadure C, et al: Continuous psoas compartment block for postoperative analgesia after total hip arthroplasty: New landmarks, technical guidelines, and clinical evaluation. Anesth Analg 2002;94:1606-1613.
8. Last RJ: Last's Anatomy: Regional and Applied, 4th ed. London, J&A Churchill, 1970.
9. Meier G, Büttner J: Atlas der peripheren Regionalanästhesie. Stuttgart, Georg Thieme Verlag, 2004, pp 183-189.
10. Hadzic A, Vloka JD: Peripheral Nerve Blocks: Principles and Practice. New York, McGraw-Hill, 2004, pp 334-335.

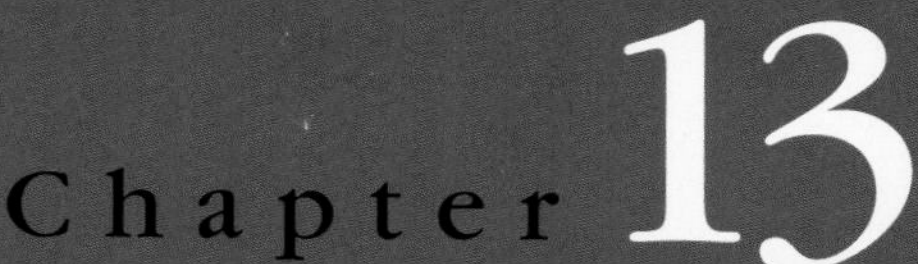

Posterior Lumbar Plexus Block

- Applied Anatomy
- Continuous Lumbar Plexus Block (Psoas Compartment)

APPLIED ANATOMY

The lumbar plexus is formed from the anterior primary rami of the first four lumbar nerve roots, and lies within the substance of the psoas major muscle (1) (Fig. 13-1). The branches of the lumbar plexus (except the iliohypogastric and ilioinguinal nerves, which are the first lumbar segmental body-wall nerve and its collateral branch, respectively) supply the lower limb, but in their passage across the posterior abdominal wall they give off branches to the parietal peritoneum. Branches of the lumbar plexus include the iliohypogastric and ilioinguinal nerves (L1), genitofemoral nerve (L1 and L2), lateral cutaneous nerve of the thigh (posterior divisions of L2 and L3), femoral nerve (posterior divisions of L2, L3, and L4), and obturator nerve (anterior divisions of L2, L3, and L4) (1).

CONTINUOUS LUMBAR PLEXUS BLOCK (PSOAS COMPARTMENT)

Introduction

Because it is a relatively easy and successful block to perform, and anesthesiologists are used to placing needles at this level in the course of performing lumbar epidural blocks, the psoas compartment block is sometimes performed for improper or debatable indications (2). If the continuous femoral nerve block is performed with the catheter on the femoral nerve and deep to the fascia iliaca, and the lateral cutaneous nerve of the thigh and obturator nerve are included in the block (see Fig. 12-5), there are very few good indications left for the psoas compartment block (2,3).

Hip replacement surgery, for example, because of the surgical destruction of the joint capsule and consequent denervation of the joint, is remarkably pain free and therefore probably not a good indication for this block, although acetabular fracture may be an excellent indication. Lumbar epidural block may be a better choice for intraoperative and postoperative analgesia in primary total hip replacement because patients can become very uncomfortable in the decubitus intraoperative position if the "down" leg is not anesthetized and if the patient's torso is not blocked. Also, the epidural catheter may be removed the day after surgery because severe pain seldom persists after 24 hours and patients are often started on thromboprophylaxis; in addition, the hip joint gets its innervation from the entire lumbosacral plexus, which is not fully covered by a lumbar plexus block.

Similarly, for lower leg surgery, a more distal saphenous nerve block combined with a sciatic nerve block is almost always a better choice than a lumbar plexus block combined with a sciatic nerve block. Another common indication for lumbar plexus block that should be questioned is inguinal hernia repair (4). An iliohypogastric and ilioinguinal nerve block combined with a field block is probably a safer alternative than an L1-L2 lumbar paravertebral block (5), but this is outside the scope of this atlas.

Specific Anatomic Considerations

The psoas compartment is a relatively large and vascular compartment, and large volumes of local anesthetic agent are necessary to fill it (6). This brings the issue of local anesthetic toxicity into the equation—the more so because it is such a vascular compartment, which also predisposes to retroperitoneal hematoma formation in case of vascular trauma by the needle or catheter.

Large volumes of local anesthetic agent in the vicinity of the epidural space are also potentially problematic, and many cases of wide epidural spread have been reported (3).

Other problems, such as intra-abdominal placement of needles and catheters, kidney and ureter injury, and subarachnoid injection, have also been reported (3).

Because the nerve roots are covered with dura, sharp or thin needles should probably not be used for this block (see Chapter 3). Even 22-gauge B-bevel needles should probably not be used because of the danger of dural penetration or intra-root injection and subsequent large-volume subarachnoid block. As a general principle, large-bore Tuohy needles (16- to 18-gauge) are the best choice here because they are the least likely to penetrate the dura or nerve root (7).

Nerves
1. Subcostal nerve (T12)
2. Iliohypogastric nerve (L1)
3. Ilioinguinal nerve (L1)
4. Lateral femoral cutaneous nerve (L2,3)
5. Femoral branch of genitofemoral nerve (L1,2)
6. Genital branch of genitofemoral nerve (L1,2)
7. Femoral nerve (L2,3,4)
8. Sciatic nerve
   a. Common peroneal nerve (L4,5,S1,2)
   b. Tibial nerve (L4,5,S1,2,3)
9. Posterior femoral cutaneous nerve (S1,2,3)
10. Nerve to Sartorius muscle (L2,3,4)
11. Saphenous branch of the Femoral nerve
12. Obturator nerve (L2,3,4)
13. Pudendal nerve (S1,2,3)
14. Sympathetic trunk
15. Lumbosacral trunk

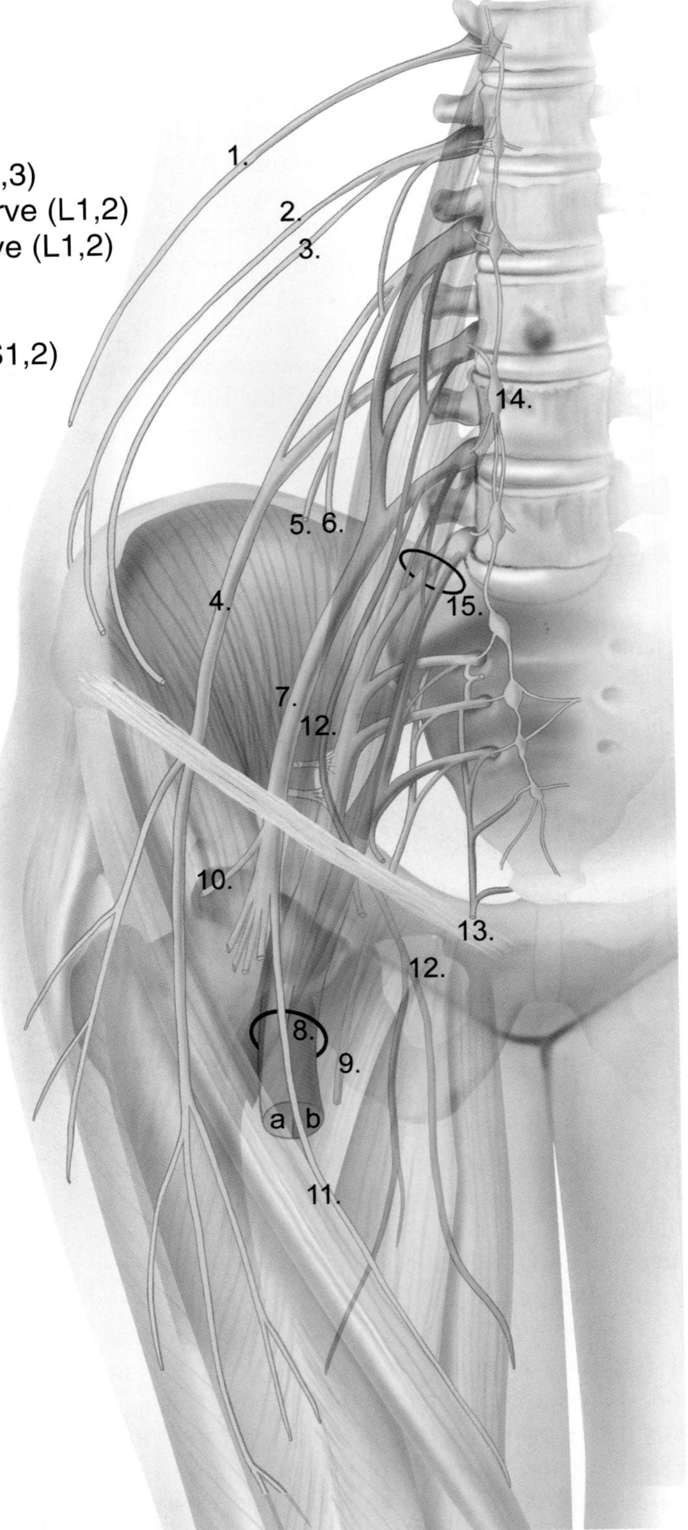

FIGURE 13-1 The lumbosacral plexus.

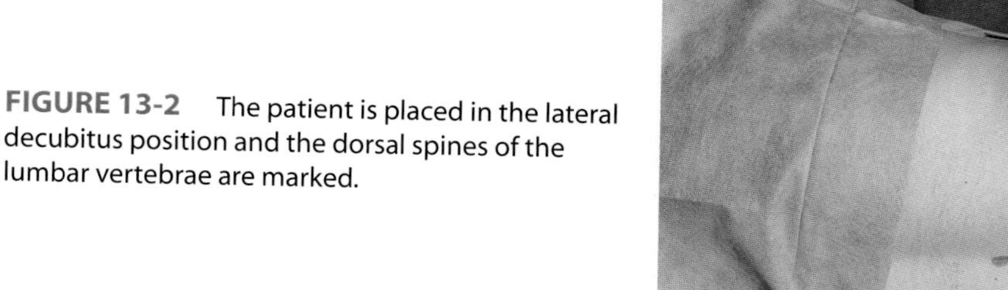

FIGURE 13-2 The patient is placed in the lateral decubitus position and the dorsal spines of the lumbar vertebrae are marked.

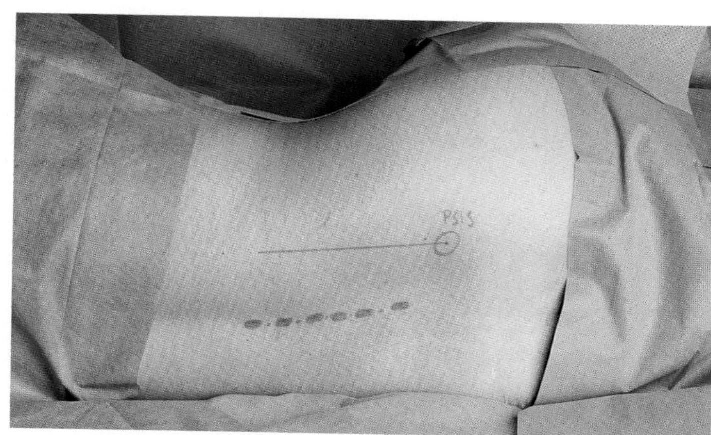

FIGURE 13-3 The posterior superior iliac spine is identified and a line drawn from it parallel to the dorsal spines.

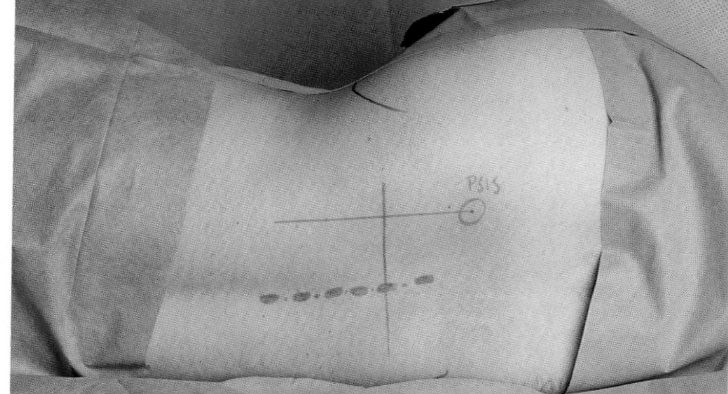

FIGURE 13-4 The intercristal line (Tuffier's line) is drawn.

Technique

With the patient in the lateral decubitus or sitting position and the lumbar spine flexed, a line is drawn marking the dorsal spines of the lumbar vertebrae in the midline (3) (Fig. 13-2).

The posterior superior iliac spine is palpated and marked, and a line drawn parallel to the midline from its midpoint (Fig. 13-3).

The intercristal line is now drawn, and the dorsal spine of the vertebra palpable on this line is the dorsal spine of the fourth lumbar vertebra (Fig. 13-4).

The distance between the two parallel lines is now measured, and this distance is divided into thirds. Needle entry is two thirds of the distance from the midline on the intercristal line, as indicated in Figure 13-5.

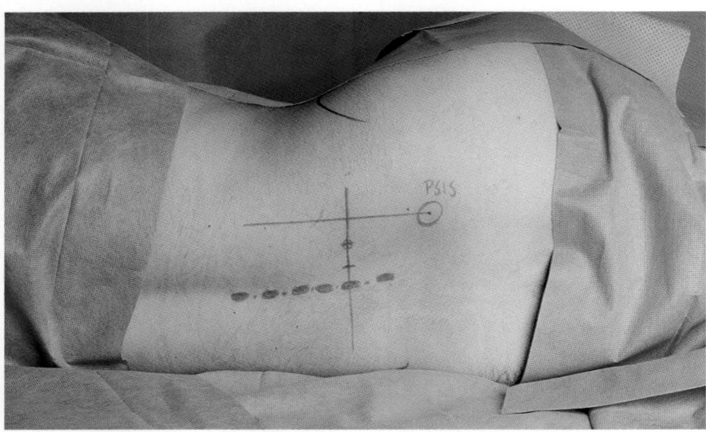

FIGURE 13-5 The distance between the two parallel lines is measured, and needle entry is two thirds of this distance from the midline.

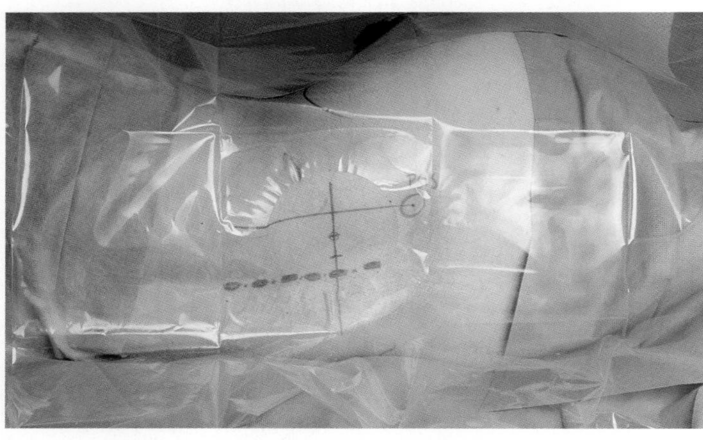

FIGURE 13-6 After skin preparation, a sterile, fenestrated drape is placed over the lumbar spine.

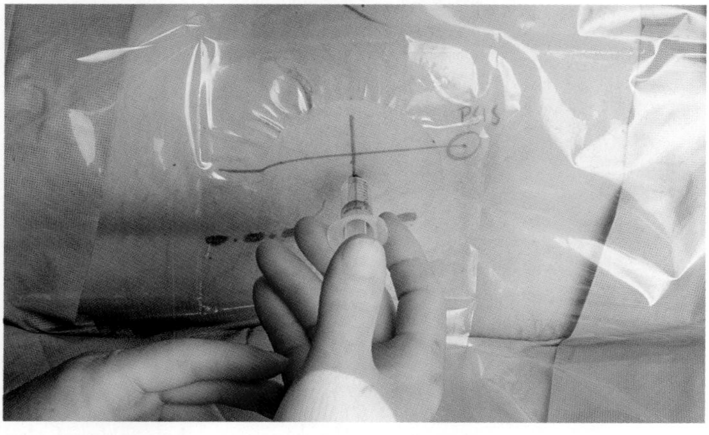

FIGURE 13-7 The skin and subcutaneous tissues are anesthetized thoroughly, all the way down to the transverse process or articular column of L4.

The skin is prepared with an appropriate antiseptic solution and the area covered with a transparent, fenestrated, sterile plastic drape (Fig. 13-6).

The skin and subcutaneous tissue are thoroughly anesthetized with a lidocaine and 1:200,000 epinephrine solution (Fig. 13-7). The anticipated path for tunneling the catheter is also anesthetized. Note the slight medial angulation of the needle, and that the tissue all the way down to the bony pars intervertebralis, articular column, or transverse process is anesthetized.

For some patients it may be necessary to use a longer needle to reach the bony parts. It is always handy to measure the depth to the bony

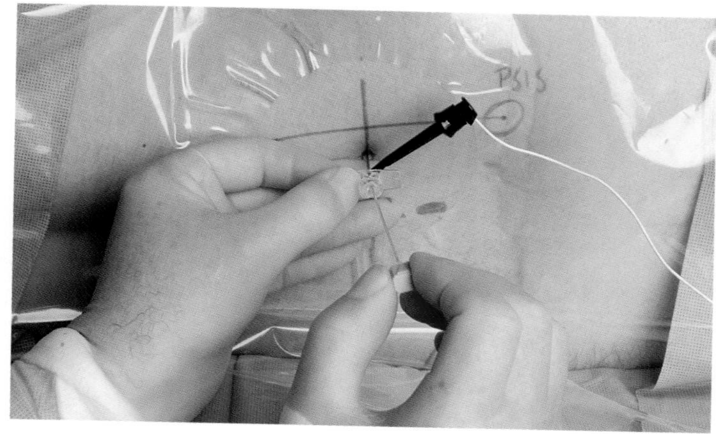

FIGURE 13-8 An insulated Tuohy needle connected to a nerve stimulator is advanced slightly mesiad, aiming for the anterior midline until contact with the transverse process or articular column is made.

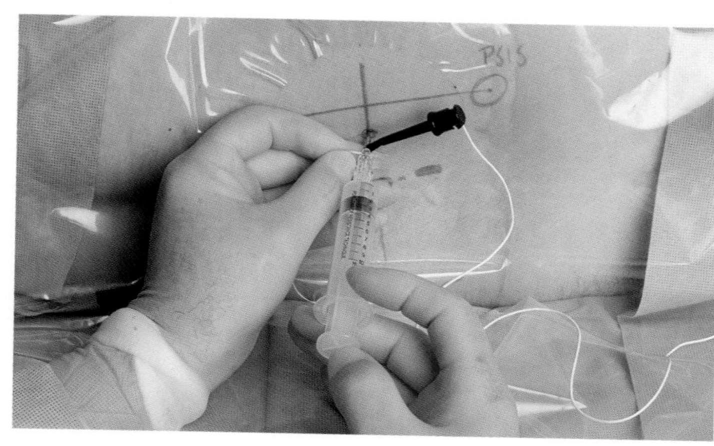

FIGURE 13-9 A loss-of-resistance-to-air syringe is attached to the needle and the needle is walked off the bony part in a caudal and lateral direction.

parts with ultrasonography before needle entry. It is, however, important to inject local anesthetic agent only after contact with the bone has been established. This is to minimize the theoretical but dangerous possibility of intrathecal injection of local anesthetic agent. Again, note the slightly medial angulation of the needle to ensure contact with the bony structures. (For all paravertebral blocks—cervical, thoracic, lumbar, and sacral—the needle is aimed at the anterior midline to ensure contact with the bony structures.)

The nerve stimulator, set to a current output of 1 to 1.5 mA, a pulse width of 200 to 300 μsec, and a frequency of 2 Hz, is clipped to the 100-mm insulated 17- or 18-gauge Tuohy needle (or a longer needle, if required), which enters the skin aiming slightly mesial toward the anterior midline (Fig. 13-8). The needle stylet is removed when contact with the bone is established.

A loss-of-resistance-to-air syringe is attached and the needle tip is walked off the bone in an inferolateral direction (obliquely lateral and caudal; Fig. 13-9).

The needle is advanced gently and, as with all types of paravertebral block, loss of resistance to air and the motor response—quadriceps muscle twitches in this instance—appear simultaneously. The nerve stimulator output is turned down and clear, brisk twitches should still be present at 0.3 to 0.5 mA.

It is important not to inject normal saline or local anesthetic agent through the needle at this stage because this will make stimulating catheter placement impossible or very difficult. The notion of "opening up the space" with saline for easier catheter passage is not based on scientific fact. In living tissue this practice causes edema, which makes further nerve stimulation through the catheter difficult or impossible. If the anesthesiologist believes that it is important to "open up the space," it should be done with 5% dextrose in water, which does not

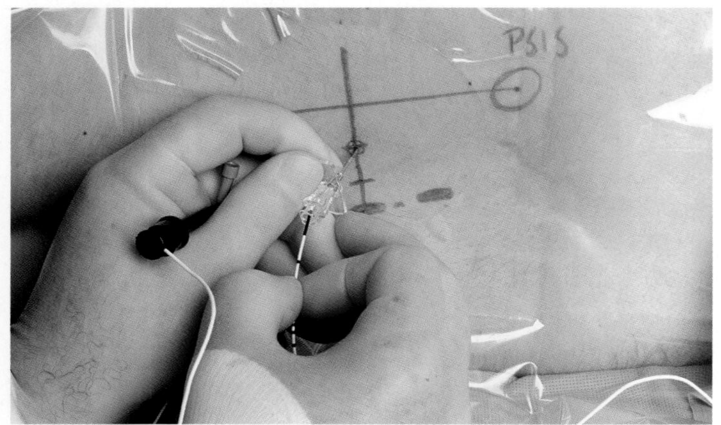

FIGURE 13-10 Once contact with the lumbar plexus is made, indicated by an ipsilateral quadriceps motor response, the nerve stimulator is attached to the proximal end of the stimulating catheter, which is advanced through the needle. If the motor response weakens or disappears during catheter advancement, the catheter is retracted carefully to within the needle shaft, the needle manipulated slightly—in this case turned 45 degrees counterclockwise—and the catheter advanced again.

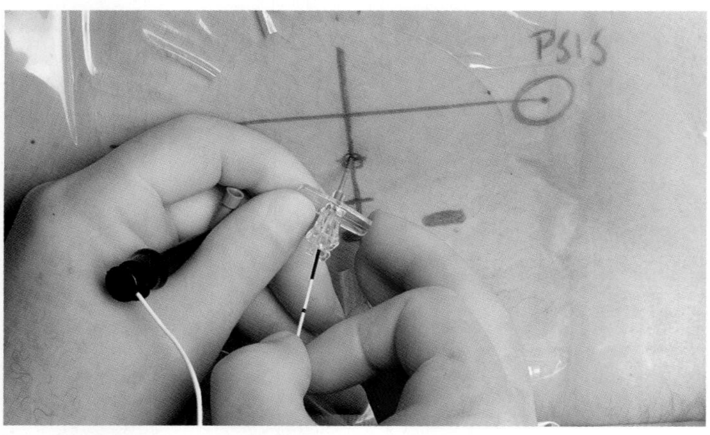

FIGURE 13-11 The special marking on the catheter indicates that the catheter has not yet protruded beyond the needle tip, and the needle can be manipulated safely.

conduct electricity and hence will not abolish the stimulated motor response.

The nerve stimulator is now attached to the proximal end of the stimulating catheter and the catheter tip placed in the needle shaft (Fig. 13-10). Notice the special mark on the catheter, which indicates that the tip of the catheter is now situated at the tip of the needle.The catheter is advanced beyond the tip of the needle and the motor response should remain unchanged during catheter advancement. If, however, the motor response changes or the twitches stop, it simply means that the catheter is advanced away from the nerves, possibly into the psoas muscle or even intra-abdominally.

Carefully withdraw the catheter tip to within the needle shaft, make a slight adjustment to the needle, such as turning it a quarter-turn clockwise or counterclockwise, or advancing or withdrawing it slightly, and advance the catheter again (Fig. 13-11). Repeat this maneuver until brisk motor twitches in the quadriceps muscles are observed during catheter advancement. The needle should never be manipulated if the broad black mark on the catheter is not completely visible, which indicates that the catheter is fully inside the needle shaft. Care should also be taken not to turn the bevel of the needle medially toward the epidural space; this may lead to epidural catheter placement.

Advance the catheter 3 to 5 cm (Fig. 13-12). The motor response should remain unchanged during catheter advancement.

The needle is now removed without disturbing the catheter (Fig. 13-13).

The catheter can be tunneled subcutaneously by using a dedicated tunneling device or by inserting the inner stylet of the needle 1 to 2 cm from the catheter exit site to the previously marked and anesthetized spot. This is not always necessary for a lumbar paravertebral block. The

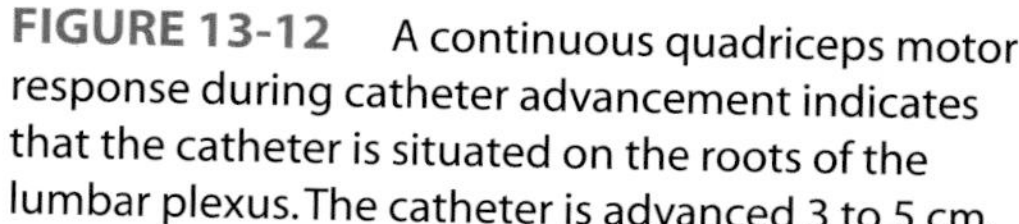

FIGURE 13-12 A continuous quadriceps motor response during catheter advancement indicates that the catheter is situated on the roots of the lumbar plexus. The catheter is advanced 3 to 5 cm.

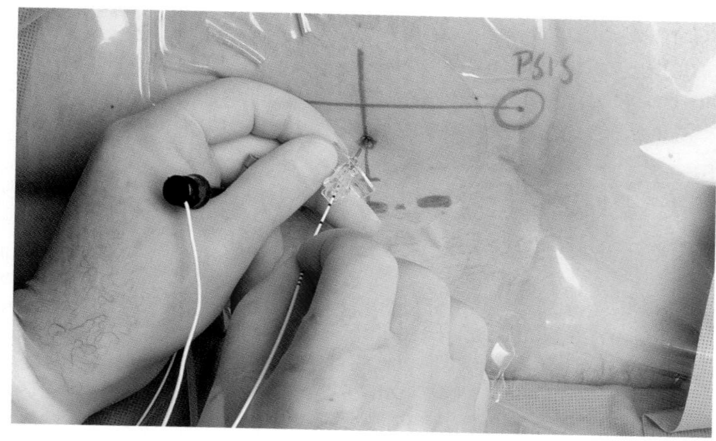

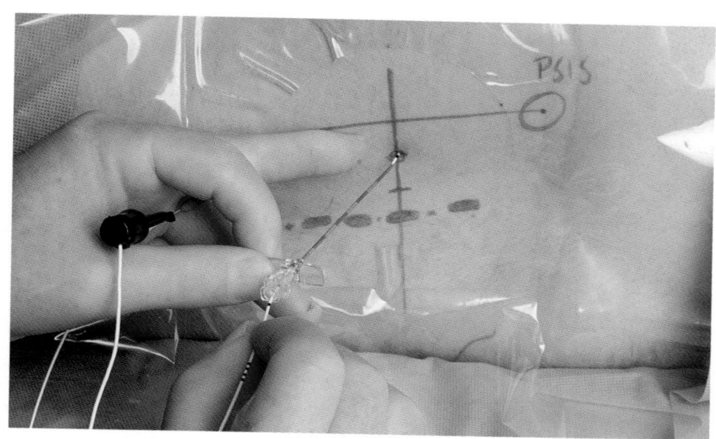

FIGURE 13-13 The needle is removed without disturbing the catheter.

tunneling technique is similar to that demonstrated previously (see Chapter 12).

Clip the Luer lock connecting device to the catheter and the nerve stimulator to the connecting device. Turn the nerve stimulator output up until a brisk motor response can just be seen.

With brisk quadriceps muscle twitching observed, inject a test dose of 2 mL lidocaine 2% in 1/200,000 epinephrine through the catheter. Notice that the motor response stops immediately on injection of the normal saline. This constitutes a positive Raj test, which gives final assurance that the primary and secondary block will be successful. Bilateral numbness in the legs or buttocks indicates intrathecal catheter placement, and tachycardia indicates intravascular injection.

The catheter and connecting device are attached to the fixation device, which is applied to a convenient position on the patient's flank or other convenient place. The catheter and exit wounds are covered with a transparent dressing to facilitate daily inspection of the site.

The catheter is removed when the patient no longer needs the continuous nerve block and full motor and sensory function has returned to the limb (see Chapter 12).

Local Anesthetic Agent Choice

Almost all local anesthetic agents in various concentrations, volumes, and combinations have been used successfully for this block. The author's choice is to use 20 to 40 mL of ropivacaine 0.5% to 0.75% as an initial bolus. This is followed by a continuous infusion of 5 to 10 mL/hour of ropivacaine 0.2% and patient-controlled regional anesthesia boluses of 5 to 10 mL of ropivacaine 0.2%. Relatively large volumes of local anesthetic agent are usually required for psoas compartment block. It is likely that use of a stimulating catheter placed next to the lumbar plexus roots may permit injection of smaller volumes, but this notion has not yet been substantiated by research.

(See continuous lumbar paravertebral block movie on DVD.)

REFERENCES

1. Last RJ: Last's Anatomy: Regional and Applied, 4th ed. London, J&A Churchill, 1970.
2. Capdevila X, Macaire P, Dadure C, et al: Continuous psoas compartment block for postoperative analgesia after total hip arthroplasty: New landmarks, technical guidelines, and clinical evaluation. Anesth Analg 2002;94:1606-1613.
3. Capdevila X, Nadeau M-J: Lumbar paravertebral (psoas compartment) block. In Boezaart AP (ed): Anesthesia and Orthopaedic Surgery. New York, McGraw-Hill, 2006, pp 358-370.
4. Hadzic A, Kerimoglu B, Loreio D, et al: Paravertebral blocks provide superior same-day recovery over general anesthesia for patients undergoing inguinal hernia repair. Anesth Analg 2006;102:1076-1081.
5. White PF: Choice of peripheral nerve block for inguinal herniorrhaphy: Is better the enemy of good? [Editorial]. Anesth Analg 2006;102:1073-1075.
6. Huet O, Eyrolle LJ, Mazoit JX, et al: Cardiac arrest after injection of ropivacaine for posterior lumbar plexus blockade. Anesthesiology 2003;99:1451-1453.
7. Boezaart AP, Franco CD: Thin sharp needles around the dura. Reg Anesth Pain Med 2006;31:388-389.

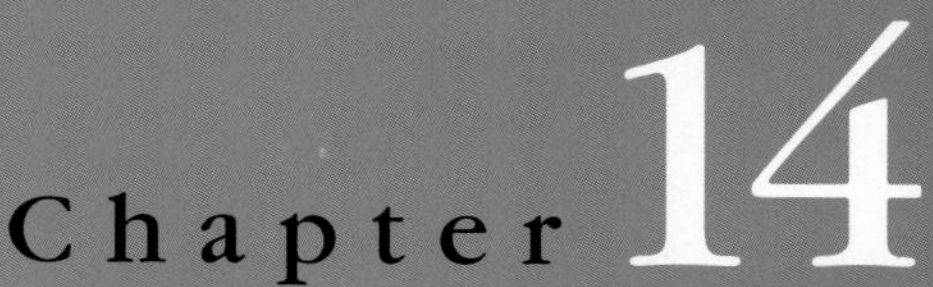

Sacral Plexus Nerves: Applied Anatomy

- Sciatic Nerve: Subgluteal Area
- Sciatic Nerve: Popliteal Area

Most of the L4 and L5 fibers enter the sacral plexus (Fig. 14-1). After the L4 root has given off its branches to the lumbar plexus, it joins the anterior primary ramus of L5 to form the lumbosacral trunk (see Fig. 13-1). This large nerve passes over the ala of the sacrum and crosses the pelvic brim, separated from the obturator nerve by the iliolumbar artery and veins (see Fig. 12-17). It descends to join the anterior primary rami of the upper four sacral nerves in the formation of the sacral plexus (see Fig. 13-1). This broad triangular structure lies between the strong membrane of parietal pelvic fascia anteriorly and the piriformis muscle posteriorly (1).

SCIATIC NERVE: SUBGLUTEAL AREA

Anatomy

The sciatic nerve is the longest nerve in the body and runs in the posterior aspect of the leg toward the knee. It consists of two branches or segments, the tibial and the common peroneal. The tibial or medial popliteal part of the sciatic nerve is a large branch formed by the union of branches from all five anterior divisions (L4, L5, S1, S2, and S3) of the sacral plexus. This segment of the sciatic nerve is destined for the flexor compartment of the lower limb. It joins the extensor compartment segment, the common peroneal nerve, in the pelvis, and leaves the pelvis as the sciatic nerve below the lower border of the piriformis muscle (cut away in Fig. 14-2), lying on the ischium in the greater sciatic notch, lateral to the ischial spine. It then passes vertically down over the obturator internus and quadratus femoris muscles to the hamstring compartment of the thigh, where it disappears under the biceps femoris muscle. In the buttock it lies deep to the gluteus maximus muscle midway between the greater trochanter and the ischial tuberosity (see Fig. 14-2). It gives sensory innervation to the areas illustrated in Figure 14-3, and in addition to motor innervation to the flexor compartment of the lower leg, the tibial component (L5 and S1) supplies motor innervation to the hamstrings and the ischial part of the adductor magnus muscle. The short head of the biceps femoris muscle is supplied by the common peroneal branch of the sciatic nerve, which is the nerve to the extensor compartment of the leg, yet the segments are the same (L5 and S1). This is because the short head of the biceps femoris muscle developed embryologically in the

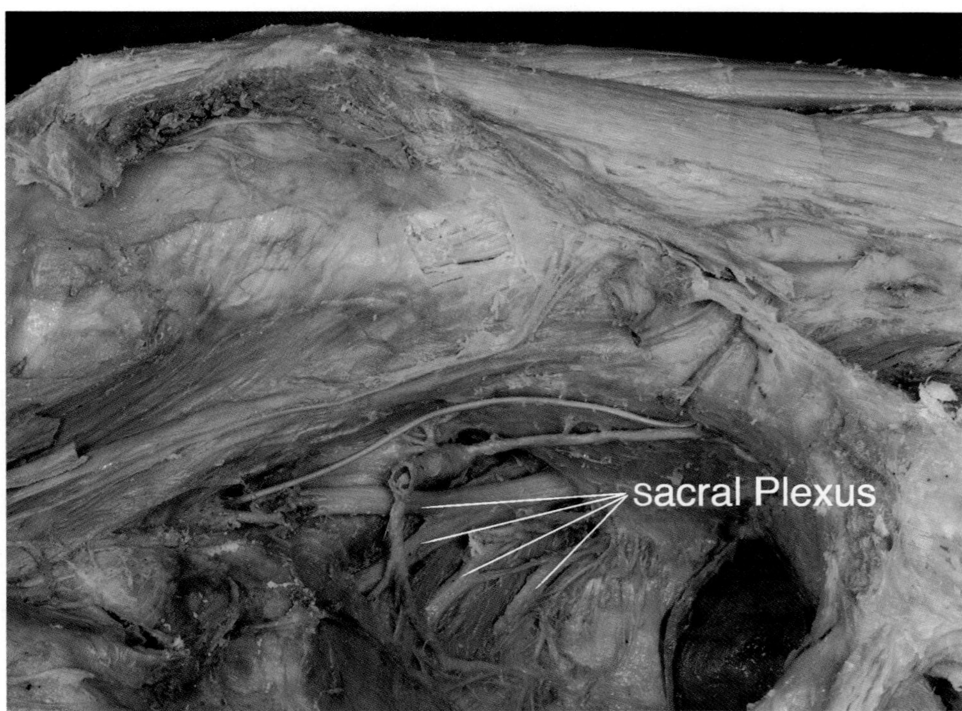

FIGURE 14-1 Dissection showing the sacral plexus.

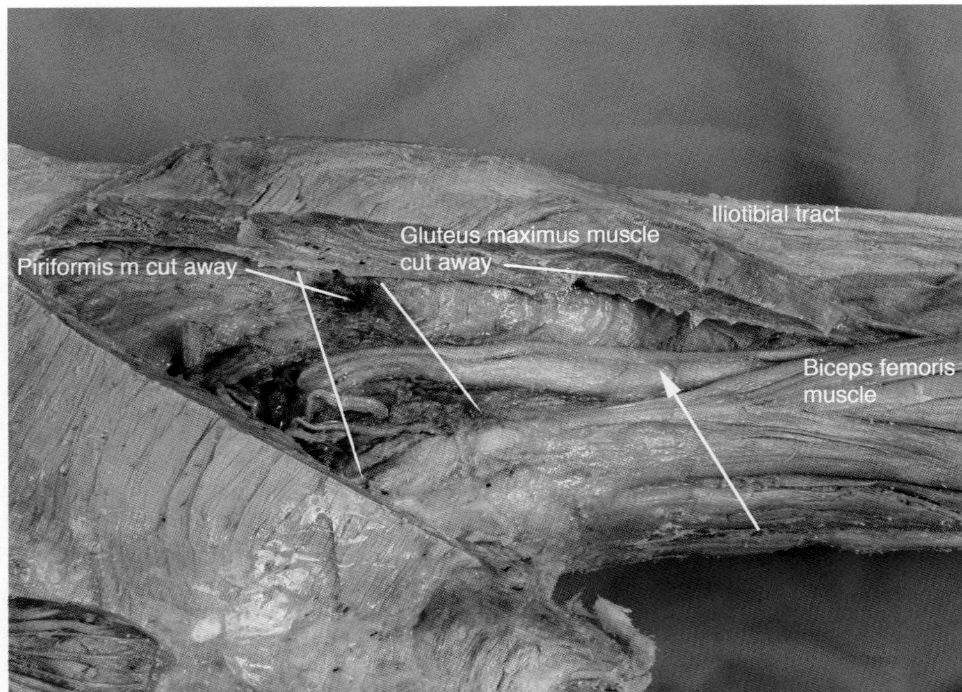

FIGURE 14-2 In this dissection, the piriformis and gluteus maximus muscles are cut away. The *dark arrow* indicates the sciatic nerve and the *two lines* indicate the position of the piriformis muscle. Note the area of compression of the sciatic nerve by the piriformis muscle.

extensor compartment but migrated to the flexor compartment for functional reasons, retaining its nerve supply. The nerve to the biceps femoris splits off the sciatic nerve in the mid-femoral area as the sciatic nerve passes deep to this muscle.

Branches that pass backward from S2 and S3, and a small contribution from S1 form the posterior cutaneous nerve of the thigh. This nerve passes lateral to the lower border of the piriformis muscle behind the sciatic nerve. It passes distally close to the sciatic nerve, but it is often separated from the sciatic nerve by a fascia plane. It is not truly a branch of the sciatic nerve, although they share common roots (S1, S2, and S3) and travel together through the greater sciatic foramen. Because both nerves may be blocked together with a subgluteal approach, for practical purposes the posterior cutaneous nerve of the thigh can be considered with the sciatic nerve.

The sciatic nerve (Fig. 14-2, *arrow*) is a long and thick nerve. It is surrounded by a rich blood supply proximally and is in a closed compartment as it exits the greater sciatic foramen, where it is situated deep to the piriformis muscle (cut away in Fig. 14-2) (1).

In the dissection illustrated in Figure 14-2, the gluteus maximus muscle has been cut away to illustrate the course of the sciatic nerve. Note the area where the nerve had been compressed by the piriformis muscle, as indicated by the yellow lines in Figure 14-2.

The sciatic nerve courses down between the biceps femoris muscle medially and the iliotibial tract, which is lateral to the sciatic nerve. The nerve to the biceps femoris muscle branches off the medial aspect of the sciatic nerve in the mid-femoral area. This fact is important in making the electromyographic distinction between, for example, needle injury to the nerve during subgluteal block from nerve injury due to tourniquet use.

Figure 14-3 illustrates the neurotomal distribution for the sensory innervation of the sciatic nerve.

Surface Anatomy of Subgluteal Sciatic Nerve

The surface anatomy of the sciatic nerve at the subgluteal and transgluteal levels is illustrated

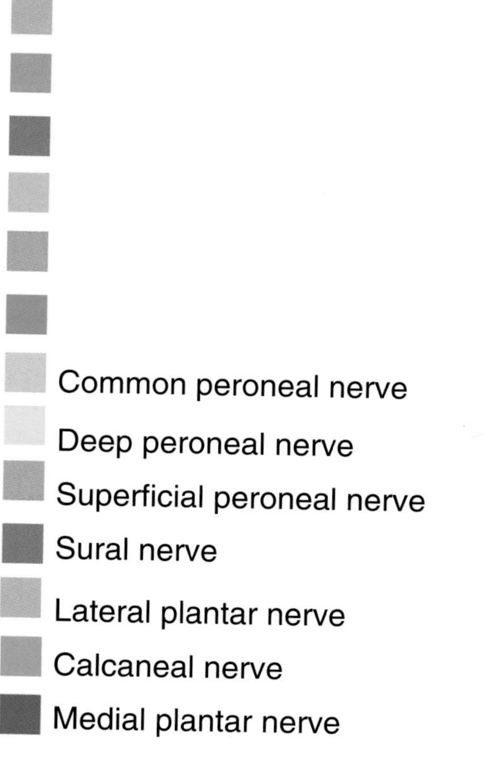

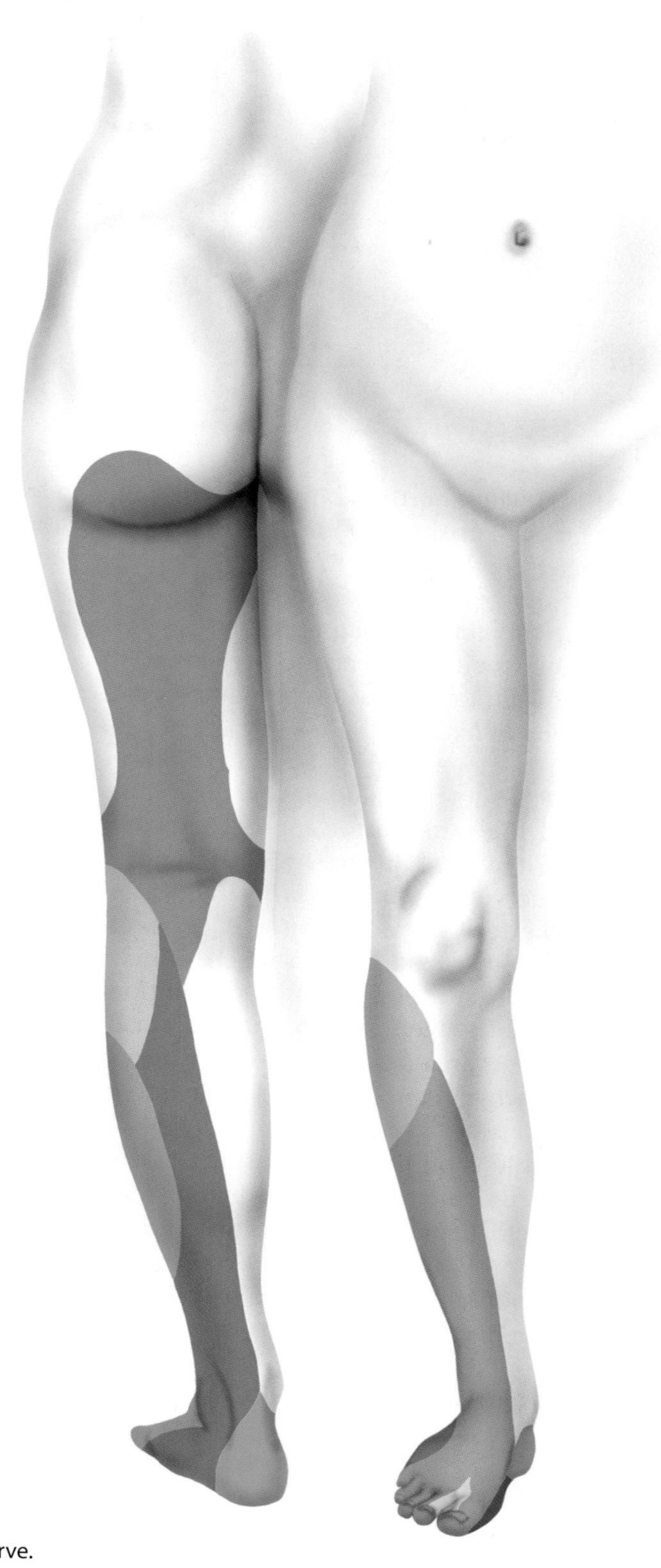

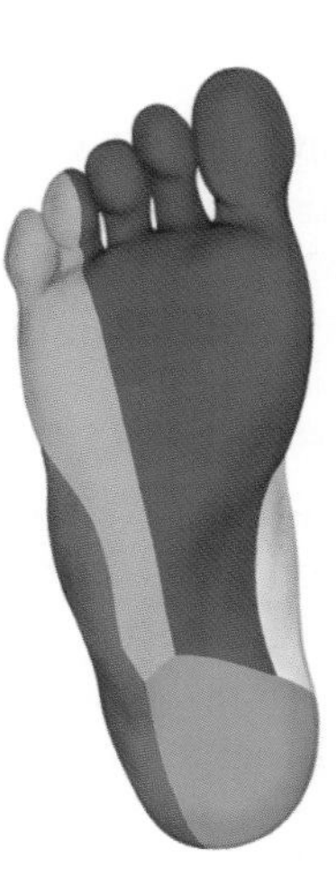

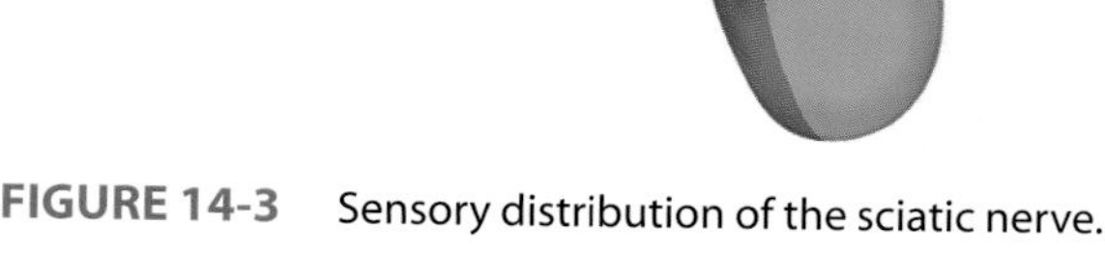

FIGURE 14-3 Sensory distribution of the sciatic nerve.

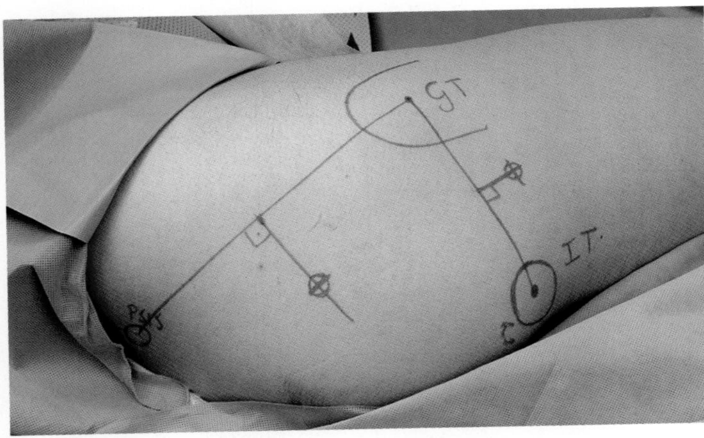

FIGURE 14-4 Surface landmarks for sciatic nerve blocks. PSIS, posterior superior iliac spine; GT, greater trochanter; IT, ischial tuberosity.

in Figure 14-4. The line that joins the midpoint of the ischial tuberosity (IT) and the midpoint of the greater trochanter (GT) of the femur is bisected by another line at 90 degrees. This line indicates the subgluteal position of the nerve in the groove between the biceps femoris muscle and the iliotibial tract and vastus lateralis. Needle entry is in the *circled* area.

A line that joins the posterior superior iliac spine (PSIS) to the midpoint of the GT is bisected, and the transgluteal approach to the sciatic nerve (Labat's approach) is through a point 5 cm down this line (*small circle*). The needle encounters the sciatic nerve deep to the piriformis muscle, in an area where it may be compressed (see Fig. 14-2). The addition of local anesthetic agent and perhaps a small hematoma in this area may cause further nerve compression, which can lead to ischemic nerve injury.

If the needle is on the medial aspect of the sciatic nerve, the motor response in the foot will be plantar flexion or inversion. Lateral placement on the nerve causes eversion of the foot. If a motor response of the hamstrings is evoked, the needle is medial to the sciatic nerve.

(See sciatic nerve movie on DVD.)

SCIATIC NERVE: POPLITEAL AREA

Applied Anatomy

Tibial Nerve

The tibial nerve is a major branch of the sciatic nerve, which splits into a median tibial nerve and a lateral common peroneal nerve in the popliteal fossa, approximately 7 to 9 cm above the crease behind the knee.

Figure 14-5 illustrates the sensory innervation of the tibial branch of the sciatic nerve.

The sciatic nerve splits into a number of branches in the popliteal fossa. The largest of these are the tibial nerve medially (Fig. 14-6, *arrow*) and the common peroneal nerve (also called the common fibular nerve) laterally. The sural nerve usually branches from both these nerves in the distal popliteal fossa.

Surface Anatomy of the Tibial Nerve

The posterior tibial nerve (Fig. 14-7, *arrow*) and the common peroneal nerve diverge approximately 7 to 9 cm above the crease behind the knee. This fact is important if a popliteal sciatic nerve block is done because both nerves are important for a successful block.

Electrical stimulation of the tibial nerve causes plantar flexion of the foot and toes.

(See tibial nerve movie on DVD.)

Common Peroneal Nerve

Figure 14-8 illustrates the sensory distribution of the common peroneal nerve.

The common peroneal nerve (Fig. 14-9, *arrow*) splits laterally from the tibial nerve in the popliteal fossa and courses around the head of the fibula, where it is often prone to injury.

Surface Anatomy of the Common Peroneal Nerve

The split in the sciatic nerve occurs approximately 7 - 9 cm from the crease behind the knee (Fig. 14-10).

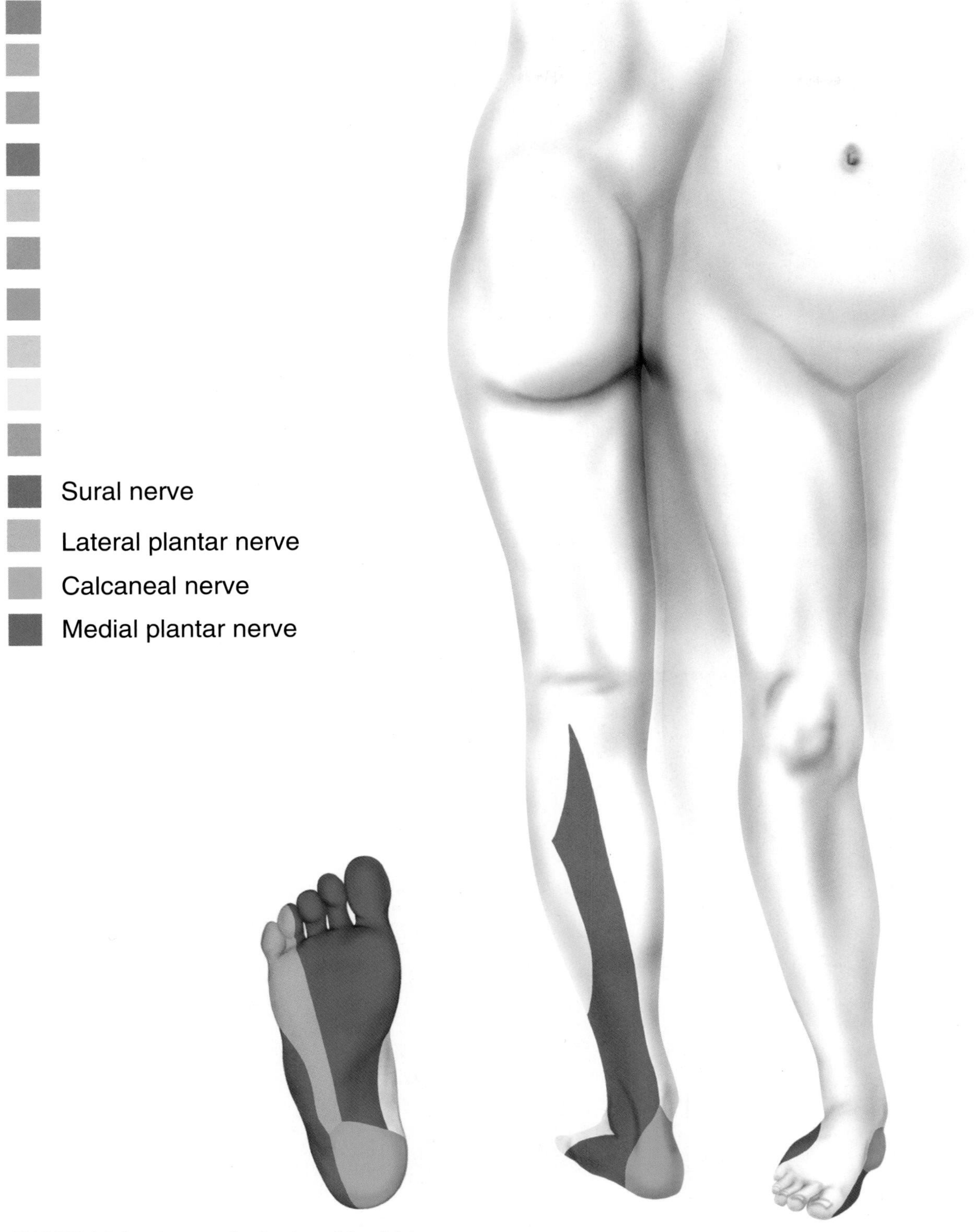

FIGURE 14-5 Sensory distribution of the tibial nerve.

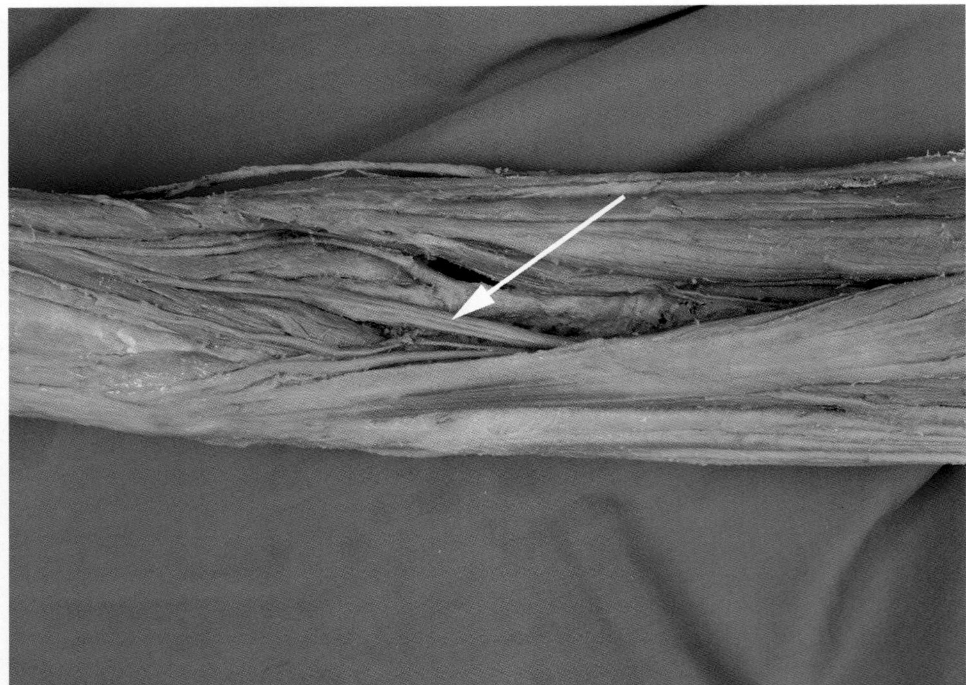

FIGURE 14-6 The *arrow* indicates the tibial nerve in the popliteal fossa.

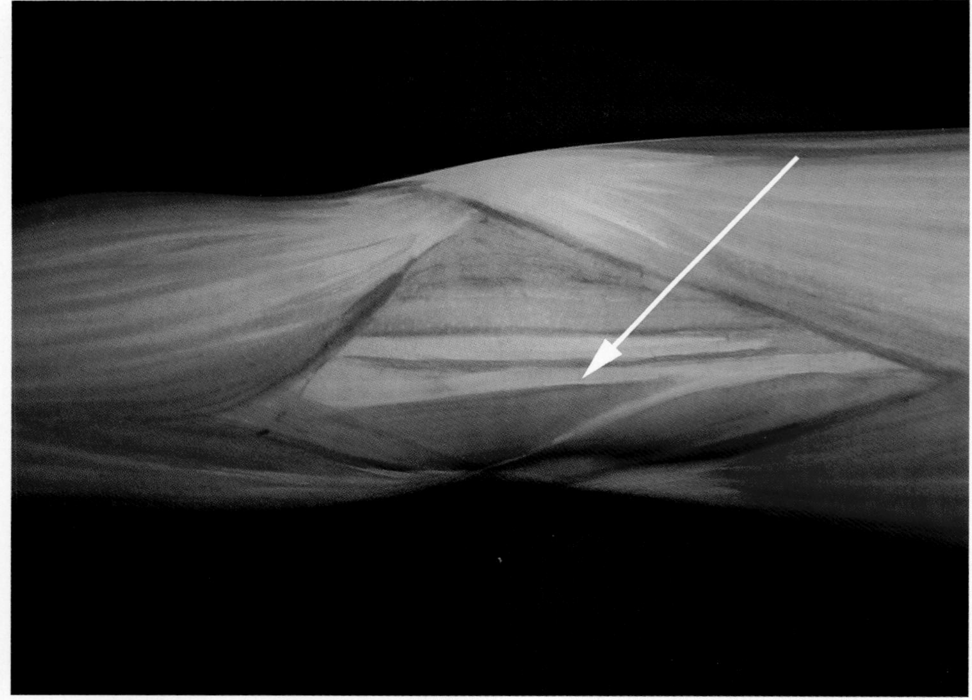

FIGURE 14-7 Surface anatomy of the tibial nerve.

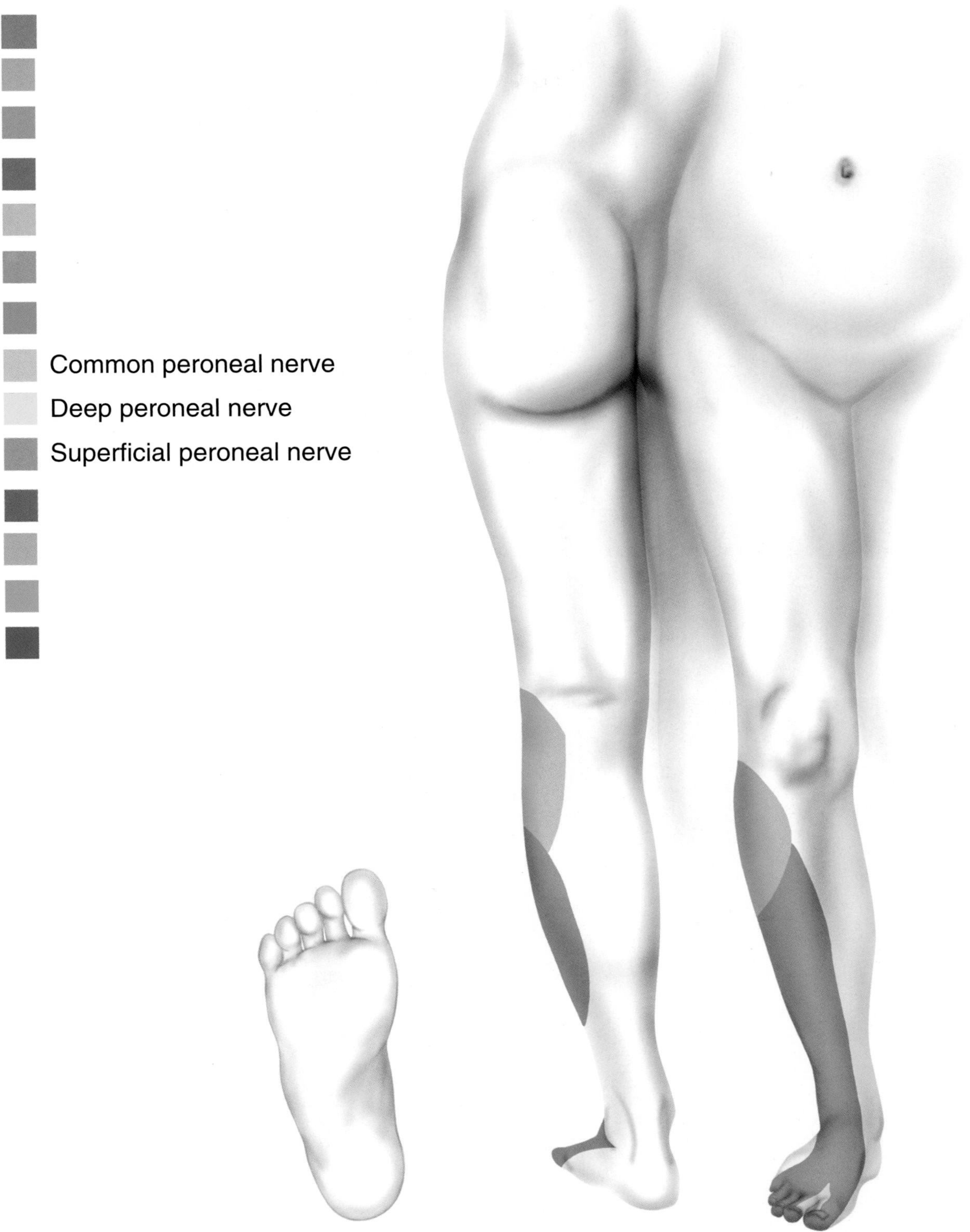

FIGURE 14-8 Sensory distribution of the common peroneal nerve.

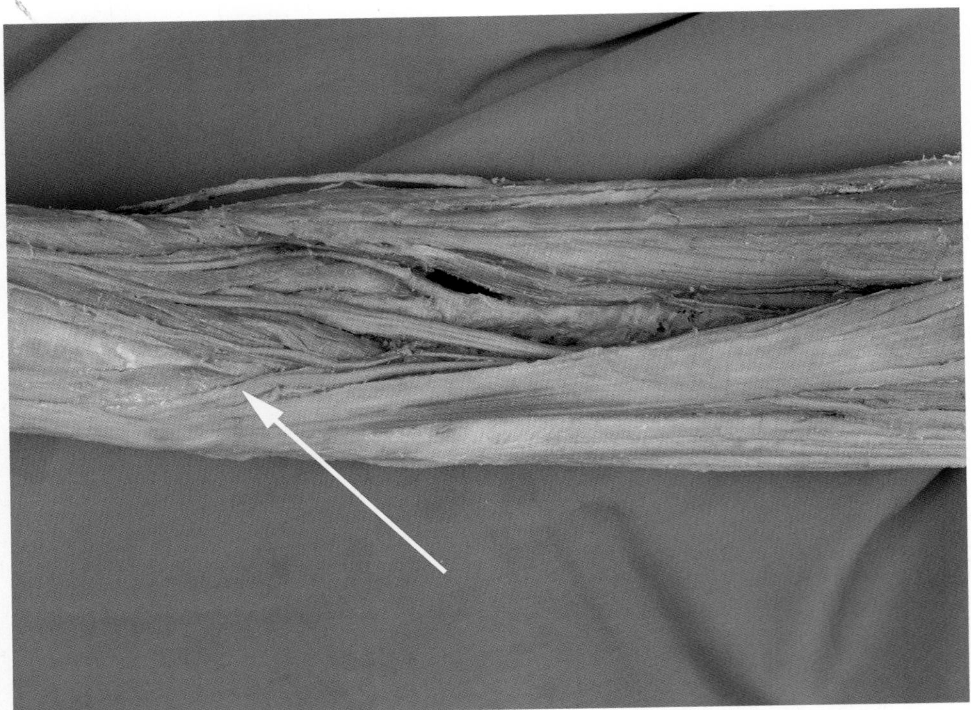

FIGURE 14-9 The *arrow* indicates the common peroneal nerve in the popliteal fossa.

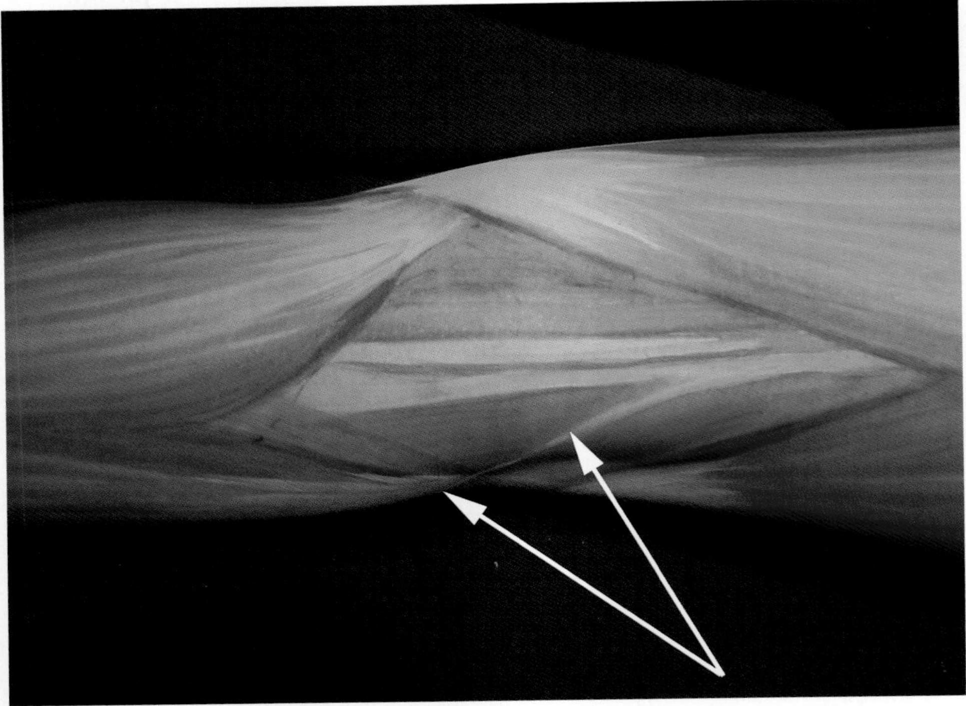

FIGURE 14-10 Surface anatomy of the common peroneal nerve.

The common peroneal nerve can easily be stimulated electrically at any point of its course around the fibular head, and such stimulation gives rise to eversion of the foot.

(See common peroneal nerve movie on DVD.)

Figure 11-8 depicts the osteotomes of the lower extremity, Figure 11-9 the dermatomes, and Figure 11-10 the neurotomes.

SUGGESTED FURTHER READING

1. Last RJ: Last's Anatomy: Regional and Applied, 4th ed. London, J&A Churchill, 1970.
2. Gray's Anatomy: The Anatomical Basis of Clinical Practice, 39th ed. Philadelphia, Elsevier, 2005.
3. Netter FH: Atlas of Human Anatomy, 2nd ed. East Hanover, NJ, Novartis, 1997.
4. Abrahams PH, Marks SC Jr, Hutchings RT: McMinn's Color Atlas of Human Anatomy, 5th ed. Philadelphia, Elsevier Mosby, 2003.
5. Boezaart AP: Anesthesia and Orthopaedic Surgery. New York, McGraw-Hill, 2006.
6. Hadzic A, Vloka JD: Peripheral Nerve Blocks: Principles and Practice. New York, McGraw-Hill, 2004.
7. Rathmell JP, Neal JM, Viscomi CM: Regional Anesthesia: The Requisites in Anesthesia. Philadelphia, Elsevier Mosby, 2004.
8. Brown DL: Atlas of Regional Anesthesia, 3rd ed. Philadelphia, Elsevier, 2006.
9. Barret J, Harmon D, Loughnane B, et al: Peripheral Nerve Blocks and Peri-operative Pain Relief. Philadelphia, WB Saunders, 2004.
10. Meier G, Büttner J: Atlas der peripheren Regionalanästhesie. Stuttgart, Georg Thieme Verlag, 2004.
11. Hahn MB, McQuillan PM, Sheplock GJ: Regional Anesthesia: An Atlas of Anatomy and Technique. St. Louis, Mosby, 1996.
12. Franco CD, Borene SC: Sciatic nerve block. In Boezaart AP (ed): Anesthesia and Orthopaedic Surgery. New York, McGraw-Hill, 2006, pp 343-351.

Chapter 15

Sciatic Nerve Blocks

- **Single-Injection Subgluteal Sciatic Nerve Block**
- **Continuous Subgluteal Sciatic Nerve Block**
- **Single-Injection Popliteal Sciatic Nerve Block**
- **Continuous Popliteal Sciatic Nerve Block**

SINGLE-INJECTION SUBGLUTEAL SCIATIC NERVE BLOCK

Introduction

The single-injection sciatic nerve block can last from 12 to 36 hours and is indicated for foot and ankle surgery, as well as painful conditions of the lateral aspect of the lower leg and the posterior aspect of the upper leg (1).

It is almost always necessary to block the saphenous branch of the femoral nerve or the entire femoral nerve when this block is performed. The single-injection subgluteal block to the sciatic nerve gives approximately the same block as the popliteal block, which is the mainstay of foot and ankle surgery, but if a thigh tourniquet is required, the subgluteal approach is preferable because it may not be wise to perform a block at the same location where a tourniquet is applied.

Specific Anatomic Considerations

The sciatic nerve arises from the fifth lumbar root to the fourth or fifth sacral roots. The bony involvement of this block includes the small posterior parts of the femur, the lateral aspect of the tibia and ankle joints, the fibula, and the entire foot, with the exception of its medial aspect (see Fig. 11-8).

The neurotomes covered with complete subgluteal sciatic nerve block include the posterior cutaneous aspect of the thigh and knee, the lateral aspect of the lower leg and ankle, and the sole and lateral aspect of the foot (see Fig. 11-10).

Technique

The patient is positioned in the lateral position. The *semicircle* in Figure 15-1 outlines the greater trochanter (GT) of the femur. The midpoint of the greater trochanter is marked and the midpoint of the ischial tuberosity (IT) is palpated and marked. A line is drawn joining these two points and the midpoint of this line is measured and marked. A line perpendicular to this line through the midpoint is drawn, and this line indicates the position of the sciatic nerve.

After disinfecting the skin, the skin and subcutaneous tissues are liberally infiltrated with local anesthetic agent (Fig. 15-1). Ultrasound can be used very effectively for this book (Fig. 15-2).

The 22-gauge, 100-mm stimulating needle enters perpendicular to the skin until the sciatic nerve is encountered (Fig. 15-3). A rule of thumb is that the nerve lies at a depth approximately 43% of the vertical distance from the surface on which the patient is lying supine to the midpoint of the inguinal crease.

If the medial or central aspect of the sciatic nerve is stimulated, the motor response is plantar flexion or inversion of the foot. More lateral stimulation elicits eversion of the foot. Injection of local anesthetic agent or normal saline causes the muscle twitches to stop immediately.

Local Anesthetic Agent Choice

Most local anesthetics have been used for this block. The author prefers to use 15 to 40 mL of ropivacaine 0.5% to 0.75%.

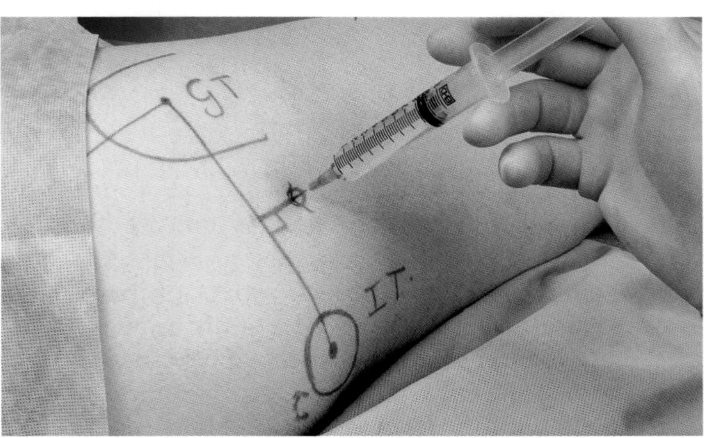

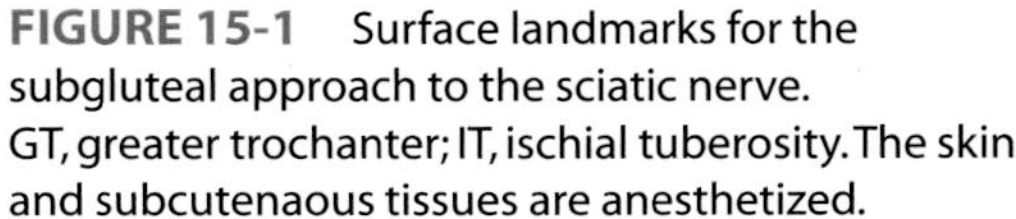
FIGURE 15-1 Surface landmarks for the subgluteal approach to the sciatic nerve. GT, greater trochanter; IT, ischial tuberosity. The skin and subcutenaous tissues are anesthetized.

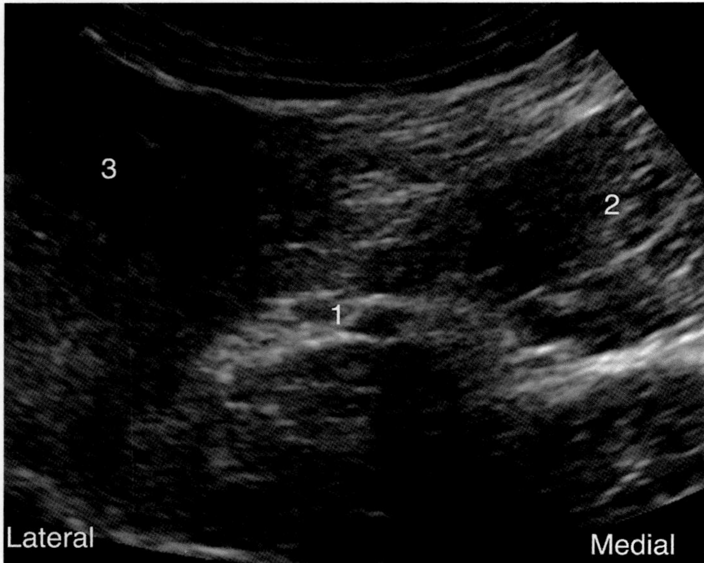

FIGURE 15-2 Transverse sonogram of subgluteal area. 1 = Sciatic nerve; 2 = Biceps femoris muscle; 3 = Vastus lateralis muscle.

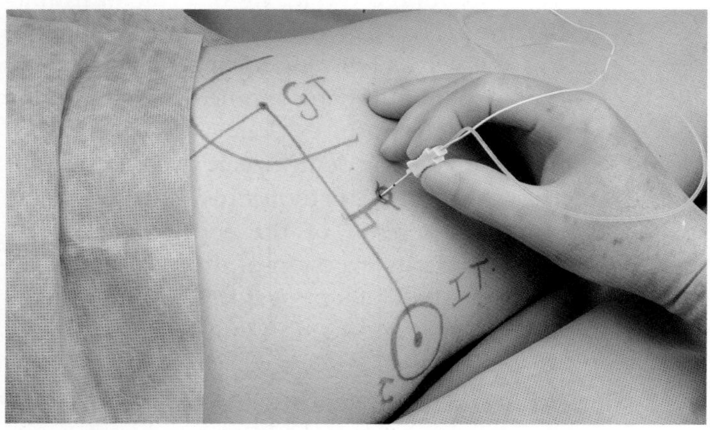

FIGURE 15-3 Needle entry with a 50- to 100-mm stimulating needle is on a line perpendicular to the midpoint of a line joining the greater trochanter with the ischial tuberosity.

(See single-injection subgluteal nerve block movie on DVD.)

CONTINUOUS SUBGLUTEAL SCIATIC NERVE BLOCK

Introduction

The continuous sciatic nerve block is indicated for painful foot and ankle surgery, as well as painful conditions of the lateral aspect of the lower leg and the posterior aspect of the upper leg (1). It is almost always necessary to also block the saphenous branch of the femoral nerve or the entire femoral nerve when this block is performed. It is advisable to perform a continuous femoral nerve block for surgeries such as triple arthrodesis of the ankle, ankle arthroplasty, and other major ankle operations. When a midthigh tourniquet is applied, the catheter can be directed cephalad. If instead a lower calf tourniquet is being used, continuous sciatic nerve block through the popliteal approach is an alternative.

Specific Anatomic Considerations

The sciatic nerve arises from the fifth lumbar root to the fourth or fifth sacral root of the sacral plexus, and the bony involvement of this block includes a small posterior part of

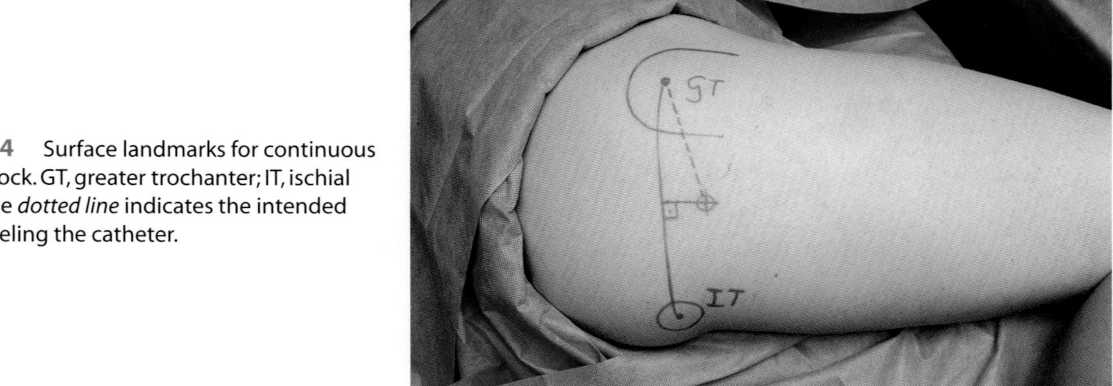

FIGURE 15-4 Surface landmarks for continuous subgluteal block. GT, greater trochanter; IT, ischial tuberosity. The *dotted line* indicates the intended path for tunneling the catheter.

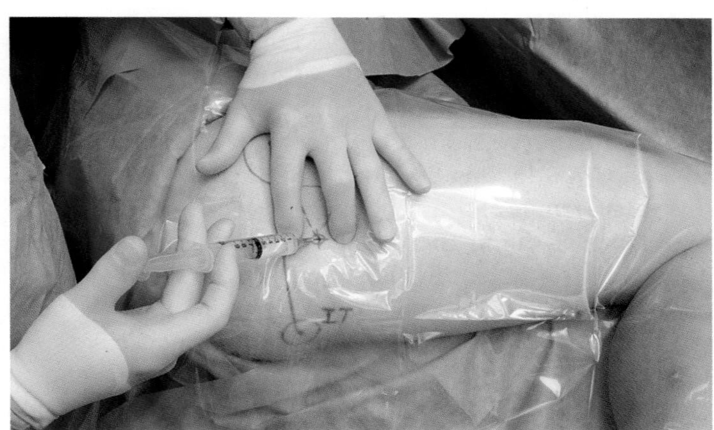

FIGURE 15-5 After preparation of the skin, a sterile fenestrated drape is placed over the area and the skin and subcutaneous tissues are thoroughly anesthetized. Note that the index and middle fingers of the nonoperative hand separate the iliotibial tract and vastus lateralis muscle from the biceps femoris muscle.

the femur, the lateral aspect of the tibia, the fibula, ankle joint, and the entire foot, with the exception of the medial part (see Fig. 11-8).

The neurotomes covered with complete subgluteal sciatic nerve block include the posterior aspect of the thigh and knee (if the posterior cutaneous nerve of the thigh is involved), the lateral aspect of the lower leg and ankle, and the sole and lateral aspect of the foot (see Figs. 11-10).

Technique

The patient is positioned in the lateral position, and the landmarks are identical to those for the single-injection subgluteal block (see Fig. 15-1).

The *dotted line* in Figure 15-4 indicates the intended path of the catheter after tunneling.

After disinfection of the skin and application of a sterile, fenestrated, transparent plastic drape, the skin, subcutaneous tissue, and intended path for tunneling the catheter are anesthetized with a fine needle using a solution of lidocaine and epinephrine 1:200,000 (Fig. 15-5).

A 17- or 18-gauge insulated Tuohy needle attached to a nerve stimulator set to an output of 1 to 1.2 mA, a frequency of 2 Hz, and a pulse width of 100 to 300 μsec, enters the skin at an angle of approximately 45 degrees (Fig. 15-6). The needle is aimed caudally in this illustration, but if the intended placement of the catheter is cephalic, the needle is aimed 45 degrees cephalically. As a general principle, catheters for continuous nerve blocks are placed pointing toward the point of convergence of nerve branches into a single nerve, rather than toward the direction of divergence into many branches.

Contact with the sciatic nerve is indicated by a brisk plantar flexion motor response of the foot. More lateral stimulation of the sciatic nerve results in eversion of the foot. The nerve stimulator output is now turned down, and

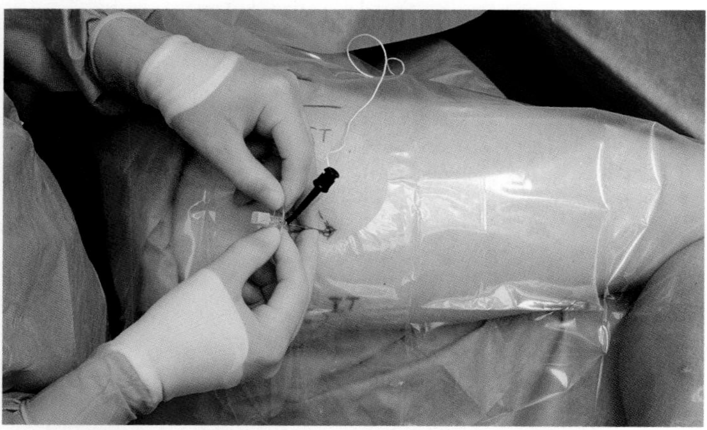

FIGURE 15-6 A 17- or 18-gauge insulated Tuohy needle, attached to a nerve stimulator, is advanced until the sciatic nerve is encountered.

brisk plantar flexion or dorsiflexion of the foot at a nerve stimulator output setting of 0.3 to 0.5 mA indicates that the needle tip is placed close to the nerve. Do not inject normal saline or any other conducting fluid through the needle at this stage. The notion of "opening up the space" with normal saline to advance the catheter is not based on scientific fact because in living tissue the saline only infiltrates the tissue, making it edematous and rendering further nerve stimulation through the catheter difficult or impossible. If, however, the anesthesiologist prefers to use this technique, 5% dextrose in water should be used because this solution does not conduct electricity and will not obliterate the motor response during placement of the stimulating catheter.

The proximal end of the stimulating catheter is now attached to the nerve stimulator (Fig. 15-7A). This part of the catheter is placed in the palm of the anesthesiologist's left hand. The catheter tip is then placed into the shaft of the needle; the muscle twitches should remain brisk and unchanged. Note that a mark on the catheter indicates that the catheter tip is situated at the tip of the needle, but it is not yet protruding from the needle tip. The needle should not be manipulated if this mark is not visible.

If the twitches disappear, the catheter is carefully withdrawn inside the shaft of the needle such that the entire mark is visible again. A small adjustment to the needle is made by rotating it one quarter-turn clockwise or counterclockwise or by withdrawing or advancing it slightly, then advancing the catheter again (Fig. 15-7B). Repeat this maneuver as many as times as necessary to ensure correct and accurate catheter placement and successful secondary block.

The catheter is advanced 3 to 5 cm while the foot twitches remain brisk at a nerve stimulator output of 0.3 to 0.5 mA.

The needle is removed without disturbing the catheter (Fig. 15-8).

The catheter can now be tunneled subcutaneously as previously described (see Chapter 12).

The Luer lock connecting device is attached to the catheter and the nerve stimulator to the connecting device. The nerve stimulator output is turned up until brisk muscle twitches can just be seen. Immediately on injection of local anesthetic agent or saline, the twitches will disappear. This constitutes a positive Raj test, which gives final confirmation that the secondary block will be successful.

The catheter and connecting device are placed in the fixation device, which is placed in a convenient position on the patient's hip or abdomen. The catheter exit sites are covered with a transparent dressing to allow daily inspection.

The catheter is removed as previously described (see Chapter 12).

Local Anesthetic Agent Choice

Almost all local anesthetic agents have been used for this block, but the author prefers to use 20 to 40 mL of ropivacaine 0.5% to 0.75% for intraoperative analgesia, followed by an infusion of 0.2% ropivacaine at a rate of 5 to 10 mL/hour for postoperative pain management. Patient-controlled boluses of 5 to 10 mL are allowed, with a lockout time of 30 to 60 minutes. If pre-

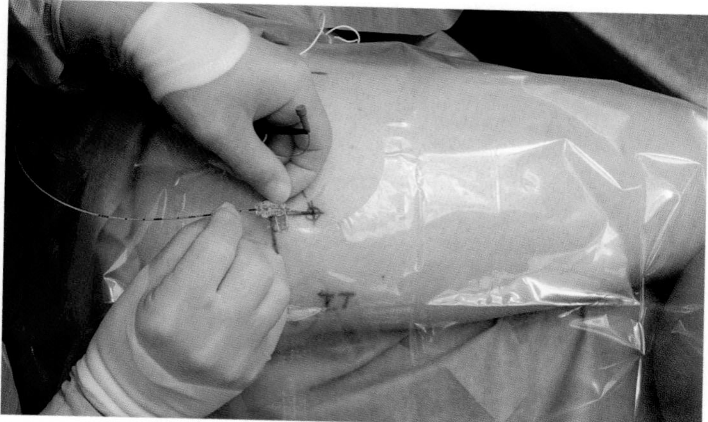

A

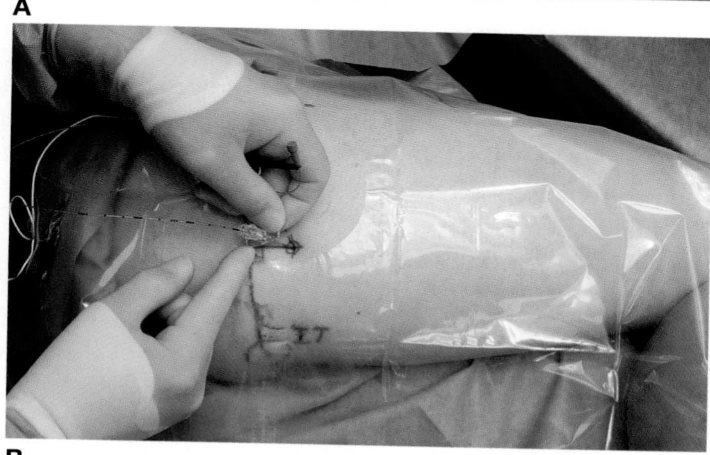

B

FIGURE 15-7 **A,** After the nerve is encountered, indicated by plantar flexion of the foot, the nerve stimulator is attached to the proximal end of a stimulating catheter, and the distal end of the catheter is advanced through the needle. **B,** If, during advancement of the catheter, the motor response is lost, the catheter is withdrawn to inside the needle shaft and the needle is manipulated as indicated.

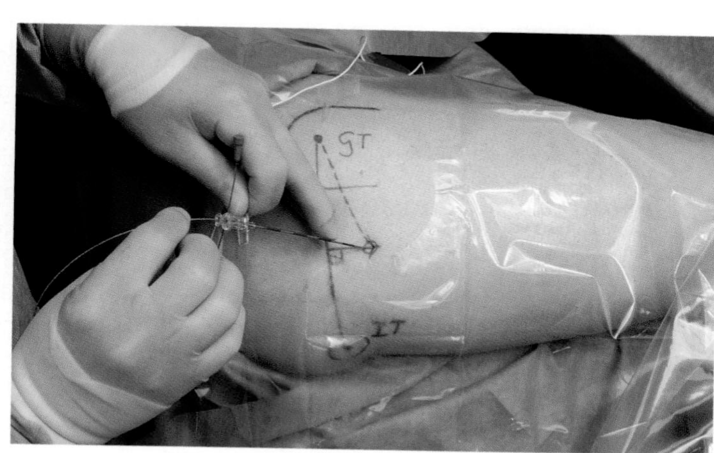

FIGURE 15-8 The catheter is advanced 3 to 5 cm through the needle with unchanged motor responses still visible. The needle is then removed without disturbing the position of the catheter.

servation of motor function is essential, the drug concentration can be decreased to 0.1% or 0.05% and infused at 1 to 3 mL/hour, with patient-controlled boluses of, for example, 10 mL, locked out at 60 minutes.

(See continuous subgluteal sciatic nerve block movie on DVD.)

SINGLE-INJECTION POPLITEAL SCIATIC NERVE BLOCK

Introduction

Just as the single-injection infraclavicular block is the mainstay of hand, wrist, forearm, and elbow

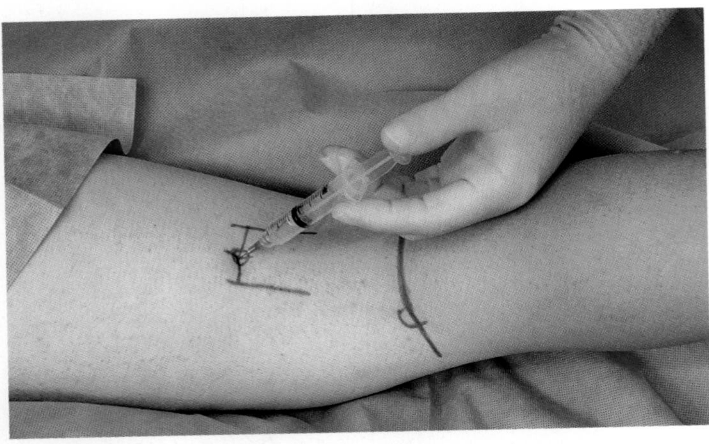

FIGURE 15-9 The patient is positioned prone and the knees slightly bent. The surface landmarks are the tendons of the biceps femoris laterally and the semitendinous/semimembranous muscles medially. A line joining these two muscles is drawn 7 to 9 cm proximal of the crease behind the knee, and the midpoint of this line indicates the position of needle entry. The skin and subcutaneous tissues are anesthetized.

surgery, the single-injection popliteal approach to the sciatic nerve is the mainstay of foot and ankle surgery. If it is combined with a block of the saphenous branch of the femoral nerve at the knee or ankle level or a complete femoral nerve block, this block is suitable for all foot and ankle surgery. Although this block can last up to 24 or even 36 hours, it is advisable to place a catheter for continuous nerve block in case of more major surgery such as triple arthrodesis of the ankle, ankle fusion, or ankle replacement. In such instances, it is almost always necessary to place a continuous femoral nerve block as well. The positioning of the tourniquet for the surgery should influence the choice of sciatic nerve block. As a general principle, a block should not be placed in the same area where a tourniquet is applied.

Specific Anatomic Considerations

The sciatic nerve innervates the lateral aspect of the lower leg, the lateral part of the ankle, and the entire foot with the exception of the medial part, which is innervated by the saphenous branch of the femoral nerve.

Technique

The patient is placed in the prone position with the knee slightly flexed. The tendons of the biceps femoris and the semitendinous/semimembranous muscles are palpated and marked (Fig. 15-9). These tendons usually meet to form the apex of a triangle, the base of which is the skin crease behind the knees. Note, however, that this feature is not consistent. Needle entry is approximately 7 to 9 cm above the posterior knee crease at the midpoint between these tendons.

This book canvery effectively be handled with ultrasound (Fig. 15-10).

The skin and subcutaneous tissue are anesthetized after skin disinfection (Fig. 15-9).

A 22-gauge, 50- to 100-mm stimulating needle with a B-bevel is attached to a nerve stimulator set at an output of 1.0 to 1.5 mA, a frequency of 2 Hz, and a pulse width of 100 to 300 μsec (Fig. 15-11). The needle enters at a slightly cephalic direction and is advanced until the sciatic nerve is encountered.

Brisk plantar flexion twitches of the foot indicate that the tibial component of the sciatic nerve is being stimulated. If the nerve is missed, it is usually missed medially, and the needle needs to be redirected laterally. The current of the nerve stimulator is turned down until brisk twitches can still be observed at a stimulator output of 0.3 to 0.5 mA. If the muscle twitches are still brisk at less than 0.2 mA, it may indicate intraneural needle placement and the needle should probably be withdrawn slightly. This notion has not yet been substantiated by research, but it is prudent to err on the side of safety.

Eversion of the foot is seen when the common peroneal fibers of the sciatic nerve are stimulated.

Local anesthetic agent or any other electrically conducting fluid such as normal saline can be injected and the muscle twitches will stop immediately. This gives final assurance that the block will be successful.

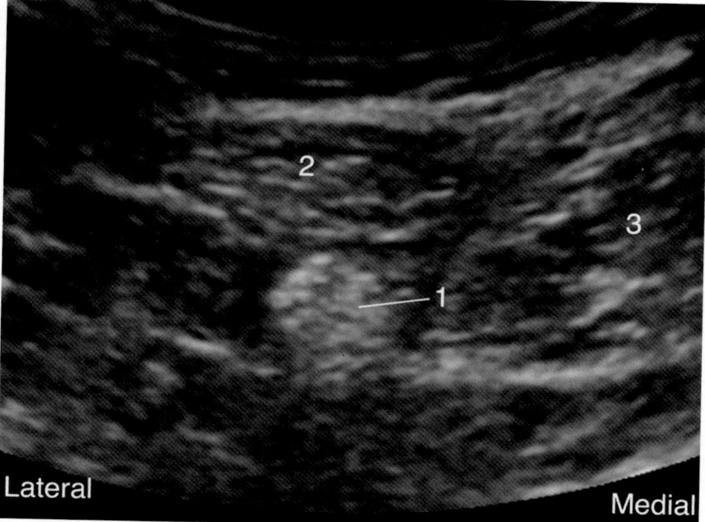

FIGURE 15-10 Ultrasound image of popliteal area. 1 = Sciatic nerve; 2 = Biceps femoris muscle; 3 = Semimembranosus and Semitendinosus muscles.

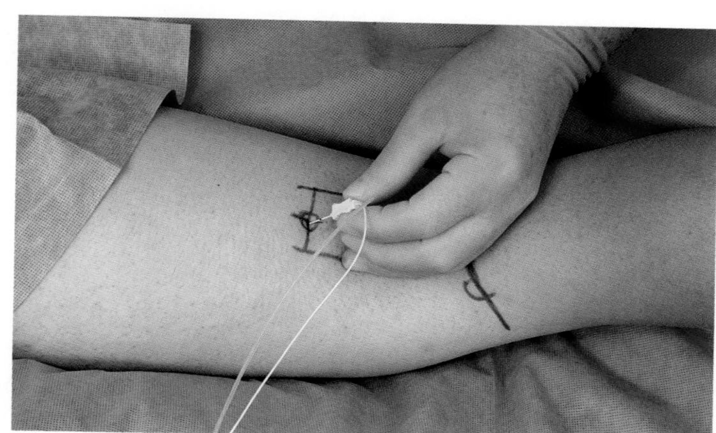

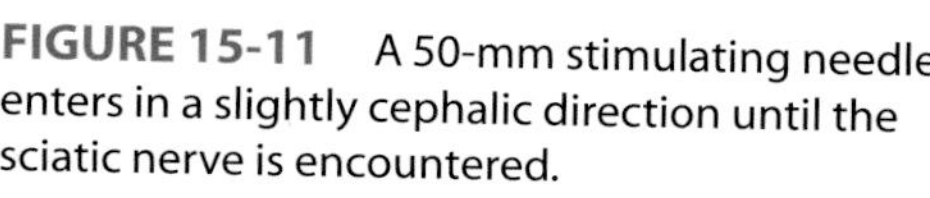

FIGURE 15-11 A 50-mm stimulating needle enters in a slightly cephalic direction until the sciatic nerve is encountered.

Local Anesthetic Agent Choice

Almost all local anesthetic agents and combinations have been used for this block. The author prefers to use 15 to 40 mL of ropivacaine 0.5% to 0.75%. The duration of the block can probably be extended by a factor of three if 0.3 mg buprenorphine is added to 20 to 40 mL of ropivacaine 0.5%. It should be obvious that if long-lasting local anesthetic agents are used, the possible complications of this block will also be long lasting. It is therefore advisable instead to place a catheter for continuous nerve block if a long-lasting block is required.

(See single-injection popliteal sciatic nerve block movie on DVD.)

CONTINUOUS POPLITEAL SCIATIC NERVE BLOCK

Introduction

The continuous popliteal approach to the sciatic nerve is the mainstay of postoperative pain control after major foot and ankle surgery, and it is almost always necessary to combine this block with a continuous femoral nerve block, which will cover the medial aspect of the lower leg and the medial aspect of the ankle and foot. Note that the saphenous branch of the femoral nerve down to and including the ankle joint also innervates the medial aspect of the tibia, especially the ankle joint. The intended

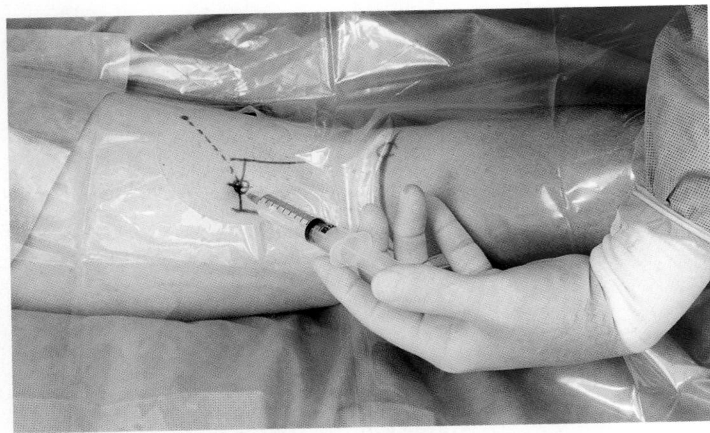

FIGURE 15-12 After preparation of the skin, a sterile fenestrated drape is placed over the popliteal fossa. The subcutaneous tissues and intended path for tunneling the catheter are thoroughly anesthetized.

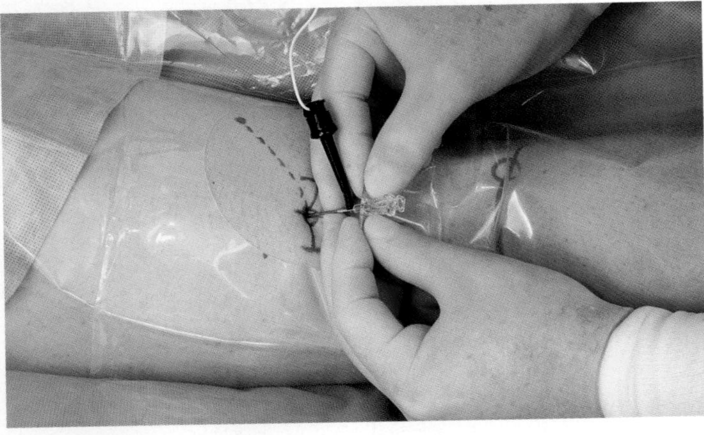

FIGURE 15-13 An insulated Tuohy needle attached to a nerve stimulator enters the skin and is advanced in a slightly cephalic direction until the sciatic nerve is encountered.

position of the tourniquet helps in making the choice between this block and the subgluteal approach.

Specific Anatomic Considerations

The sciatic nerve innervates the lateral aspect of the lower leg, the lateral part of the ankle, and the entire foot with the exception of the medial part, which is innervated by the saphenous branch of the femoral nerve.

Technique

The patient is positioned in the prone position with the knee slightly flexed (see Fig. 15-9). The tendons of the biceps femoris and the semimembranous muscles are palpated and marked (see Fig. 15-9). Needle entry is approximately 7 to 9 cm above the posterior crease of the knee, midway between these tendons.

After the skin has been disinfected and the area covered with a clear fenestrated drape, the skin, subcutaneous tissue, and intended path for tunneling the catheter are anesthetized with a fine needle using a solution of lidocaine and epinephrine 1:200,000 (Fig. 15-12).

A 17- or 18-gauge insulated Tuohy needle is attached to a nerve stimulator set to a current of 1.0 to 1.5 mA, a frequency of 2 Hz, and a pulse width of 100 to 300 μsec (Fig. 15-13).

The needle enters the skin at an angle of approximately 45 to 60 degrees, pointing cephalically, with the bevel pointing upward to facilitate easy catheter placement. It is advanced until the sciatic nerve is encountered. Contact with the tibial component of the sciatic nerve is indicated by a brisk plantar flexion motor response at a nerve stimulator output of 0.3 to 0.5 mA. This indicates accurate needle placement, which can also be ultrasonographically (Fig. 15-10), but not necessarily accurate catheter

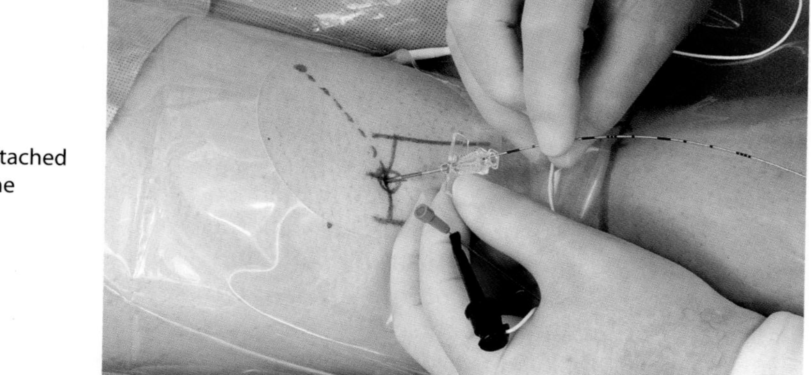

FIGURE 15-14 A stimulating catheter attached to a nerve stimulator is advanced through the needle.

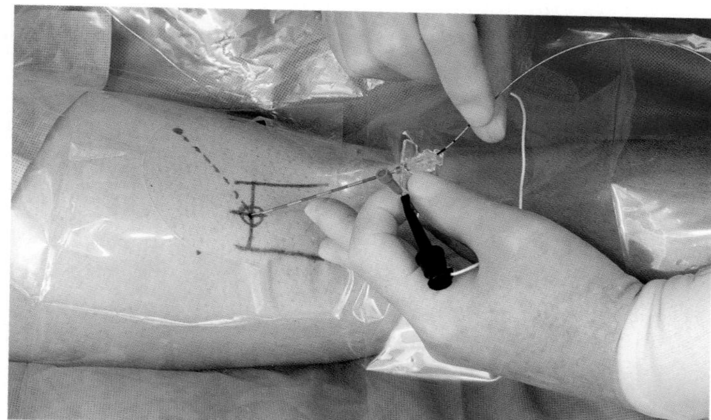

FIGURE 15-15 The catheter is advanced 3 to 5 cm beyond the needle tip and the needle is removed without disturbing the position of the catheter.

placement later. Do not inject any local anesthetic or saline through the needle at this stage. The notion of "opening the space" with normal saline to make catheter advancement easier is not based on scientific evidence, but if desired, 5% dextrose in water may be used for this purpose because it does not conduct electricity and therefore will not abolish the motor response when the stimulating catheter is placed. Saline injection at this stage serves only to make the tissue edematous and renders further nerve stimulation through the catheter very difficult or impossible.

The stylet of the needle is removed, the nerve stimulator is attached to the proximal end of the catheter, and the distal end of the catheter is placed inside the needle shaft (Fig. 15-14). The anesthesiologist holds the proximal end of the catheter in the palm of the left hand. A special mark on the catheter indicates that the catheter tip is at the tip of the needle. Advance the catheter. If the motor response stops, it simply means that the catheter is moving away from the nerve. Carefully withdraw the catheter to within the needle shaft, rotate the needle a quarter-turn clockwise or counterclockwise, and advance the catheter again. If the motor response again ceases, withdraw the catheter once more to within the needle shaft and advance or withdraw the needle slightly before advancing the catheter again. Repeat these maneuvers until the motor response remains positive and brisk during advancement of the catheter. Make sure that the catheter is always withdrawn to inside the needle shaft (i.e., the special mark on the catheter is visible) before manipulating the needle. The catheter can be advanced 3 to 5 cm. Advancing it further than 5 cm may cause the catheter to coil and even curl around the nerve. This possibility has been suggested but never clearly described.

Remove the needle without disturbing the catheter (Fig. 15-15). If the catheter is now left in this position, it will almost certainly dislodge, and it should be tunneled subcutaneously.

Tunneling can be accomplished with a special tunneling device or by using the available equipment, as described previously (see Chapter 12).

The Luer lock connecting device is attached to the proximal end of the catheter and the nerve stimulator is attached to the connecting device. The nerve stimulator output is set to zero and slowly turned up until muscle twitches can just been seen. The local anesthetic agent or any other fluid that conducts electricity is injected through the catheter. The motor response disappears immediately on injection, which constitutes a positive Raj test and a further indication that the primary and secondary blocks will be successful.

The catheter exit site is covered with a transparent dressing to allow daily inspection. The connecting device and catheter are placed in the fixation device, which is in turn attached to a convenient place on the leg. The main dose for the block can now be injected through the catheter.

The catheter is removed as previously described (see Chapter 12).

Local Anesthetic Agent Choice

The author prefers to use 15 to 40 mL of ropivacaine 0.5% to 0.75% as the initial bolus of this block. This is followed by a continuous infusion of 3 to 10 mL/hour of ropivacaine 0.2% for postoperative pain management. Patient-controlled bolus injections of 5 to 10 mL can be allowed every 30 to 60 minutes. This regimen is adjusted over the next few days as the clinical situation dictates.

(See continuous popliteal sciatic nerve block movie on DVD.)

REFERENCE

1. Franco CD, Borene SC: Sciatic nerve block. In Boezaart AP (ed): Anesthesia and Orthopaedic Surgery. New York, McGraw-Hill, 2006, pp 343-351.

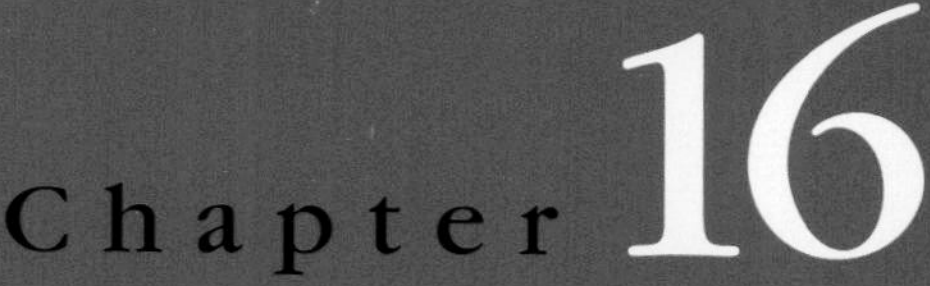
Chapter 16

The Ankle: Applied Anatomy

Figure 16-1 illustrates the five nerves of the foot at the ankle in the context of the fascial layers in which they lie.

To ensure successful ankle block, it is important to understand that two of the nerves are deep to the fascia layer and three nerves are superficial to it. Electrical current can readily cross fascia, but local anesthetics cannot. Therefore, it is important to deposit the local anesthetic on the correct side of the fascia. The deep nerves are the posterior tibial nerve and the deep peroneal nerve. The superficial nerves are the sural nerve, the saphenous nerve, and the superficial peroneal nerve. If the name of the nerve starts with an "S," it lies superficial to the fascia.

The posterior tibial nerve is the terminal branch of the tibial nerve. It innervates most of the sole of the foot and is also the only motor nerve at the ankle, and can thus be identified with a nerve stimulator. Figure 16-2 shows the sensory distribution of the foot.

The posterior tibial nerve (Fig. 16-3, *arrow*) is deep to the fascia of the ankle and lies posterior to the posterior tibial artery.

1. Superficial peroneal nerve
2. Deep peroneal nerve
3. Saphenous nerve
4. Posterior tibial nerve
5. Sural nerve
6. Achilles tendon
7. Fascia layers
8. Extensor hallucis longus tendon
9. Anterior tibialis tendon

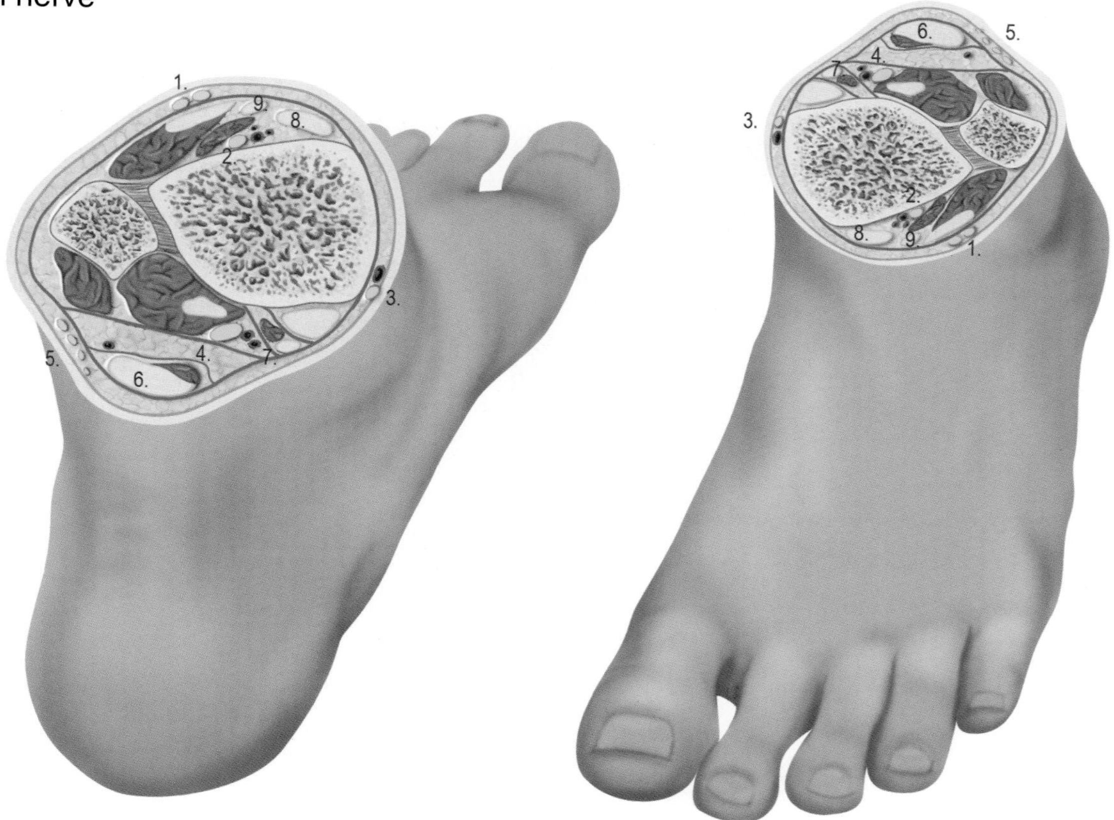

FIGURE 16-1 Transectional anatomy of the nerves around the ankle. The *purple lines* indicate the fascial planes.

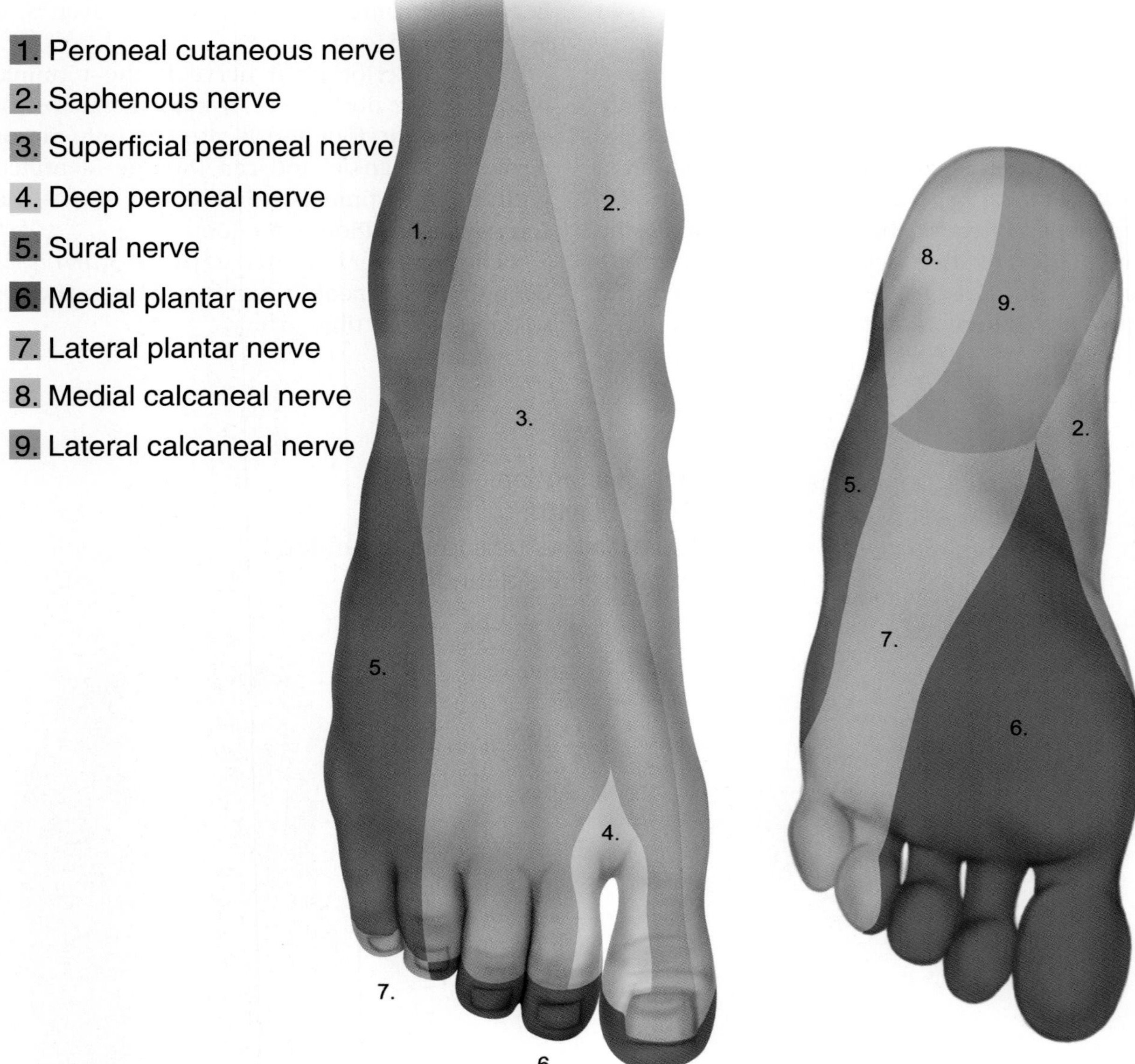

FIGURE 16-2 Sensory distribution of the nerves of the foot and ankle.

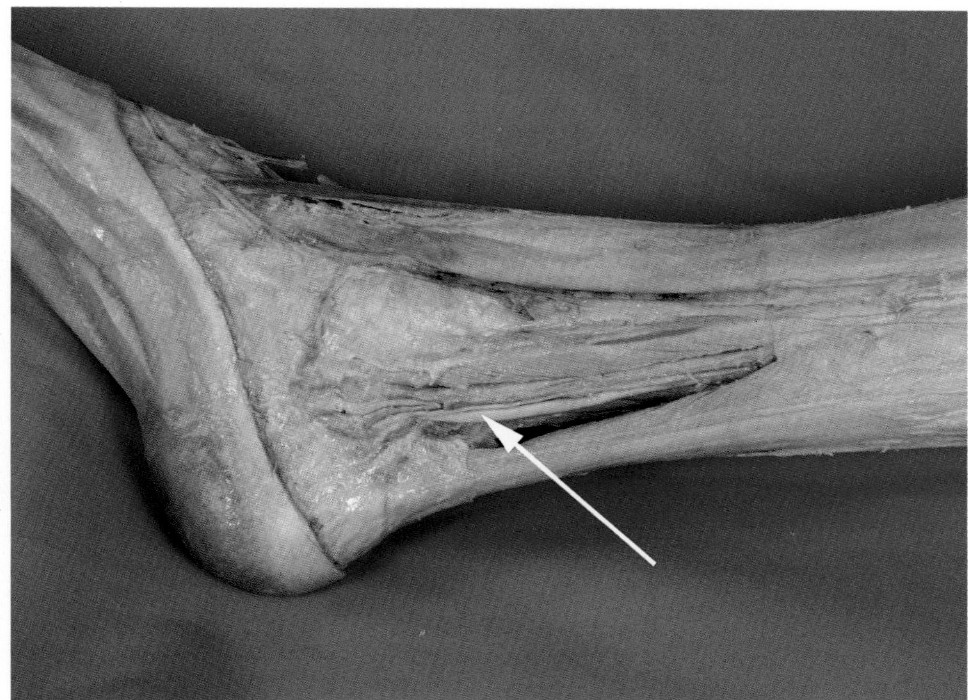

FIGURE 16-3 Dissection of the medial aspect of the ankle. The *arrow* indicates the posterior tibial nerve.

Stimulation of the posterior tibial nerve causes unmistakable plantar flexion of the toes. This is often not present in diabetic patients.

(See posterior tibial nerve movie on DVD.)

Figure 16-4 illustrates all five of the nerves innervating the foot at the ankle region.

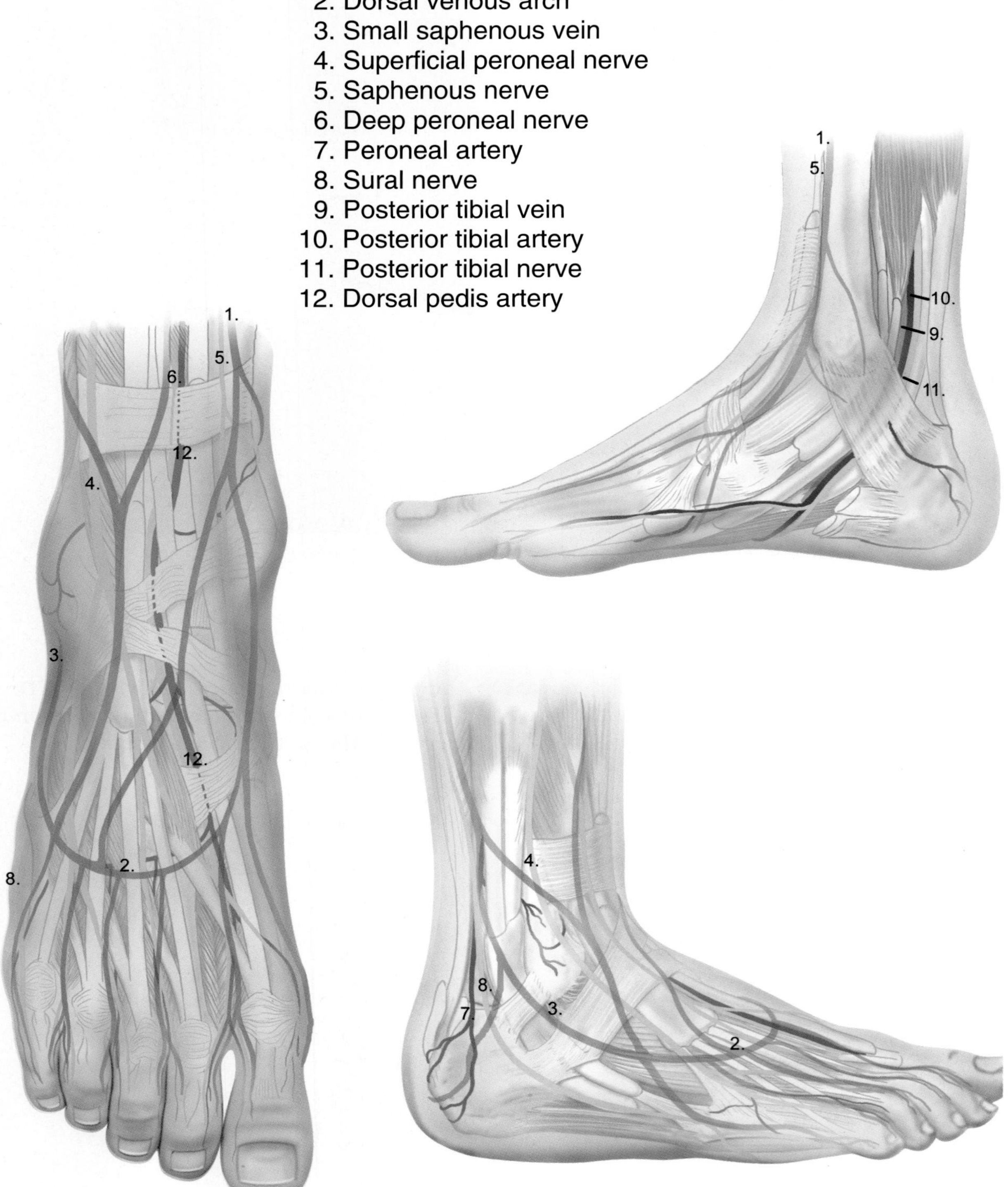

FIGURE 16-4 Surface anatomy of the nerves around the ankle.

SUGGESTED FURTHER READING

1. Gray's Anatomy: The Anatomical Basis of Clinical Practice, 39th ed. Philadelphia, Elsevier, 2005.
2. Netter FH: Atlas of Human Anatomy, 2nd ed. East Hanover, NJ, Novartis, 1997.
3. Abrahams PH, Marks SC Jr, Hutchings RT: McMinn's Color Atlas of Human Anatomy, 5th ed. Philadelphia, Elsevier Mosby, 2003.
4. Boezaart AP: Anesthesia and Orthopaedic Surgery. New York, McGraw-Hill, 2006.
5. Hadzic A, Vloka JD: Peripheral Nerve Blocks: Principles and Practice. New York, McGraw-Hill, 2004.
6. Rathmell JP, Neal JM, Viscomi CM: Regional Anesthesia: The Requisites in Anesthesia. Philadelphia, Elsevier Mosby, 2004.
7. Brown DL: Atlas of Regional Anesthesia, 3rd ed. Philadelphia, Elsevier, 2006.
8. Barret J, Harmon D, Loughnane B, et al: Peripheral Nerve Blocks and Peri-operative Pain Relief. Philadelphia, WB Saunders, 2004.
9. Meier G, Büttner J: Atlas der peripheren Regionalanästhesie. Stuttgart, Georg Thieme Verlag, 2004.
10. Hahn MB, McQuillan PM, Sheplock GJ: Regional Anesthesia: An Atlas of Anatomy and Technique. St. Louis, Mosby, 1996.
11. Rickelman T, Boezaart AP: Ankle block. In Boezaart AP (ed): Anesthesia and Orthopaedic Surgery. New York, McGraw-Hill, 2006, pp 253-257.

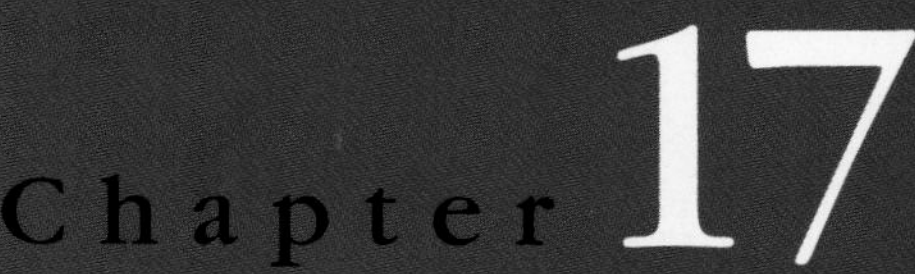

Ankle Block

- Ankle Block

ANKLE BLOCK

Introduction

Ankle block is very widely practiced for distal foot surgery (1). It is also a commonly failed block, for two main reasons: first, the fascia layers and the relative positions of the five nerves to these layers around the ankle are not widely understood; second, practitioners sometimes neglect to block all five nerves in disregard of the fact that the areas of the foot's sensory nerve supply overlap, and this overlap is not consistent.

The most common indication for ankle block is diabetic foot surgery. Practitioners should be careful in diabetic patients because the skin around the ankle tends to be fragile, and ankle block often leads to skin necrosis. Furthermore, these patients often have neuropathy, which gives the anesthesiologist a false sense of success with this block until he or she attempts an ankle block for bunion or rheumatoid arthritis surgery on a patient with normal nerves.

The other common indications for ankle block are for the management of postoperative pain after bunion surgery, and for surgery for rheumatoid arthritis. The ankle block can be used for most distal foot surgery, but it is not suitable for ankle surgery.

It can be painful to place an ankle block, and liberal use of skin infiltration with a fast-acting local anesthetic agent such as lidocaine, injected slowly through a fine needle, is advised. There should be no problem placing an ankle block in a heavily sedated or even anesthetized patient.

Specific Anatomic Considerations

Figure 11-8 shows that the nerve supply of the bones of the foot originates from all the lumbar and most of the sacral roots. Selective nerve blocks around the ankle therefore almost always result in some degree of failure. The diagram demonstrates that all five nerves around the ankle should be blocked for every foot operation except the most superficial skin surgery, for which local field blocks may in any case be a better choice.

It can also be seen that the dermatomal supply of the foot originates from an extensive area in the lumbar and sacral spine—from L4 to S2, at least (see Fig. 11-9).

The medial aspect of the foot receives its sensory supply from the saphenous nerve, which is a branch of the femoral nerve (see Fig. 16-2). The deep peroneal nerve supplies the area between the first and second toe, whereas most of the dorsal aspect of the foot gets its sensory nerve supply from the superficial peroneal nerve.

The lateral aspect of the foot is supplied by the lateral dorsal cutaneous and lateral calcaneal branches of the sural nerve, which in turn originates from the tibial nerve in the popliteal fossa behind the knee. The medial and posterior aspects of the heel receive their sensory nerve supply from the medical calcaneal branch of the tibial nerve.

Figure 16-1 shows that three nerves run superficial to the fascia, which is represented by a *purple line* in the image. These nerves are the superficial peroneal nerve, the saphenous nerve, and the sural nerve. Note that the names of all three of these nerves start with the letter "S."

Anterior, deep to this fascia and between the tendons of the hallucis longus and anterior tibial muscles, is the deep peroneal nerve running close to the tibia, and posterior, adjacent to the tibial artery and vein, in a complex array of fascia compartments, is the tibial nerve. The tibial nerve is a motor nerve, which makes its identification with a stimulating needle and nerve stimulator relatively easy. The anesthesiologist must keep in mind that local anesthetic agents do not cross fascia layers readily, and it is thus important to place the needle in the same fascial compartment as the nerve. The method, described in many older textbooks, of approaching the tibial nerve from posterior until the tibia itself is encountered, and then withdrawing the needle slightly, is outdated and possibly an important reason why many ankle blocks fail. The tibial nerve supplies nearly the entire sole of the foot.

Technique

With the patient in the supine position, the knee slightly flexed, and the foot externally rotated, the posterior tibial artery can usually be palpated behind the medial malleolus (Fig. 17-1). The tibial nerve is just posterior to the artery. If the artery

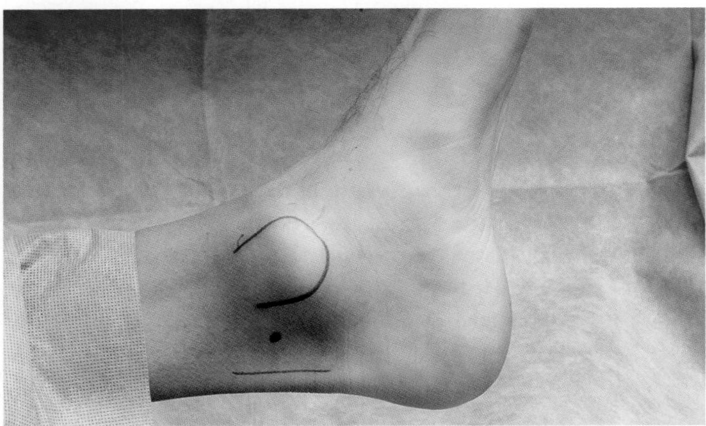

FIGURE 17-1 The medial malleolus and Achilles tendon are marked. Needle entry is halfway between these two landmarks for blockage of the posterior tibial nerve.

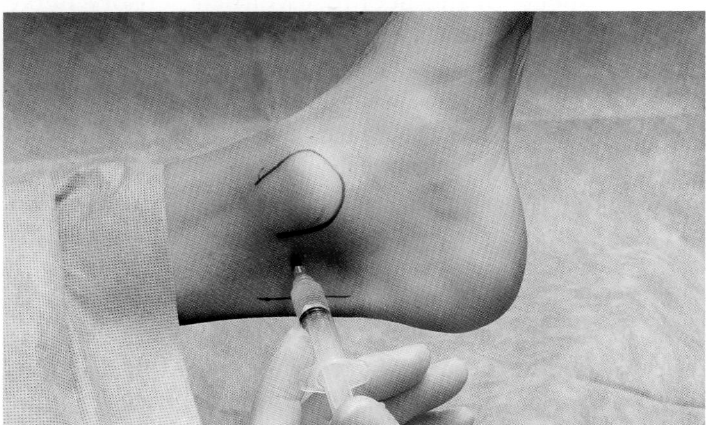

FIGURE 17-2 A small skin wheal is raised, taking care not to penetrate the fascia with this needle.

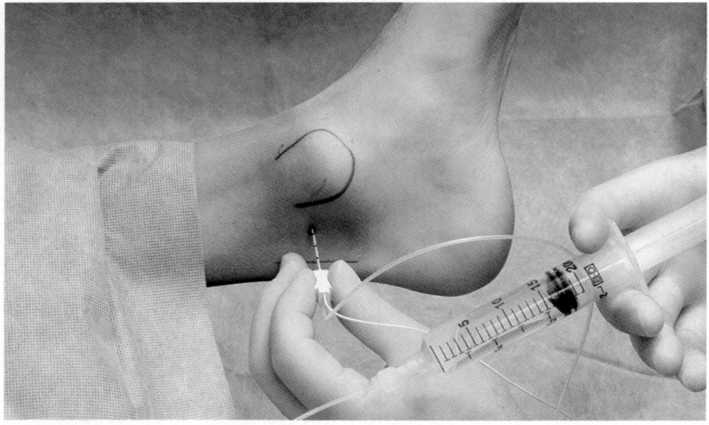

FIGURE 17-3 A 50-mm stimulating needle attached to a nerve stimulator is now advanced through the fascia until plantar flexion of the toes is caused by stimulation of the posterior tibial nerve.

cannot be palpated, the surface landmark of the nerve is usually halfway between the medial malleolus and the Achilles tendon.

The skin and subcutaneous tissue is infiltrated with 1% to 2% lidocaine, with care taken not to penetrate the fascia with the fine needle at this stage (Fig. 17-2).

A 22-gauge, 2-inch stimulating needle, attached to a nerve stimulator set at a current output of 1 to 2 mA, a frequency of 2 Hz, and a pulse width of 200 to 300 μsec, is used to locate the nerve (Fig. 17-3). Ultrasound can also be used. Toe flexion indicates that the nerve has been encountered. The nerve stimulator is now turned down until

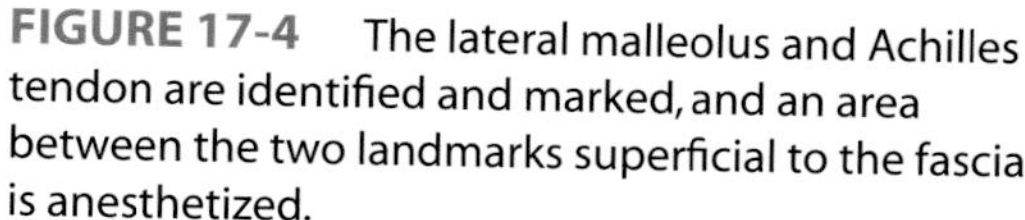

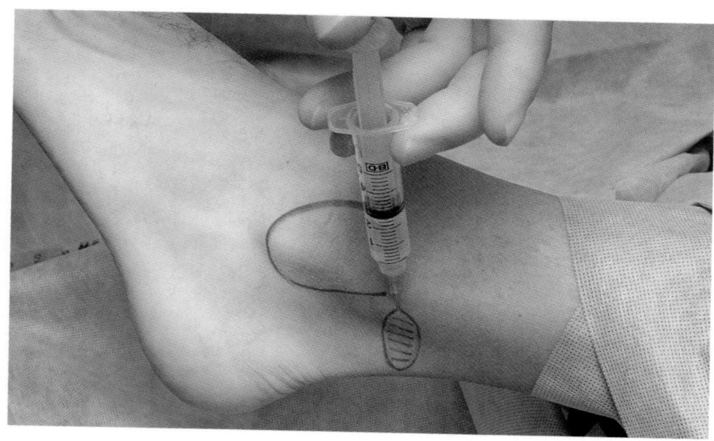

FIGURE 17-4 The lateral malleolus and Achilles tendon are identified and marked, and an area between the two landmarks superficial to the fascia is anesthetized.

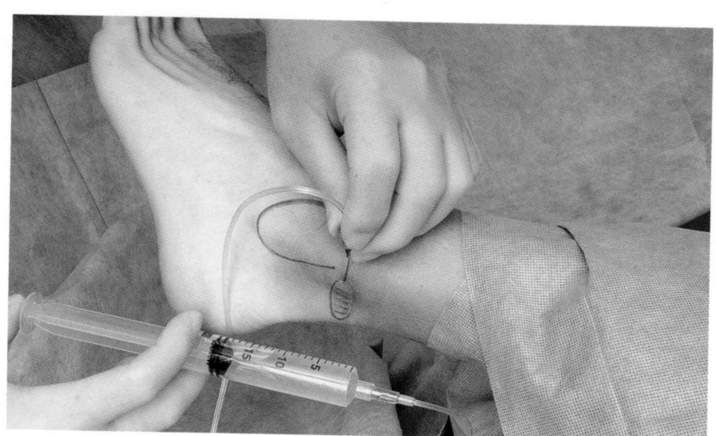

FIGURE 17-5 The area is now injected with local anesthetic agent to block the sural nerve.

brisk motor twitches of the toes can still be observed at a current output of 0.3 to 0.5 mA. This may not be possible in diabetic patients because of diabetic neuropathy, and higher currents may be required.

The motor response will immediately cease on injection of local anesthetic agent.

The foot is internally rotated, and the "valley" from the lateral malleolus to the Achilles tendon on the lateral side of the ankle is turned into a "hill" (Fig. 17-4). It is necessary to remain superficial to the fascia with the needle and to ensure that a skin wheal is observed when the sural nerve is blocked. This is a pure sensory nerve and it does not matter if the skin infiltration also blocks the nerve.

The main dose of the local anesthetic agent is now injected subcutaneously and superficial to the fascia, again ensuring that a skin wheal is raised (Fig. 17-5).

With care taken to remain proximal to the retinaculum that approximately joins the medial and lateral malleoli, the tendons of the anterior tibial muscle and extensor of the big toe are palpated (Fig. 17-6). Lidocaine is injected all the way down to the bone of the tibia between these two tendons.

The same needle entry site is used to inject lidocaine to the subcutaneous area lateral to the fibula (Fig. 17-7).

The area around the saphenous vein is also anesthetized using the same needle entry point (Fig. 17-8).

A 25-gauge needle attached to a syringe with local anesthetic agent is inserted between the tendons of the anterior tibial muscle and the extensor hallucis longus until it encounters the tibia (Fig. 17-9). It is then slightly withdrawn and 3 to 7 mL of local anesthetic agent is injected.

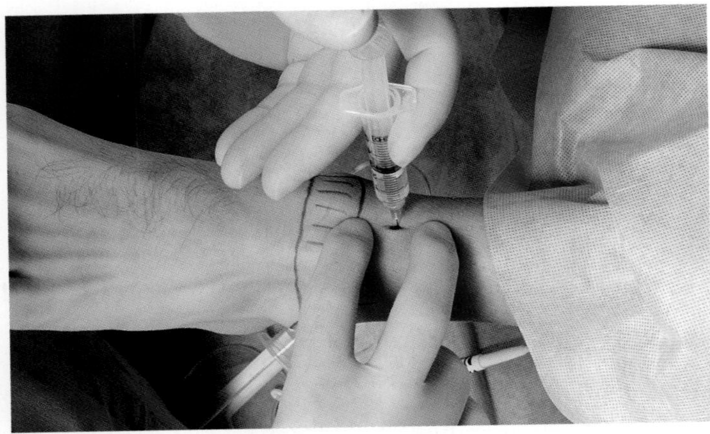

FIGURE 17-6 The two tendons are separated by the index and middle fingers of the nonoperative hand, and the skin and subcutaneous tissues are anesthetized.

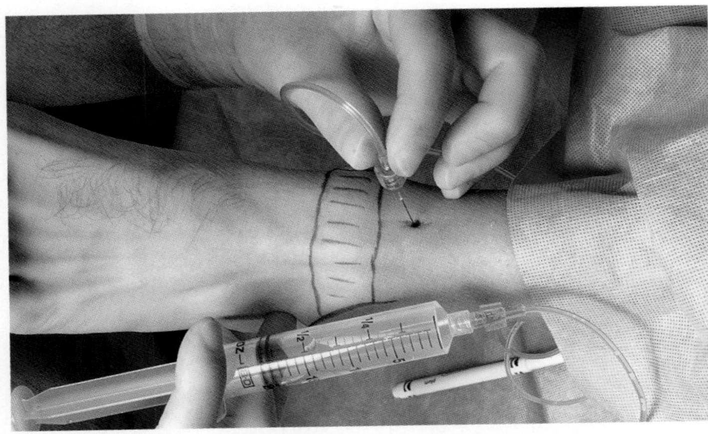

FIGURE 17-7 The local anesthetic is injected all the way down to the tibia to anesthetize the deep peroneal nerve.

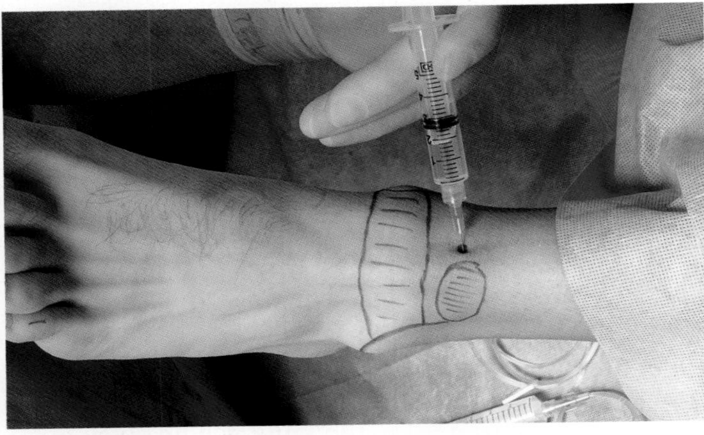

FIGURE 17-8 The area from the approach to the deep peroneal nerve to the fibula is anesthetized.

Without withdrawing the needle from the skin, it is now directed laterally between the skin and fascia layer toward the fibula (Fig. 17-10). The skin wheal raised during injection indicates that the injection is subcutaneous, yet superficial to the fascia. Like injection deep to the fascia, intradermal injection will lead to failed block.

The needle is now directed medially and subcutaneously toward the anterior aspect of the medial malleolus (Fig. 17-11). A skin wheal should be observed during injection on the

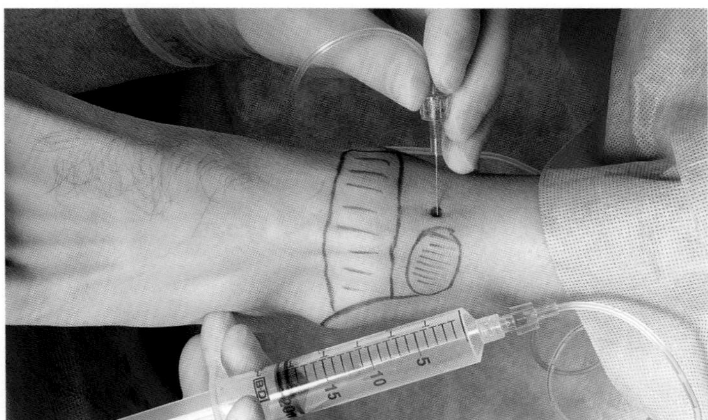

FIGURE 17-9 Local anesthetic agent is injected superficial to the fascia in the area indicated.

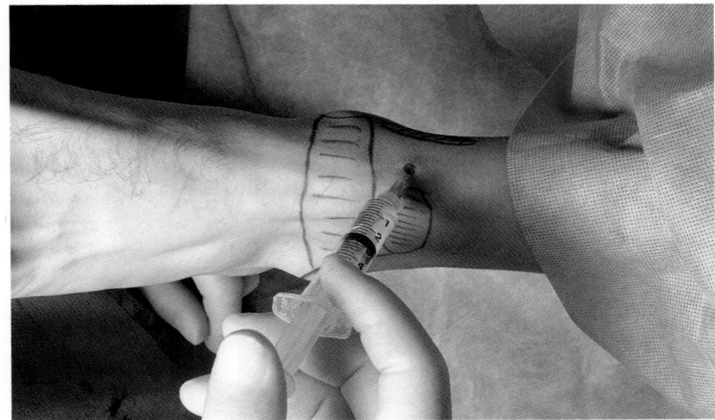

FIGURE 17-10 The area of the medial malleolus is anesthetized.

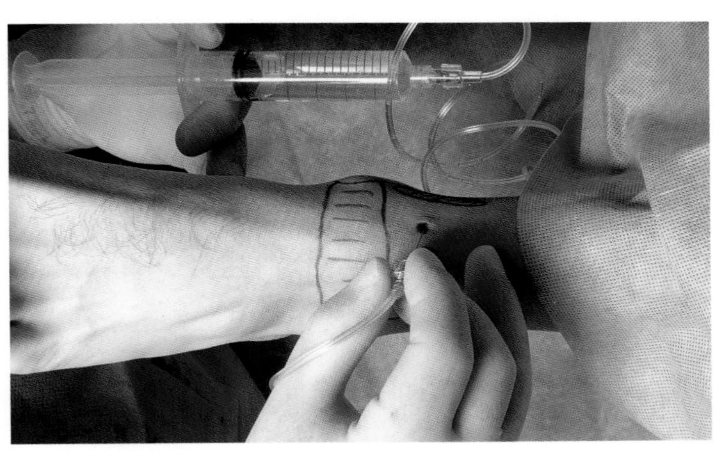

FIGURE 17-11 Local anesthetic is injected around the saphenous vein to anesthetize the saphenous nerve.

saphenous nerve subcutaneously and superficial to the fascia, around the saphenous vein.

Local Anesthetic Agent Choice

If a nerve stimulator is used to identify the tibial nerve at the ankle, 5 to 7 mL of 0.75% or 0.5% ropivacaine, or 0.5% bupivacaine, can be injected on each of the five nerves. It is important to remember that addition of epinephrine to the local anesthetic agent is absolutely contraindicated with an ankle block because this can seriously threaten the integrity of the blood supply to the foot, with devastating effects. Figure 16-1 shows that the main blood supply to the foot (i.e., the dorsal pedal artery and the posterior tibial artery) is situated close to the tibial nerve and the deep peroneal nerve.

(See ankle block movie on DVD.)

REFERENCE

1. Rickelman T, Boezaart AP: Ankle block. In Boezaart AP (ed): Anesthesia and Orthopaedic Surgery. New York, McGraw-Hill, 2006, pp 253-257.

Chapter 18

Thoracic Paravertebral Block

- **Single-Injection and Continuous Thoracic Paravertebral Blocks**

SINGLE-INJECTION AND CONTINUOUS THORACIC PARAVERTEBRAL BLOCKS

Introduction

The indications for thoracic paravertebral block for orthopedic surgery are relatively few, but include multiple rib fractures and flail chest. Other, nonorthopedic indications include unilateral mastectomy, unilateral thoracotomy, and unilateral laparotomy or retroperitoneal surgery.

The three potential problems with this block are intrapleural catheter placement with or without pneumothorax formation, and epidural or subarachnoid injection. Pneumothorax is not always a consequence of intrapleural needle or catheter placement and is a rare complication. Pneumothorax follows only if the visceral pleura is penetrated.

As is the case with all paravertebral blocks (cervical, thoracic, lumbar, and sacral), two principles apply with this block:

1. Because the nerve roots are covered with dura, sharp or thin needles should not be used for thoracic paravertebral or any other paravertebral block. Even a 22-gauge B-bevel needle is not advisable because of the danger of dural (or pleural) penetration and large-volume subarachnoid injection. As a general principle, large-bore Tuohy needles (16- to 18-gauge) are the best choice. Because of their design, these needles are the least likely to penetrate the dura or the pleura.
2. The indication for this block should be carefully selected and weighed against the possibility of doing a thoracic epidural block.

Figure 18-1, a postmortem photograph in a pig, the catheter can be seen coiled up in the paravertebral space.

When 1 mL of India ink is injected through a thoracic paravertebral catheter, spread is mainly localized (Fig. 18-2).

After a 10-mL India ink injection, however, it is clear that the spread is largely local but also

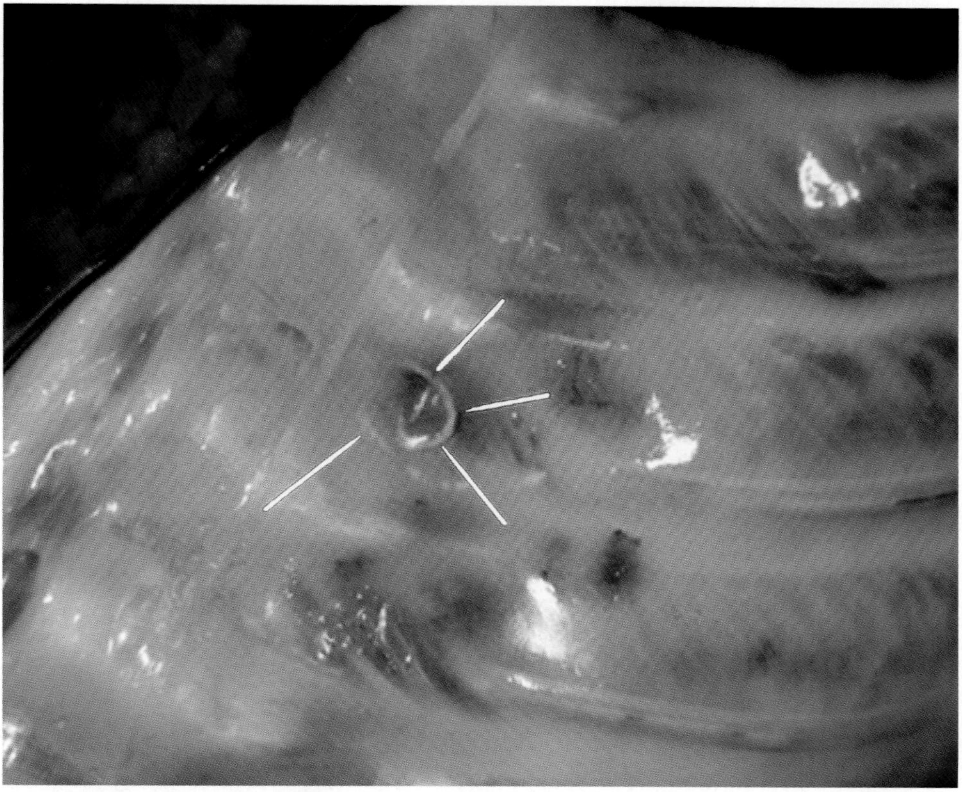

FIGURE 18-1 Postmortem dissection. The *arrows* indicate the coiling of a thoracic paravertebral catheter placed in an anesthetized pig. (Photographs courtesy Alex Fraser, MD.)

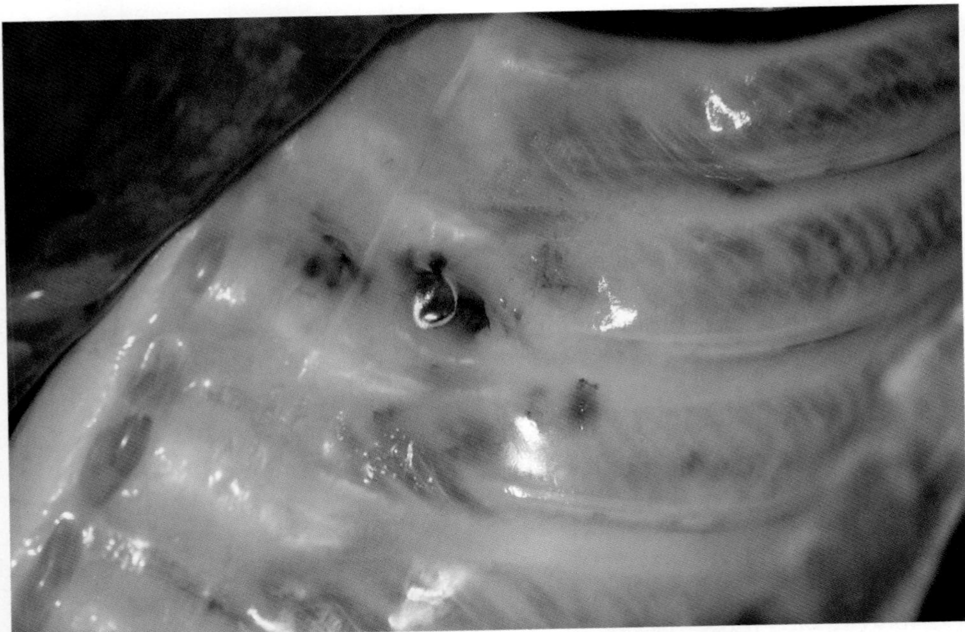

FIGURE 18-2 One milliliter of India ink is injected through the catheter.

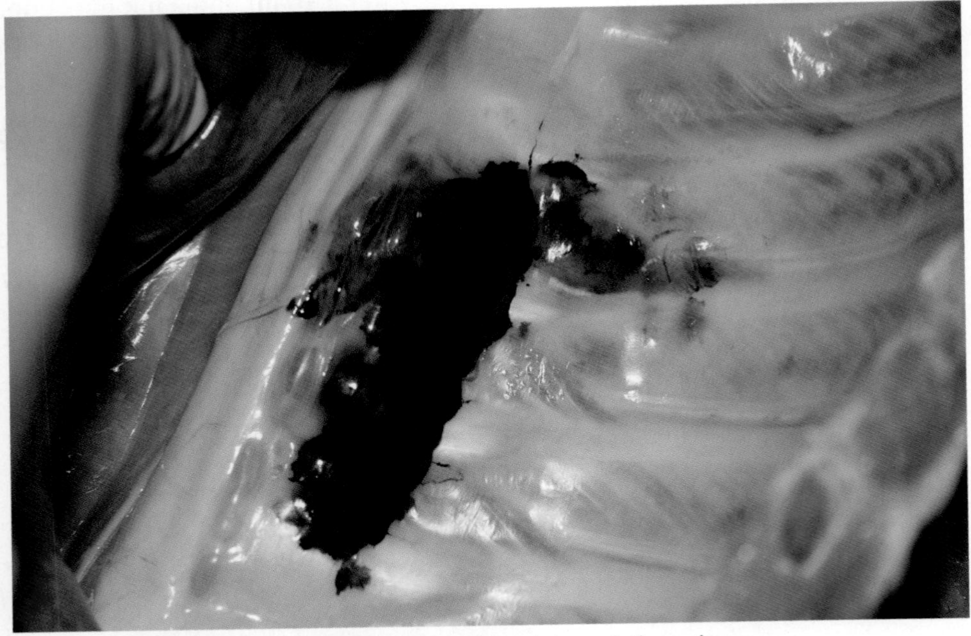

FIGURE 18-3 Ten milliliters of India ink is injected through the catheter.

cephalic and caudal (Fig. 18-3). Spread is also along the intercostal nerve. If the pleura were injured, as in the case with rib fractures, spread will also be intrapleural.

The noncontinuous block techniques using multiple-level injection sites have been the subject of controversy and contradictory research findings. Cheema and colleagues demonstrated a spread of approximately 4.6 segments after a 15-mL, one-level injection, whereas Naja and colleagues recently demonstrated that multiple-level injections provide wider and more reliable spread. A continuous thoracic paravertebral block placed at one level has the obvious advantage of long-term analgesia into the postoperative period, yet it may block insufficient levels to function as the sole anesthetic for major breast and other unilateral thoracic and upper abdominal surgery.

Specific Anatomic Considerations

The thoracic paravertebral space is wedge-shaped and bounded above and below by the heads and necks, respectively, of adjoining ribs (Fig. 18-4). The posterior wall is formed by the superior costotransverse ligament, which runs from the lower border of the transverse process above, to the upper border of the rib below. The posterolateral aspect of the vertebral body and the intervertebral foramen and its contents forms the base of this wedge. Anterolaterally, the space is limited by the parietal pleura.

Medially, the space communicates with the epidural space through the intervertebral foramen and, lateral to the tips of the transverse processes, it is continuous with the intercostal space.

Technique

The patient is placed in the lateral decubitus or sitting position (Fig. 18-5). Needle entry is approximately 3–4 cm lateral of the midpoint of the most appropriate thoracic vertebral dorsal spine—the fourth thoracic vertebra (T4) in the case of major breast surgery.

After thorough local anesthetic agent infiltration of the skin and subcutaneous tissue, a 17- or 18-gauge insulated Tuohy needle is advanced directly perpendicular to the skin until contact with the pars intervertebralis, articular column, or transverse process of the particular vertebra is established. This is typically at a depth of 4 to 6 cm from the skin surface (Fig. 18-6).

A nerve stimulator and loss-of-resistance-to-air syringe is attached to the needle and, while continuously testing for loss of resistance to air or 5% dextrose in water (D_5W), the needle is walked off the bony structure in an inferolateral (lateral and caudal) direction and advanced approximately 1 cm (but no more than 1.5 cm), ensuring that the bevel of the needle points laterally, away from the medial structures (Fig. 18-7). As the costotransverse ligament is penetrated, a "pop" can usually be felt, and there is loss of resistance to air or D_5W simultaneously with an intercostal muscle motor response. The "pop," however, is not consistently reliable. If saline is used to test for loss of resistance, the capacity for nerve stimulation is lost; D_5W is likely the better choice because it does not conduct electricity and hence preserves the ability to perform nerve stimulation. In theory, D_5W should provide a more distinct loss of resistance.

The nerve stimulator is set to a current output of 1 to 3 mA, a frequency of 2 to 5 Hz, and a pulse width of 200 to 300 μsec. Because the nerve roots are covered by dura, the paravertebral block is in essence an extradural or epidural block, and all the precautions used for epidural needle and catheter placement should be applied. Similarly, as for all the paravertebral blocks, relatively fine and sharp needles, such as 21-G needles should probably not be used because these are more likely to puncture the dura or pleura. A 17- or 18-G Tuohy needle is ideal for this application because they are designed to preclude dural puncture. When the tip of the needle nears the roots of an intercostal nerve, as indicated by loss of resistance, a "pop" as it penetrates the superior costotransverse ligament, and an intercostal muscle motor response, the needle is held steady while the syringe is removed. If a continuous nerve block is not required, the local anesthetic agent can now be injected through the needle.

When placing a T4 thoracic paravertebral block for breast surgery, it is helpful to ask an assistant to place his or her hand in the patient's ipsilateral axilla to detect the intercostal muscle motor response, which is obvious and easy to feel. The patient will also report the sensation of a pulsating electrical stimulus in the nipple.

The nerve stimulator lead is now attached to the proximal end of a 19- or 20-G stimulating catheter and its distal end inserted into the needle shaft (Fig. 18-8). With the nerve stimulator output kept constant at a current output that provides brisk twitching of the intercostal muscle, the catheter tip is advanced beyond the tip of the needle. If the muscle twitches stop or decrease during catheter advancement, the catheter tip has moved away from the nerves. The catheter is then carefully withdrawn so that its distal end is once again inside the needle shaft. A small adjustment is made to the needle (e.g., the needle is turned 45 degrees clockwise

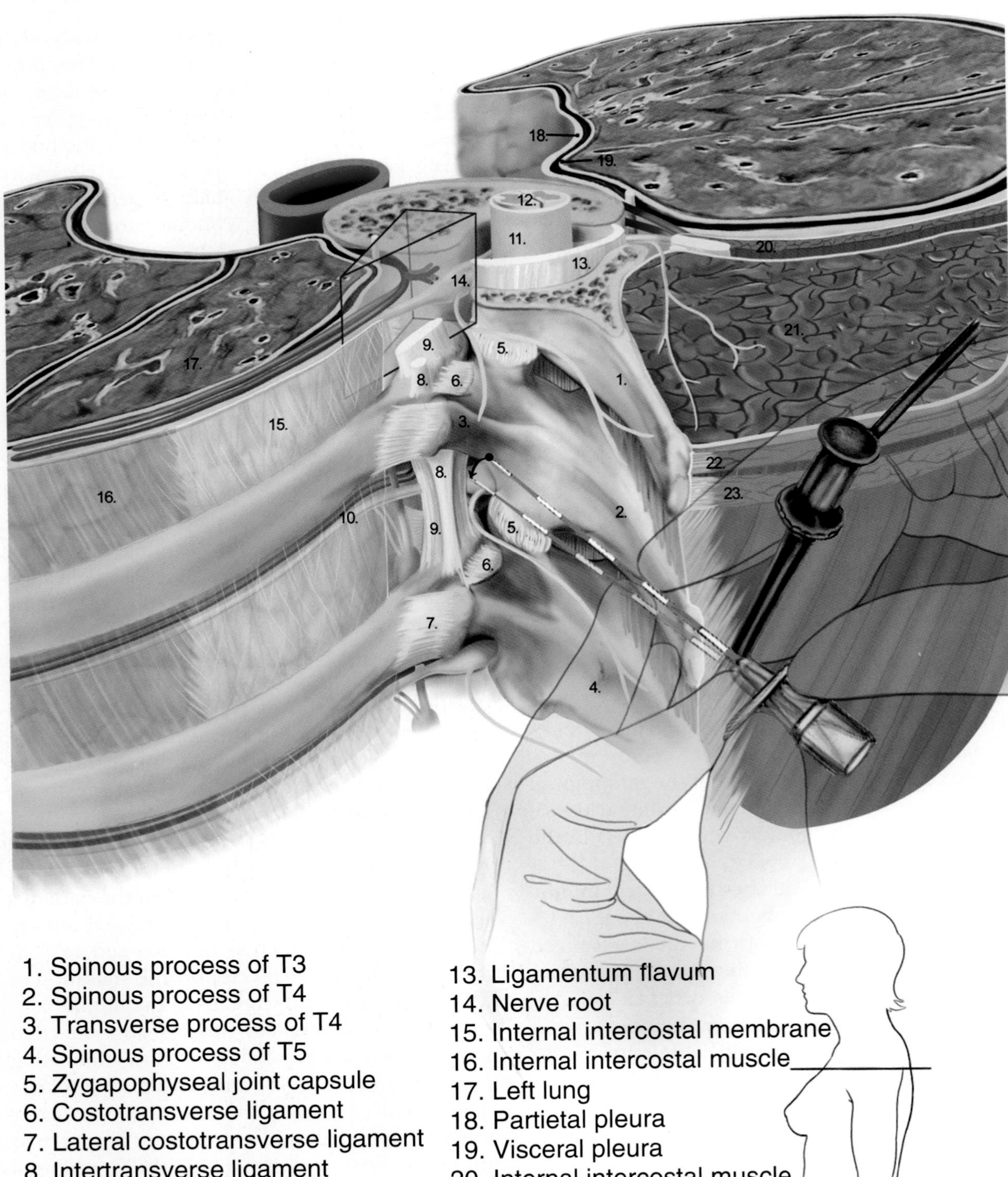

1. Spinous process of T3
2. Spinous process of T4
3. Transverse process of T4
4. Spinous process of T5
5. Zygapophyseal joint capsule
6. Costotransverse ligament
7. Lateral costotransverse ligament
8. Intertransverse ligament
9. Superior costotransverse ligament
10. Intercostal vein, artery and nerve
11. Dura mater
12. Spinal cord
13. Ligamentum flavum
14. Nerve root
15. Internal intercostal membrane
16. Internal intercostal muscle
17. Left lung
18. Partietal pleura
19. Visceral pleura
20. Internal intercostal muscle
21. Erector spinae muscle
22. Rhomboid major muscle
23. Trapezius muscle

FIGURE 18-4 Anatomy of the thoracic paravertebral space.

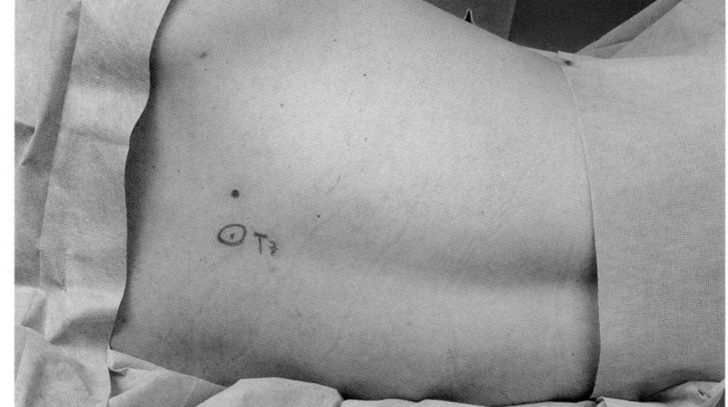

FIGURE 18-5 Surface anatomy for the thoracic paravertebral block. The *circle* indicates the dorsal spine of the seventh thoracic vertebra.

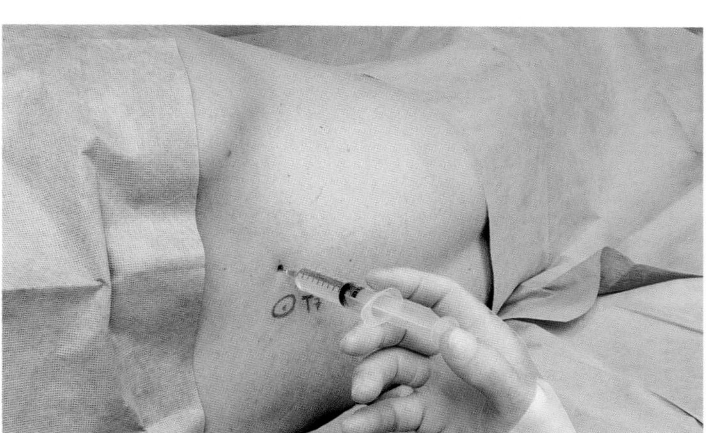

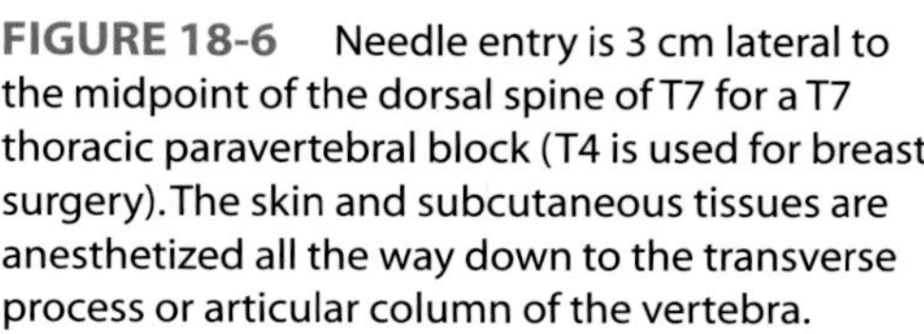

FIGURE 18-6 Needle entry is 3 cm lateral to the midpoint of the dorsal spine of T7 for a T7 thoracic paravertebral block (T4 is used for breast surgery). The skin and subcutaneous tissues are anesthetized all the way down to the transverse process or articular column of the vertebra.

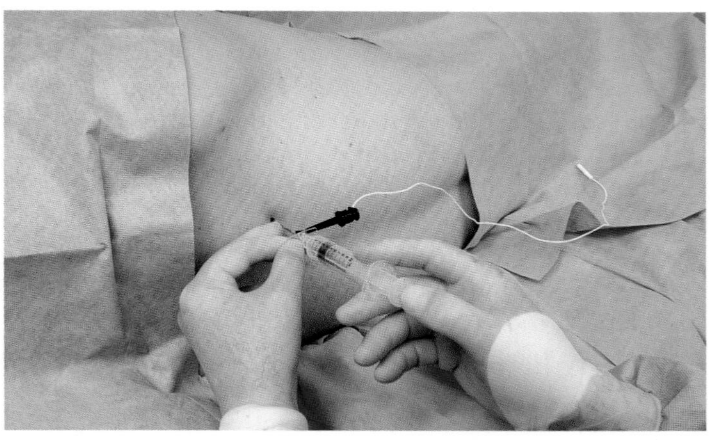

FIGURE 18-7 An insulated, 17- or 18-gauge Tuohy needle attached to a nerve stimulator and a loss–of–resistance-to-air syringe is advanced until contact is made with the transverse process or articular column of the vertebra. The needle is walked off the bony part in a caudal and lateral direction.

or counterclockwise, or moved 1 mm outward or inward), and the catheter is readvanced while the appropriate nerve stimulation is monitored. These maneuvers may be repeated until the intercostal muscles twitch briskly throughout catheter advancement. The advisability of withdrawing and readvancing the catheter is unclear and controversial, but the benefits of doing this outweigh the potential risk of catheter shearing. If it proves difficult to withdraw the catheter carefully, the needle should be removed with the catheter and the process restarted.

Too easy advancement of the catheter may suggest that the catheter does not lie within

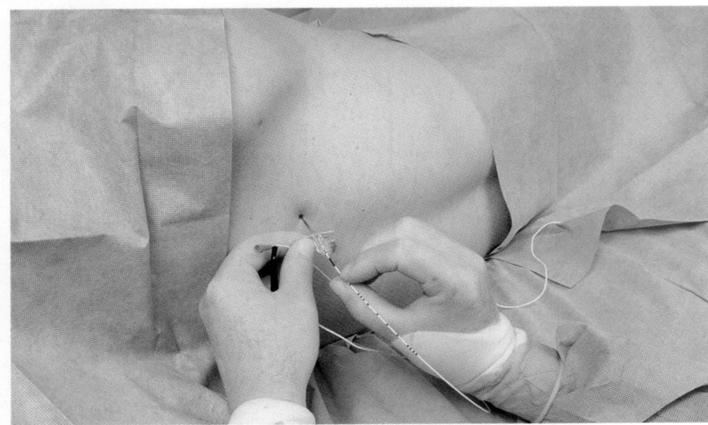

FIGURE 18-8 Once contact with the nerve root is made, a clear intercostal muscle motor response can usually be seen. Loss of resistance to air is also demonstrated. A stimulating catheter attached to a nerve stimulator is advanced through the needle while the operator continues to observe the intercostal motor response.

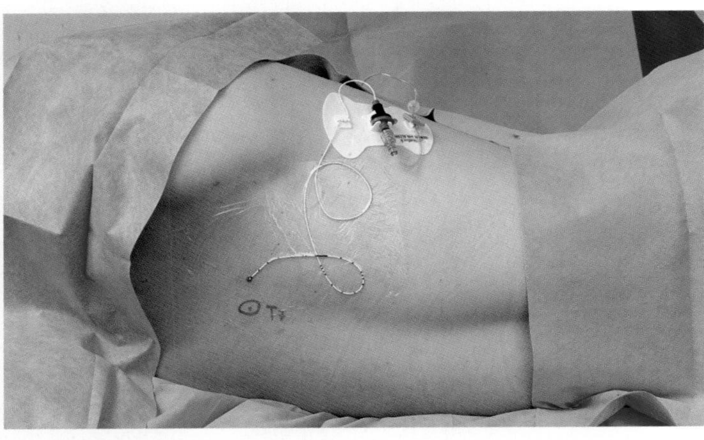

FIGURE 18-9 The needle is removed and the catheter is placed in a fixation device attached to the patient in an appropriate and comfortable position.

the paravertebral space. Advancement in the paravertebral space seems to be associated with more resistance than anesthesiologists are used to in the epidural space. Although this observation has never been quantified or scientifically confirmed, easy advancement may imply that the catheter is situated intrapleurally, epidurally, or intrathecally. If, during nerve stimulation, the motor response is lost, intrapleural placement is likely. If the motor response becomes bilateral or bizarre, the anesthesiologist should be suspect intrathecal or epidural catheter placement. A normal unilateral intercostal muscle motor response is strongly indicative of pure paravertebral catheter placement. The catheter is typically advanced 2 to 3 cm beyond the tip of the needle against some resistance, which invariably causes the catheter to coil up in the paravertebral space (see Fig. 18-1). Spread of injectant is first local (see Fig. 18-2), and then along the intercostal nerve (see Fig. 18-3). Finally, the injectant spreads up and down the paravertebral "gutter" (see Fig. 18-3).

To prevent dislodgement, the catheter may be tunneled subcutaneously to a convenient and stable position, although in the thoracic area this usually is not required. Leaving a small, 1- to 3-mm skin bridge after tunneling, as described previously (see Chapter 12), may make catheter removal easier.

After tunneling and securing the catheter, the Luer lock attachment device with a stimulator lead attachment may be attached to the catheter, and the nerve stimulator attached to the fixation device, which in turn is attached to a convenient position (Fig. 18-9).

While stimulating the nerve with the minimum current that produces appropriate muscle twitches, a test dose of 2 mL short-acting local anesthetic agent such as lidocaine 2% with epinephrine 1/200,000 is injected through the catheter. This should cause the muscle twitches to stop immediately, which is a further indicator of the proximity of the catheter to the nerve root. Inadvertent intrathecal injection should present with subarachnoid block, whereas intravascular injection should present with tachycardia. Because paravertebral block is essentially an epidural block, all the precautions for epidural block, including test dosing as described previously, should be used. There is no known low-dose test to distinguish true epidural block from paravertebral block. The main bolus dose should therefore be injected in 5-mL increments, followed by hemodynamic evaluation after each increment.

Local Anesthetic Agent Choice

Many local anesthetic combinations and dosages have been used for this block. The author prefers to use 20 mL of ropivacaine 0.5% to 0.75% or bupivacaine 0.5% as 5-mL incremental injections for intraoperative and postoperative analgesia if the block is combined with general anesthesia. Naja and colleagues proposed 0.26 mL/kg, but a dose per kilogram is probably not appropriate because body mass may not necessarily relate to paravertebral space size and longitudinal spread. Because Cheema and colleagues demonstrated a spread of approximately 4.6 segments after an injection of 15 mL, which is equivalent to a spread of approximately 1 segment per 2.5 to 3 mL, 20 mL should provide a spread of approximately 6 to 8 segments. However, segmental spread per volume injected is not consistent. Therefore, if it used as the sole anesthetic, larger volumes of up to 30 mL of the 0.5% solution may be required. If after 30 minutes the dermatomal spread of the bock is insufficient to cover the surgical area, a single-injection block can be done a few segments cephalic or caudal from the catheter as appropriate for the clinical situation.

Catheter placement and bolus injection is typically followed by a continuous infusion of bupivacaine 0.25% or ropivacaine 0.2% at an infusion rate of 5 mL/hour. Slow, incremental injection is strongly encouraged.

Although there is controversy about performing blocks in heavily sedated or anesthetized patients, and the literature is unclear on the relative or absolute risks of injury, blocks in awake patients may be preferable. When appropriate, this block may safely be placed under light sedation with midazolam in adult patients. General anesthesia may facilitate block placement in selected settings, such as in children, very anxious patients, or very painful preexisting conditions. A potent analgesic agent such as remifentanil 0.3 to 0.5 µg/kg, with careful respiratory monitoring, is sometimes indicated if painful conditions such as fractured ribs are present.

(See thoracic paravertebral block movie on DVD.)

SUGGESTED FURTHER READING

Boezaart AP, Raw RM: Thoracic paravertebral block: Sleeping Beauty or Big Bad Wolf. Reg Anesth Pain Med 2006;31:189-191.

Boezaart AP, Raw RM: Continuous thoracic paravertebral block for major breast surgery. Reg Anesth Pain Med 2006;31:470-476.

Naja ZM, El-Rajab M, Al-Tannir MA, et al: Thoracic paravertebral block: Influence of the number of injections. Reg Anesth Pain Med 2006;31:196-201.

Eason MJ, Wyatt R: Paravertebral thoracic block: A reappraisal. Anaesthesia 1979;34:638-642.

Greengrass R, O'Brian F, Lyerly K, et al: Paravertebral block for breast cancer surgery. Can J Anaesth 1996; 43:858-861.

Karmaker MJ: Thoracic paravertebral block. Anesthesiology 2001;95:771-780.

Lang SA: The use of a nerve stimulator for thoracic paravertebral block. Anesthesiology 2002;97:521.

Cheema SP, Ilsley D, Richardson J, Sabanathan S: A thermographic study of paravertebral analgesia. Anaesthesia 1995;50:118-121.

Lönnqvist P-A: Entering the paravertebral space age again. Acta Anaesthesiol Scand 2001;45:1-3.

Naja ZM, Lönnqvist P-A: Somatic paravertebral nerve blockade: Incidence of failed block and complications. Anaesthesia 2001;56:1184-1188.

Klein SM, Bergh A, Steele SM, et al: Thoracic paravertebral block for breast surgery. Anesth Analg 2000;90:1402-1405.

Buckenmaier CC 3rd, Klein SM, Nielsen KC, Steele SM: Continuous paravertebral catheter and outpatient infusion for breast surgery. Anesth Analg 2003;97:715-717.

Buckenmaier CC 3rd, Steele SM, Nielsen KC, et al: Bilateral continuous paravertebral catheters for reduction mammoplasty. Acta Anaesthesiol Scand 2002;46:1042-1045.

Cheema S, Richardson J, McGurgan P: Factors affecting spread of bupivacaine in the adult thoracic paravertebral space. Anaesthesia 2003;58:684-687.

Naja MZ, Zaide MF, El Rajab M, et al: Varying anatomical injection points within the thoracic paravertebral space: Effect on spread of solution and nerve blockade. Anaesthesia 2004;59:459-463.

Lang SA, Saito T: Thoracic paravertebral nerve block, nerve stimulator guidance and the endothoracic fascia. Anaesthesia 2005;60:930-931.

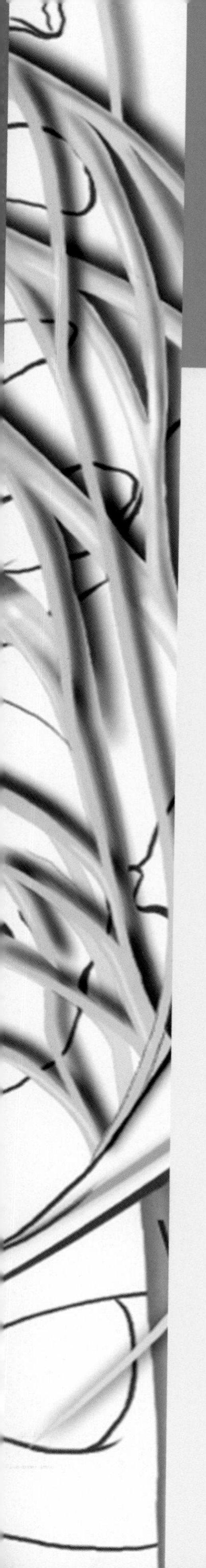

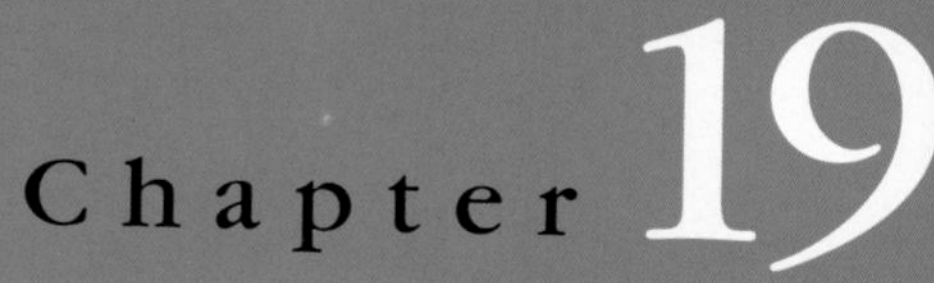

PITFALLS IN REGIONAL ANESTHESIA (and how to avoid them)

INTRODUCTION

While Regional Anesthesia (RA) is undoubtedly the most effective and efficient modality for the management of acute postoperative pain following most orthopedic and other surgery, it is not without pitfalls. The first important step in avoiding these pitfalls is to acknowledge their existence.

Because the shoulder joint in particular is such a complex joint, and the brachial plexus has to accommodate the complex movements of the upper limb, fixed only at the sterno-clavicular joint, it should not be surprising that blocks of the brachial plexus are responsible for the majority pitfalls in RA. This chapter is based on the existing literature, but also on the opinion of the author following experience over a number of years dealing with patients undergoing orthopedic surgery, and with medico-legal challenges. Some of the author's opinions may be perceived as controversial, but readers will hopefully find a few concepts that are useful—even if it is only to provoke them into identifying potential sources of complications based on their own training and experience.

To be successful with RA, there are four criteria that have to be met:

1. Valid indications for peripheral nerve blocks
2. The correct block(s) for the particular surgery
3. The correct nerve block technique
4. The correct equipment

Ignoring any one of these factors may lead to complications.

Indications

Indications for regional anesthesia (RA) are often the subject of debate, but if legal cases are reviewed, and the subject is discussed with people with experience in dealing with lawsuits, it often becomes clear that the patient did not need the block in the first place, or the block was of no benefit to the patient. Although there are many examples, and opinions vary greatly, a few common misconceptions exist. The two surgical procedures that most commonly fall into this category are subacromial decompression (SAD) or acromioplasty of the shoulder and arthroscopy and meniscectomy of the knee joint. These are typically not very painful procedures, which are easily managed with systemic analgesics. Yet they often lead to dissatisfaction, because of minor complications of the blocks. Furthermore, the indications for SAD are not always pure, and patients scheduled for this operation may actually have shoulder pain due to existing brachial plexopathy. In such cases a brachial plexus block, if anything, will make the condition worse.

The Correct Block

Hilton's Law

Hilton was a British surgeon and anatomist, born in 1804 in Castle Hedingham, Essex, and died in 1878. Hilton's law states, *"The nerve trunk innervating a joint also supplies the overlying skin and the muscles that move that joint."* Conversely, when a nerve innervates the muscles that move a joint, or the overlying skin of the joint, that nerve also innervates that joint. For RA it is important to understand this law of anatomy.

For example, the most perfect interscalene block will not provide anesthesia and analgesia for severe acute wrist pain. Neither would the perfect femoral nerve block provide complete anesthesia and analgesia for pain following total knee arthroplasty. There are many other examples. For the upper limb, the most common mistakes are interscalene block for anything other than shoulder surgery (because the C8 and T1 dermatomes are often not blocked). Other examples are supra- and infraclavicular block for shoulder surgery, suprascapular nerve block for gleno-humeral surgery, incomplete axillary block for any upper limb surgery, elbow block not involving the musculocutaneous or antebrachial cutaneous nerves for lower arm surgery, continuous infraclavicular nerve block for elbow and wrist surgery, etc. The entire brachial plexus innervates the elbow, wrist and shoulder.

Similarly, the entire lumbosacral plexus innervates all the major joints of the lower limb. Common mistakes in the lower limb are to do a femoral or lumbar plexus block for hip or knee surgery, a sciatic nerve block without saphenous nerve block for ankle surgery, etc. There is no single nerve block in the lower limb to treat the pain associated with surgery to any joint. An interscalene block may take care of the entire shoulder. This is because all the nerves are grouped together in the upper limb. This is not the case with the lumbosacral plexus, where the nerves are distributed over a wide area and a single nerve block cannot block the entire plexus. Unlike lower jaw surgery, for example, where a single block of the mandibular nerve will provide analgesia for lower jaw surgery, there is no single injection peripheral nerve block that will take care of any orthopedic surgical procedure. Epidural and spinal blocks for lower limb surgery and interscalene, supra and infraclavicular blocks in the upper limb are exceptions. But these are neuraxial or plexus blocks and not peripheral nerve blocks.

The Correct Technique

It is important to choose a technique, become familiar and confident with it and stay with this technique. It probably does not matter whether one routinely uses nerve stimulation, ultrasound, paresthesia or a combination of these techniques, as long as the technique is sound. The best block is most often the block one can do best.

Correct Equipment

The author joins Chelly in his plea for blunt large bore needles for nerve blocks (1,2). This is especially true for blocks around the dura and other fascia layers like the pleura. Also, blunt large bore needles cannot penetrate nerve fascicles, and extra-fascicular intraneural injections are probably harmless. The Tuohy needle has been specifically designed not to penetrate tissue like the dura and it has certainly stood the test of time. Anesthesiologists have been using these needles successfully for many decades now, and most anesthesiologists would feel very uncomfortable in using anything but a 16- to 18-guage Tuohy needle for epidural blocks. Yet, the same anesthesiologists will not hesitate to use a 22-guage B-beveled needle to perform a single-injection paravertebral block, whether at the cervical, thoracic, lumbar or sacral level. This ignores the fact, or perhaps signifies ignorance of the fact, that the dura extends well down the nerve roots into the paravertebral space. Put differently, the perineuriums of all the nerve fascicles join together at the root level to form the dura. An intra-root injection, therefore, becomes an intra-fascicular (or subdural) injection, of which the extracellular fluid is similar to the cerebrospinal fluid (CSF) and connects to it. High pressure will cause the injectate not only to spread to the CSF but also to the spinal cord. Paravertebral blocks are performed just outside the dura, or extradural, or peridural or epidural and the same rules applying to epidural blocks (large bore Tuohy needles, lidocaine test dose, fractionated injection, etc.) should therefore apply to any paravertebral block. Neglect of this fact has lead to many tragic complications in RA, mainly spinal cord injuries (3,4), although most of these cases never reach the anesthesia literature, since they are engulfed by the legal system and usually settled out of court. Defense lawyers generally do not allow their clients to publish the cases in fear of incrimination, and because these cases do not reach closure in the courts, they do not reach the closed claim studies and publications.

WHERE NOT TO DO BLOCKS

There are several areas in the body where blocks are traditionally done, but which may be wise to avoid unless there are no alternatives and thus absolutely necessary.

Injury to a nerve can be due to direct trauma to the nerve, toxicity, or due to ischemia (5,6,7). Ischemia, in turn, may be due to pressure or traction on the nerve or vasoconstriction. If we avoid direct trauma to the nerve and avoid blocks in places where the nerves are in a confined space or closed compartment, nerve damage might be even more rare than they are. We should be careful to avoid traction and surgical trauma such as diathermy injury intra-operatively. This is especially applicable to shoulder surgery.

With blocks of nerves that are in relatively confined spaces we add volume to the space in which the nerve is situated by injecting local anesthetic agent into that space. We may also cause some bleeding and hematoma in the area. If we now further cause vasoconstriction by adding epinephrine to the injected anesthetic, we have the potential for nerve ischemia and nerve injury.

The places that we probably need to avoid are:

1. Intervertebral Neuroforamen

This is the area between vertebrae where the nerve roots exit the spinal canal. It is never necessary in RA to place needles or catheters in these foramina. In chronic pain practice is it a frequently applied technique.

Intraforaminal placement of a needle is possible during interscalene block if the incorrect technique is used. The techniques that Winnie has described in 1970 (8), does not facilitate entrance into the neuroforamen. According to the description of this technique the needle should to be advanced mesiad, posteriorly and *caudally*. If the needle enters perpendicular to the skin in slender people, and the caudal direction is ignored, it is conceivable that the neuroforamen may be entered. This latter approach may have originated from the later description of Alon Winnie (9) in which he described a technique similar to that of his previous publication, but he added "*perpendicular to the skin in all plains*." This became the standard technique for some practitioners. This is unfortunate; since the 1975 description was never intended to apply to interscalene block but to cervical plexus block. Most practitioners, however, have, converted to the longitudinal (10) or lateral (11) approach to the interscalene space. If this technique is used, it is not possible to enter the neuroforamen with the needle.

It is, however, practically possible to place a catheter into the neuroforamen during continuous paravertebral block (12). Intraforaminal catheter placement during thoracic, lumbar or sacral paravertebral block may also be possible, which is another reason why all paravertebral blocks should be regarded as epidural blocks.

2. Supraclavicular Area

Large studies have shown supraclavicular block to be safe and effective (13). Because the supraclavicular block does not usually include the suprascapular nerve, it is not used for shoulder surgery—especially if the surgery involves the rotator cuff. The reason for not advocating this block as a routine block for distal arm surgery, is that the nerves are all bundled together where they cross the first rib deep to the clavicle. The middle and anterior scalene muscles are posterior and anterior to the nerve bundle, and further anterior is the subclavian artery. While this confined space may be the very reason why this approach is so easy to perform and so successful, it may also be the cause of volume-induced pressure and ischemia to the nerve.

Although the above argument has not been tested by research, and this block has stood the test of time, it seems prudent to perform the supraclavicular block only when a fast onset and dense block is sought and not to use it as routine. The feared higher incidence of pneumothorax resulting as a complication of supraclavicular block has not been substantiated by research, and this complication may be minimized even further by the increased use of ultrasound. In the infraclavicular area the cords of the brachial plexus, however, are situated in a wide-open space and the infraclavicular block should probably be a better alternative.

3. Sulcus Ulnaris

It is obvious that the nerve here is in a very confined compartment, and performing a nerve block here almost always leads to ischemic nerve injury.

4. Carpal Tunnel at the Wrist

This is where the median nerve crosses deep to the retinaculum at the wrist. The median nerve is a large nerve in a very confined space and local anesthetic agent injected here will invariably result in ischemic nerve injury if the "roof" of the carpal tunnel is not immediately removed, as is often done following this block by hand surgeons when performing carpal tunnel release surgery.

5. Transgluteal Approach to the Sciatic Nerve

The cadaver dissection in Figure 14-2 shows the area of the nerve where the piriformis muscle has been removed and it clearly shows the compression to the sciatic nerve by the piriformis muscle (Figure 14-2). The subgluteal approach to the sciatic nerve is probably a better approach, since the nerve in this area is not in a confined space. At the popliteal area the nerve is also not in a confined compartment and these two blocks should be better alternatives than the classical transgluteal or "Labat" or "Winnie" approaches. The only exception would be if the surgeon were to convert the subgluteal or popliteal areas into confined compartments by applying a tourniquet for a long period of time to these areas. The transgluteal approach may be a better choice if it is essential to also block the posterior cutaneous nerve of the thigh.

The best choices for sciatic nerve block are probably the popliteal and the subgluteal approaches, and the choice between these two should probably be dictated by the planned position of the tourniquet.

6. Common Peroneal Nerve

The common peroneal nerve crosses the head of the fibula, and in this area it is very prone to injury. Not only is the nerve in a tight compartment, it is also prone to traction injury (for example after valgus knee repair) and external pressure (for example by leg braces—especially in the insensate leg after a peripheral or neuraxial nerve block). There is not many clinical applications for this block, as there is no clinical use for a pure ulnar nerve block.

To summarize, the places to avoid for routinely doing nerve blocks are anywhere where the nerves are bundled together in a tight compartment. These locations are the very places where blocks are usually easy to do, and the blocks are successful, due to the very fact that the nerves are in a tight compartment. Furthermore, ultrasound studies have taught us that it is difficult to place a needle intrafascicular if the nerve is not fixed. In these tight compartments the nerves are usually fixed.

Patients are especially vulnerable to nerve injury after shoulder surgery. It is now becoming clear that the nerve block is very seldom the cause of nerve injury and surgery, especially shoulder, hip and knee surgery, is increasingly being recognized as a cause of nerve injury (14,15,16,17).

EPINEPHRINE (ADRENALINE)

Addition of 1/200,000 to 1/400,000 epinephrine to the local anesthetic solution shortens the onset time of the block, make the block last longer when short-acting drugs are used, and increases the density of the block. The reason for these actions is nerve ischemia.

In a classical experiment on rat sciatic nerve, Selander (18) demonstrated in 1985 that intraneural injection of saline and 0.5% bupivacaine caused no permanent axonal degeneration. On the other hand, bupivacaine 1% without epinephrine or bupivacaine 0.5% with 1/200,000 epinephrine caused axonal degeneration in almost 100% of cases. These experimental findings have been verified subsequently (19, 20).

Because ischemia is the main cause of nerve injuries and decreased neural blood flow, it seems logical that whatever the reason for using epinephrine, it does nothing good for the nerve. If a shorter onset time and denser block is required, more modern or more appropriate drugs can be used. And if a longer acting block is needed, a continuous nerve block can be placed. Apart from being potentially dangerous to the nerve, epinephrine is not really necessary. This should provide a strong incentive not to use it routinely.

Epinephrine is, however, regularly used as an "intravascular marker," but the true value of this should be seriously questioned.

EXISTING NEUROPATHY

The issue of existing brachial plexitis or neuropathy is poorly understood and under appreciated, although the obvious causes of neuropathy, such as diabetes, Sharcot-Mary Tooth disease (SMT) and trauma are well understood. These conditions and others where the pathology is well documented are not contraindication to nerve block. However, undocumented and undiagnosed neuropathies can cause embarrassment.

When a nerve is already injured or under pressure in a tight compartment or area of impingement or traction, further pressure often causes persistent clinical symptoms of neuropathy. This often ranges from persistent numbness to severe neuropathic pain that is often blamed on the block.

Existing Brachial Plexopathy

Patients with clinical or sub-clinical brachial plexopathy may present with non-descript pain in the shoulder and arm. This can vary from severe shoulder pain, to paresthesia or dysesthesia in the arm and hand. The patient is typically referred to a shoulder surgeon who schedules the patient for arthroscopy of the shoulder. Patients with existing brachial plexopathy may present with pain distal to the elbow, which is not a symptom of *bona fide* shoulder pathology.

The mechanism of the brachial plexopathy is not clear, but is thought to be due to pressure, and consequently ischemia to the brachial plexus where it crosses the first rib and where the clavicle may impinge upon it. This condition is thought to be more common in females than in males. The space between the first rib and the clavicle is larger in males than in females, which probably explains the gender difference. The impingement is chronic and low-grade, usually just enough to cause pain in the shoulder, arm, and hand. It usually involves the inferior trunks of the brachial plexus more than the upper trunks or divisions. Interscalene or supraclavicular injection of a large volume of local anesthetic agent, where the brachial plexus crosses the first rib and is already under potential stress, may cause further pressure and ischemia to the nerves. If epinephrine is added it may aggravate the nerve ischemia. A small hematoma in the area would increase the pressure even more.

Since *bona fide* shoulder pathology does not typically cause pain distal to the elbow, it may be wise to ask the patient about the distribution of the pain, and other symptoms. If the patient admits to these symptoms distal to the elbow, we should be cautious and rather offer them post-operative blocks once the pathology is clear. These patients sometimes end up getting subacromial decompression surgery, while subacromial impingement has not been the original pathology.

It is relatively easy to perform continuous or single injection blocks postoperatively. If a nerve stimulator has to be used, it can be painful to evoke a motor response after surgery. It can then be helpful to use 0.3-0.5 μg/kg remifentanil as a bolus intravenous injection at 1 to 3 minute intervals as required (21). Propofol or alfentanil can also be used.

If a cervical paravertebral block is used, a single injection or a continuous block can be done with loss-of-resistance to air as the only indicator of correct placement. An 18-G insulated Tuohy needle should be used for continuous or single-injection CPVB, and not a 22-G stimulating needle designed for peripheral nerve block. An interscalene block can also be done without nerve stimulation by using ultrasound.

Frozen Shoulder

Frozen shoulder or adhesive capsulitis is a common condition of which anesthesiologists should have some understanding. It is classified as primary (idiopathic) or secondary adhesive capsulitis. The secondary form is caused by trauma, surgery, infection, etc. in the joint and is due to adhesions in the glenohumeral or subacromial joints. Because the capsule of the joint is not involved, the glenohumeral joint does not "freeze" in the anatomical or functional position. Primary adhesive capsulitis, on the other hand is due to a fibroblast proliferation of the joint capsule. Microscopically there are collagen deposits similar to that in Dupuytren's contracture of the hand. But while Dupuytren's contracture is common in males, primary frozen shoulder is more common in females (22,23,24,25). The shoulder "freezes" in the functional anatomical position of abduction, flexion and internal rotation.

Primary adhesive capsulitis is the most common and the least understood form of frozen shoulder. Lloyd and Lloyd (26), Hill (27), and Reeves (28), have all suggested three phases of primary adhesive capsulitis based on clinical observations.

- Phase I is characterized by localized shoulder pain. The patient develops painful range of motion and exhibits progressive loss of motion.
- Phase II is characterized by diffuse shoulder pain with progressive loss of motion secondary to pain or to the development of a capsular pattern described by movement limitations. Most restricted is external rotation, followed by abduction and internal rotation. This phase slowly progresses to phase III.
- In Phase III, the patient continues to have decreased range of motion. Patients with phase III adhesive capsulitis do suffer pain, but placing the arm in the functional position of abduction, internal rotation and flexion relieves this pain.

A patient may consult a shoulder surgeon at any stage of the progression of the disease, which is a self-limiting disease, and the shoulder stiffness usually subsides after three to five years (22-28). The personality profile of patients with primary adhesive capsulitis is typical with 75% being women of whom 84% falls into the 40-59 years age group. Most patients (66%) have no other medical problems (29). Hand dominance seems to have no role in the development of primary adhesive capsulitis.

Finally, and perhaps most important to anesthesiologists, because of difficulty in the physical examination of frozen shoulder, a coexisting neuropathic process may go undetected (30). Patients with primary frozen shoulder will often, when asked how they relieve the pain, say that they keep the arm on pillows in the functional position. When the arm is then carried at the side, the scapula rotates externally, and pseudo-winging of the scapula develops (personal communication Dr. J F de Beer—shoulder surgeon, Cape Shoulder Institute, Cape Town, South Africa). The net effect of this is that the distance from the cervical vertebrae to the coracoid increases (31), resulting in chronic light traction on the brachial plexus—most severely where the brachial plexus crosses the first rib. As a result, the patient presents with pain in the shoulder and arm. Doing nerve blocks, especially blocks in the area of the first rib (interscalene and supraclavicular), may cause more pressure and more ischemia to the brachial plexus, especially if epinephrine is added to the local anesthetic agent. The "double crush" mechanism of nerve injury may also explain the frequency of nerve injury in the case of frozen shoulder.

It may therefore be prudent to avoid doing blocks in the area of the first rib in the case of primary adhesive capsulitis. There should be no problem doing blocks in the case of secondary capsulitis, because the shoulder does not freeze in the functional position but with the arm at the side of the patient. There is thus no rotation of the scapula and traction to the brachial plexus in secondary adhesive capsulitis, and consequently no danger of further injury the brachial plexus.

Because of our poor results with continuous interscalene blocks in patients with primary adhesive capsulitis, we started to use the continuous cervical paravertebral block for the management of peri-operative pain and assisting with physical therapy some years ago (32). Since starting to do CCPVB for capsulotomy for primary adhesive capsulitis we have had excellent results. In theory, that could be attributed to the fact that the CCPVB is done more proximally, away from the area where the brachial plexus crosses the first rib.

Subacromial Decompression

Subacromial impingement is probably over-diagnosed and over-treated. Although this possibility has not been proven by research, there is a strong suspicion that a substantial number of patients that present for subacromial decompression (SAD) actually have existing brachial plexopathy causing the pain in their shoulders. The diagnostic test for subacromial impingement is to inject local anesthetic agent into the subacromial space. If the pain then subsides, it presumably provides "proof" of subacromial impingement and the patient is scheduled for subacromial decompression.

It has been demonstrated some time ago (33,34), that in the majority of patients, if an invasive measure, such as an injection is used for the treatment of pain, the pain will subside even if the origin of the pain is remote from the site of injection. This has been demonstrated by immediate disappearance of pain when a local anesthetic is injected around the supraspinatus muscle in patients with referred shoulder pain due to liver pathology (33). It is therefore fair to assume that referred shoulder pain caused by brachial plexopathy will, like pain due to subacromial impingement, also subside after subacromial injection of a local anesthetic agent. This notion has not been evaluated by clinical research but it may be prudent for anesthesiologists *not* to assume that all patients with positive subacromial injection tests have subacromial impingement. We have to assume that some of these patients have existing brachial plexopathy. At the very least, anesthesiologists have to be careful with these patients especially if they also present with pain and neurological symptoms distal to the elbow.

Because of this uncertainty, we have adopted the following practice:

Subacromial decompression is generally not painful surgery requiring a major nerve block. When anesthetizing a patient scheduled for SAD with no proof of other shoulder pathology, the patient should be asked about pain, or neurological symptoms distal to the elbow. If the patient does have these neurological symptoms distal to the elbow, it may be wise not to do a preoperative block on this patient. We can then offer a postoperative block to the patient, should it be necessary and the pain difficult or impossible to control with systemic analgesics.

Some practitioners may prefer to use a nerve stimulator for post-operative blocks, which is perfectly acceptable, but the patient may suffer extreme pain during a stimulated motor response. Remifentanil 0.3-0.5 μg/kg as a single or repeated bolus intravenous injection has been very successful to alleviate this pain in the experience of this author. If the choice is a single injection or continuous interscalene block, it can be done with ultrasound assistance, while CCPVB can be done with ultrasound or loss of resistance to air techniques.

Hereditary Neuropathy with Liability to Pressure Palsies (HNPP)

Hereditary neuropathy with liability to pressure palsies (HNPP) is a poorly understood condition and most anesthesiologists are not aware of its existence (35,36). It is an autosomal dominant inherited disorder characterized by a tendency to develop focal neuropathy after trivial trauma (such as nerve blocks). Studies on teased nerve fibers show sausage-shaped myelin sheaths on ultrasound (35,36). Diffusely enlarged peripheral nerves can be demonstrated outside entrapment sites with ultrasound. The incidence of HNPP has been estimated to be 1/100,000 of the population but it is probably significantly higher (37). The patient often also has hyporeflexia, talipes cavus, and a family history of peripheral nerve palsies. The condition is suspected when electrodiagnostic studies show one or more entrapment neuropathies superimposed on a background of sensimotor polyneuropathy. There are no specific electrodiagnostic criteria, but predominant slowing of distal nerve conduction velocity may indicate underlying HNPP. The diagnosis is confirmed when the genetic defect responsible for the disease is demonstrated: a deletion of chromosome 17p11.2-12 (38). A high index of suspicion exists if there is a family history of multiple pressure neuropathies such as carpal tunnel, tarsal tunnel, ulnar nerve entrapment, or a personal history of multiple entrapment neuropathies.

The motor palsy following trivial trauma to the nerve is usually permanent and there is no sensory loss. The nerve block is often blamed for this condition.

Thoracic Outlet Syndrome

There are several well-recognized peripheral neurological syndromes that affect the upper extremities. These include:

1. Herniated disk and hypertrophic spondylosis of the cervical vertebrae.
2. Brachial plexus compression by a cervical rib or elongated C7 transverse process.
3. Ulnar nerve entrapment in the cubital tunnel of the elbow or Guyton's canal in the wrist.
4. Median nerve entrapment by the pronator teres muscle in the forearm or the carpal tunnel.

Each of these conditions has characteristic location patterns or radiating pain, tenderness, and muscle weakness, and some have diagnostic radiological and electrodiagnostic features. The correct diagnosis can usually be made by history, examination, and ancillary tests and the condition can be documented. These conditions should not pose contra-indications to regional anesthesia, if the areas where the nerves are under pressure are avoided.

However, there remains a group of underdiagnosed patients who present with moderate to severe pain, paresthesia, weakness and dysfunction of the arm and hand that do not fall within these specific clinical entities. The patients are usually young and predominantly female. The pain typically radiates from the scapula down the arm to the hand—again, distal to the elbow. The pain is often generalized. The theory, which is thus far unproven, is that scalene muscles are developed out of proportion to the rest of the musculature in young females and these scalene muscles compresses the brachial plexus as it lies through them. Most of the arm and shoulder pain spontaneously disappear at the age of

25-30 years. Patients with this condition often have lax ligaments and at a young age of around 18-20 years old, present for capsulorraphy. This is usually the first of a series shoulder surgeries.

(In a small, as yet unreported personal series of 12 patients, excellent results were obtained by botulinum toxin (Botox) injections into one of the scalene muscles. All the patients remained pain free for 4-6 months and first rib resection was done after the third to fourth Botox injection. This needs further research).

Anesthesiologists should be careful when offering continuous or single injection brachial plexus blocks in young female patients scheduled for capsulorraphy, capsulotomy or other shoulder operations for which the indications are not perfectly clear. These young women, because they are in the optimal child bearing age, tend to have relatively lax ligaments and they often present for capsulorraphy or capsule plication due to "lax ligaments" and subluxation. Unfortunately, this usually does not improve the shoulder pain, but because the primary cause of the shoulder pain and pain in the arm and hand is pressure on the brachial plexus, brachial plexus blocks are often afterwards blamed for the neurological symptoms. Again, young female patients with a history of multiple shoulder surgery and pain distal to the elbow should be approached with caution when considering brachial plexus blocks (39,40,41,42,43). Subluxation per se, however, can also cause brachial plexus injury.

OTHER CONSIDERATIONS

Compartment Syndrome

Compartment syndrome occurs when excessive pressure develops within a closed fascial compartment, and renders the tissue within the affected compartment ischemic (44). In orthopedics compartment syndrome occurs in the upper extremities, lower extremities, and in the gluteal region. These syndromes have multiple causes, but they are most commonly due to trauma and fractures. Aggressive emergency treatment is essential to prevent the patient from losing a limb.

The most common cause of compartment syndrome is a fracture. The syndrome is often caused by higher energy, closed fractures, but can also occur with lower-energy forces and open fractures. There is often a history of direct blunt injury to the limb, such as a tibia struck by the bumper of a car. They occur most commonly with closed tibia fractures, and are particularly common in proximal tibia fractures.

Vascular injury can also lead to compartment syndrome. Arterial bleeding in a closed compartment can readily cause excessive intracompartmental pressure in it. Reperfusion after prolonged ischemia can cause excessive swelling leading to a compartment syndrome. This typically occurs after a revascularization procedure. Compartment syndrome can also result from external causes such as casts, constrictive dressings, or "antishock" lower extremity garments. Compartment syndrome has also been reported in patients subjected to prolonged lithotomy position in obstetric and urological reconstructive operations. The basic physiological mechanism is excessive intracompartmental pressure, which causes microcirculatory failure of perfusion of the tissues in the compartment. As the pressure increases, it eventually exceeds the arteriolar pressure causing a rapid failure of the local capillary anastamoses and blood flow to the tissues ceases. Excessive pressure inhibits venous return, further blocking flow within the compartment.

Tissue damage depends on the duration of the compartment syndrome. Muscle tissue can usually survive four hours of ischemia, but more than eight hours of ischemia causes irreversible damage. Peripheral nerves will continue to conduct normally for up to one hour of complete ischemia and will survive without injury when subjected to four hours of ischemia, but will be irreversibly damaged after eight hours.

The characteristic symptom of compartment syndrome is progressive, unrelenting pain out of proportion to the underlying condition. These patients frequently report severe increases of pain with a fairly rapid onset. This is mainly a clinical diagnosis, especially in patients at risk. The leg is firm and often shiny. The earliest and most reliable physical sign is severe exacerbation of tenderness of the affected compartment by manual compression or passive stretching of the muscles within the compartment. A gentle squeeze of the calf or passive flexion of the toe or ankle is excruciatingly painful.

Because compartment syndrome is due to a microcirculatory failure, the *peripheral pulses are usually intact*. Anesthesiologists often do not realize this extremely important fact. Some incorrectly believe that if the arterial pulses are present, compartment syndrome is ruled out. This is in direct contrast to an acute arterial thrombosis. The misconception that the legs of patients with compartment syndrome are pulseless needs to be corrected. The pulses are often bounding and only very late in a compartment syndrome, when pressures are dramatically elevated, does the affected extremity become pulseless. Due to increased perfusion to the subcutaneous tissues surrounding the compartment, the leg is pink and shiny, in contrast to a mottled, pallorous extremity seen in cases of arterial thrombosis. Early in a compartment syndrome, the peripheral nerves function normally. It is not until the compartment syndrome has advanced that patients complain of tingling and numbness. Finally, in advanced cases, the limb becomes paralytic.

In an alert patient with a firm painful leg that becomes more painful with gentle passive stretching, the diagnosis should be made immediately and emergency fasciotomy should be performed. In less obvious cases, compartment pressure can be measured. Once the diagnosis of compartment syndrome is established, the affected compartment should be decompressed immediately.

The most common compartment syndromes are those in leg and forearm. Because the crucial window of opportunity to save the limb by decompression is within four to eight hours and because most peripheral nerve blocks will last four to eight hours, regional anesthesia or peripheral nerve block must be avoided in these patients, since it will mask the most important and often only symptom of compartment syndrome namely pain. After fixation of fractures, that pain usually subsides and gets progressively less. Any exacerbation of pain after fractures have been fixed should be regarded with great caution. (This section on compartment syndrome has been adapted from reference 44).

Failed or incomplete blocks

Arguably, the most common "complication" of nerve blocks is failed or incomplete block. Possibly the most common reason for failure is not poor technique but blocking the wrong nerve or not blocking all the nerves for the planned surgery.

This might seem very basic, but to do the appropriate block or blocks for the surgery, is probably the most commonly overlooked or neglected issue in regional anesthesia. Common examples are:

1. Performing a continuous cervical paravertebral block for shoulder surgery on the C8 or T1 level accepting a triceps muscle motor response. With the initial relatively large bolus, the C5 and C6 roots needed for shoulder surgery may be reached, but the secondary block the days after surgery, with a relatively low infusion volume of say 5 ml/hr, does not reach the C5 nerve root and the block is classified as failed.
2. Cervical paravertebral block for elbow and wrist surgery accepting a biceps muscle (C5) motor response. This leads to a good initial block but the next day when the low infusion volume is used, the patient has a numb shoulder and painful elbow and wrist because the C7, C8 and T1 roots are not reached.
3. Pain in the axilla or T1 area following shoulder arthroplasty treated with continuous interscalene block. The initial block is done on the C5 root or superior trunk and the initial bolus may reach the C8 and T1 roots or inferior trunk. The continuous infusion after the initial block had worn off, does not reach the C8 or T1 roots or inferior trunk and the patient has pain in the T1 and C8 dermatome area.
4. Continuous or single injection interscalene blocks performed for elbow, wrist, and hand surgery is another example of a block with a potential to fail. The interscalene block reaches the C5, C6 roots or upper and middle trunk, but not the inferior trunk or lower cervical roots and therefore the medial part of the lower arm is not blocked.
5. Continuous infraclavicular block on the posterior cord is done for elbow and wrist surgery. If a large initial bolus is used, it usually reaches all three of the cords and the initial block is good. On infusion of a lower

volume subsequent days, the patient suffers pain because the middle and lateral cords are not reached. This block is then deemed to have failed.

6. A number of reasons can cause the axillary block to fail. Typically, the musculocutaneous nerve is blocked and all the other nerves are missed. Alternatively, all the other nerves are blocked and the musculocutaneous is missed. This leads to incomplete block. It is essential when doing an axillary block to ensure that all seven of the nerves are blocked. Two of these nerves are sensory nerves and difficult to identify in the axilla, while the musculocutaneous is a motor nerve in the upper arm and a sensory nerve in the lower arm. These nerves are often overlooked, which can lead to a failed block.
7. Lumbar plexus block is often done for hip surgery ignoring the fact that the hip joint gets its innervation from the entire lumbosacral plexus and not only from the lumbar plexus.
8. Lumbar plexus blocks for knee and ankle surgery. The lumbar plexus block involves only the anterior upper part of the leg and the medial aspect of the lower leg and is not sufficient on its own for knee or ankle surgery.
9. Femoral block is often performed for knee surgery, especially for anterior knee surgery. In an estimated 20–80% of patients pain after total knee replacement, for example, is severe in the posterior aspect of the knee. This is because the posterior aspect of the knee is supplied by the sciatic nerve and to a lesser extent by the obturator nerve (joint capsule), which nerves are not blocked with a single injection femoral nerve block. A continuous femoral nerve block reaches the femoral, obturator and lateral cutaneous nerve of the thigh. The patient can still suffer posterior knee pain due to the unblocked sciatic nerve.
10. Continuous sciatic nerve block is often performed for ankle joint surgery. This is not good enough, since the saphenous nerve (a branch of the femoral nerve) supplies the medial aspect of the ankle joint (45).
11. The sciatic nerve block is often performed for bunion surgery ignoring the fact that the saphenous nerve also innervates the medial aspect of the foot in a large percentage of patients.
12. Ankle block often fails because not all five nerves around the ankle are blocked. Because of the huge variation in neurotomes of the foot, it is almost impossible to predict which nerve supplies which part of the foot in a specific patient. It is also almost impossible to predict how deep the surgery would be. For example, the superficial peroneal nerve supplies the front part of the lateral side of the foot, while the posterior tibial nerve supplies the sole of the foot. It is not clear at which depth the nerves take over the nerve supply and most often, there is significant overlap of nerve supply frequently leading to incomplete or failed blocks.

As can be seen from the above, it is essential to understand the neurotomal, osteotomal, and dermatomal supply of each nerve and to do appropriate blocks, and to understand Hilton's Law. If a nerve block is in any case not going to have any beneficial effect, and we only have the risks and no benefits, it should be better not to do a block at all. The commonly accepted notion that a partial block may be better than no block at all, and that the deficit in blocks may be treated effectively with multimodal analgesia has not been substantiated by research, and, in the opinion of this author, is devoid of any truth.

"Over-blocking"

As said earlier in this chapter, one of the most crucial requirements for effective regional anesthesia is to have the correct indications and valid reasons for nerve blocks. There are many examples of major nerve blocks done when pain is likely to be insignificant, or easily treated with mild systemic analgesic agents. Examples of such situations are interscalene or cervical paravertebral blocks for subacromial decompression, femoral nerve blocks for diagnostic knee arthroscopy, etc. Experience has taught us that in most instances of complications leading to medico-legal action, the patient usually did not need the block in the first place. There are well-known examples in the literature of, for example, major continuous infraclavicular blocks done for carpal tunnel release (46) and major lumbar plexus or psoas compartment blocks for surgery below the knee where a simple saphenous nerve block would have been sufficient (47). Patients will tolerate a large number of complications if the indications for the block were good in the first place and the block was done solely for the benefit of the patient. If a block, however, is done for any reason other than real benefit to the patient, complications often cause legal problems.

Duration of Nerve Blocks

As continuous infraclavicular blocks for carpal tunnel syndrome is inappropriate, so is single injection interscalene block, for example, probably inappropriate for rotator cuff or shoulder arthroplasty surgery. Although the patient wakes up from the anesthesia without any pain, he or she usually wakes up in the middle of the night after surgery with excruciating unmanageable pain. A continuous nerve block would clearly be a better choice for these very painful shoulder operations. Also, a single injection infraclavicular block for total elbow, or total wrist arthroplasty would be as inappropriate as would continuous infraclavicular block be for wrist ganglion excision, for example. The one block that would cover all three major joints of the upper limb at the low infusion rate of the days after surgery, would be a continuous cervical paravertebral block done at the correct root level. For example, C5 and C6 level with biceps muscle response would be ideal for shoulder surgery whereas a triceps response (C7/8) would be ideal for wrist and elbow surgery. It is therefore important to match the duration of the block with the expected duration and severity of the surgical pain.

The continuous lumbar paravertebral block or psoas compartment block has been advocated as a way of blocking the nerves to all the joints of the lower limb. Unfortunately, this is not the case. This block has only a few good indications; the main being if a proper continuous femoral block cannot be performed. It is almost impossible to justify the use of a single-injection lumbar plexus block, since this major block should be reserved for severe pain following major surgery, and it would almost always be a better choice to do a continuous nerve block in such circumstances. It would also almost always be necessary to do a continuous infusion of the sacral plexus as well, and an epidural block should most likely be more appropriate in these circumstances. It is noteworthy that Capdevila (48), wrote, ."..unlike the femoral nerve block, which involves very few risks, side effects related to psoas compartment block are quite severe."

High Yield Blocks

A high yield block is one that gives the highest success rate and the lowest complication rate. It is therefore important for all anesthesiologists to have a serious and hard look at their practices and honestly try to calculate their expected success and complication rates. This would eliminate blocks that are unnecessary. High yield blocks could be identified and should make out the bulk of practitioners routine practice. Only in exceptional circumstances, should "low yield" blocks be performed.

Generally speaking, there are only a limited number of single injection blocks and continuous nerve blocks that would represent a sufficient repertoire, in addition to lumbar and thoracic epidural blocks, spinal anesthesia and thoracic paravertebral blocks for thoracic or other major unilateral trunk surgery. The single injection blocks should, amongst others, include interscalene, cervical paravertebral block, infraclavicular or supraclavicular, femoral block, subgluteal block, popliteal block and ankle block. Only four continuous peripheral nerve blocks are absolutely essential for orthopedic surgery. These include continuous cervical paravertebral block, continuous femoral block, continuous subgluteal block, and continuous popliteal block. The other blocks described in the literature should be done under exceptional circumstances.

Long Acting Local Anesthetic Agents

The introduction of long acting local anesthetic agents has been anticipated for some time and seems attractive. But, one must bear in mind that the complications or side effects of these blocks would also be long acting. Examples are long lasting respiratory depression, hypoxia, and nausea, vomiting and itching due to extended release epidural morphine (49,50). Also, there is usually no problem when, after performing an interscalene block, the phrenic nerve is blocked for 6 to 8 hours. Blocking the phrenic nerve for 3-5 days would, however, be totally unacceptable.

In **conclusion,** there are four basic principles for successful regional anesthesia that will help to avoid pitfalls. These are the correct indications, the correct block for the surgery, the correct technique and the appropriate equipment. Furthermore, places where nerves are in confined spaces should be avoided if possible, and conditions causing existing brachial plexopathy should be recognized and approached with caution. Nerve blocks are contra-indicated in patients who may develop compartment syndrome, and nerve blocks should be matched to the surgery and severity and duration of the pain.

REFERENCES

1. Chelly JE: How can we possibly prevent complications related to peripheral nerve blocks? [letter]. Anesth Analg 2001;93:1080.
2. Boezaart AP, Franco CD: Thin sharp needles around the dura [letter]. Reg Anesth Pain Med 2006;31:388-389.
3. Voermans NC, Crul BJ, Zwarts MJ, et al: Permanent loss of spinal cord function associated with the posterior approach. Anesth Analg 2006;102;330.
4. Boezaart AP: Please don't blame the block … [letter]. Anesth Analg 2007;104:211-212.
5. Lundborg G: Ischemic nerve injury: Experimental studies on intraneural microvascular pathophysiology and nerve function in a limb subjected to temporary circulatory arrest. Scand J Plast Reconstr Surg Suppl 1970;6:3-113.
6. Lundborg G, Dahlin LB: Anatomy, function and pathophysiology of peripheral nerves and nerve compression. Hand Clin 1996;12:185-193.
7. Lundborg, G, Dahlin LB: The pathophysiology of nerve compression. Hand Clin 1992;8:215-227.
8. Winnie AP: Interscalene brachial plexus block. Anesth Analg 1970;49:455-466.
9. Winnie AP, Ramamurthy S, Durrani, et al: Interscalene cervical plexus block: A single-injection technique. Anesth Analg 1975;54:370-375.
10. Boezaart AP, de Beer JF, du Toit C, et al: A new technique of continuous interscalene block. Can J Anesth 1999; 46:275-281.
11. Borgeat A, Dullenkopf A, Ekatodramis G, et al: Evaluation of the lateral modified approach for continuous interscalene block for shoulder surgery. Anesthesiology 2003; 99:436-442.
12. Frohm RM, Raw RM, Haider N, Boezaart AP: Epidural spread after continuous cervical paravertebral block. Reg Anesth Pain Med 2006;31:279-281.
13. Franco CD, Gloss FJ, Voronov G, et al: Supraclavicular block in the obese population: An analysis of 2020 blocks. Anesth Analg 2006;102:1252-1254.
14. Boardman ND 3rd, Cofield RH: Neurologic complications of shoulder surgery. Clin Orthop Relat Res 1999;368: 44-53.
15. McFarland EG, O'Neill OR, Hsu C-Y: Complications of shoulder arthroscopy. J South Orthop Assoc 1997;6: 190-196.
16. Bigliani LU, Flatow EL, Deliz ED: Complications of shoulder arthroscopy. Orthop Rev 1991;20:743-751.
17. Weber SC, Abrams JS, Nottage WM: Complications associated with arthroscopic shoulder surgery. Arthroscopy 2002;18:88-95.
18. Selander D, Mansson LG, Karlsson L, Svanvik J: Adrenergic vasoconstriction in peripheral nerves of the rabbit. Anesthesiology 1985;62:6-10.
19. Selander D, Brattsand R, Lundborg G, et al: Local anesthetics: Importance of mode of application, concentration and adrenaline for the appearance of nerve lesions. An experimental study of axonal degeneration and barrier damage after intrafascicular injection or topical application of bupivacaine (Marcain). Acta Anaesthesiol Scand 1979;23:127-136.
20. Tsao BE, Wilbourn AJ: Infraclavicular brachial plexus injury following axillary regional block. Muscle Nerve 2004;30:44-48.
21. Boezaart AP, Berry RA, Nell ML, et al: A comparison of propofol and remifentanil for sedation and limitation of movement during peri-retrobulbar block. J Clin Anesth 2001;13:422-426.
22. Bunker TD, Anthony PP: The pathology of frozen shoulder: A Dupuytren-like disease. J Bone Joint Surg Br 1995;77:677-683.
23. Smith SP, Devaraj VS, Bunker TD: The association between frozen shoulder and Dupuytren's disease. J Shoulder Elbow Surg 2001;10:149-151.
24. Noël E, Thomas T, Schaeverbeke T, et al: Frozen shoulder. Joint Bone Spine 2000;67:393-400.
25. Müller LP, Müller LA, Happ J: Frozen shoulder: A sympathetic dystrophy? Arch Orthop Trauma Surg 2000;120: 84-87.
26. Lloyd JA, Lloyd HM: Adhesive capsulitis of the shoulder: Arthrographic diagnosis and treatment. South Med J 1983;76:879-883.
27. Hill JJ, Bogumill H: Manipulation in the treatment of frozen shoulder syndrome. Orthopedics 1987;11: 1255-1260.
28. Reeves B: The natural history of frozen shoulder syndrome. Scand J Rheumatol 1975;4:193-196.
29. Boyle-Walker KL, Gabard DL, Bietsch E, et al: A profile of patients with adhesive capsulitis. J Hand Ther 1997;10:222-228.
30. Simatas AC, Tsairis P: Adhesive capsulitis of the glenohumeral joint with an unusual neuropathic presentation. Am J Phys Med Rehabil 1999;78: 577-581.

31. Klein AH, France JC, Mutschler A, et al: Measurement of brachial plexus strain in arthroscopy of the shoulder. Arthroscopy 1987;3:45-52.
32. Boezaart AP, Koorn R, Rosenquist RW: Paravertebral approach to the brachial plexus: An anatomic improvement in technique. Reg Anesth Pain Med 2003;28: 241-244.
33. Lemaire A: La perception des douleurs viscerales. Rev Med Louvain 1926;6:81.
34. Weiss S, Davis O: Significance of afferent impulses from the skin in the mechanism of visceral pain. Am J Med Sci 1928;176:517.
35. Beekman R, Visser LH: Sonographic detection of diffuse peripheral nerve enlargement in hereditary neuropathy with liability to pressure palsies. J Clin Ultrasound 2002;30:433-436.
36. Pareyson D: Diagnosis of hereditary neuropathies in adult patients. J Neurol 2003;250:148-160.
37. De Visser M, Vermeulen M, Wokke HJH: Neuromusculaire Zieke [Neuromuscular Disease]. Maarssen, the Netherlands, Elsevier/Bunge, 1999, p 174.
38. Keller MP, Chance PF: Inherited neuropathies: From gene to disease. Brain Pathol 1999;9:327-341.
39. Wilbourn AJ: Thoracic outlet syndrome surgery causing severe brachial plexopathy. Muscle Nerve 1988;11: 66-84.
40. Roos DB: Historical perspectives and anatomical considerations: Thoracic outlet syndrome. Semin Thorac Cardiovasc Surg 1996;8:183-189.
41. Liu JE, Tahmoush AJ, Roos DB, Schwartzman RJ: Shoulder-arm pain from cervical bands and scalene muscle anomalies. J Neurol Sci 1995;128:175-180.
42. Roos DB: Thoracic outlet syndrome is under-diagnosed. Muscle Nerve 1999;22:126-129.
43. Wilbourn AJ: Thoracic outlet syndrome is over-diagnosed. Muscle Nerve 1999;22:130-136.
44. McKinley T, Boezaart AP: Common fractures, compartment syndrome and crush injuries. In: Boezaart AP (ed): Anesthesia and Orthopedic Surgery. New York, McGraw-Hill, 2006, pp 209-213.
45. Sarrafian SK: Anatomy of the Foot and Ankle: Descriptive, Topographical and Functional, 2nd ed. Philadelphia, JB Lippincott, 1993, p 396.
46. Rawal N, Allvin R, Axelsson K, et al: Patient-controlled regional analgesia (PCRA) at home. Anesthesiology 2002;96:1290-1296.
47. Buckenmaer C, McKnight G, Winkley J, et al: Continuous peripheral nerve block for battlefield anesthesia and evacuation. Reg Anesth Pain Med 2005;30:202-205.
48. Capdevila X, Coimbra C, Choquet O: Approaches to the lumbar plexus: Success, risks, and outcome. Reg Anesth Pain Med 2006;30:150-162.
49. Hartrick GT, Martin G, Kantor, et al: Evaluation of a single-dose, extended-release epidural morphine formulation for pain after knee arthroplasty. J Bone Joint Surg Am 2006;88:273-281.
50. Viscusi E, Martin G, Hartrick C, et al: Forty-eight hours of postoperative pain relief after total hip arthroplasty with a Novel, extended-release epidural morphine formulation. Anesthesiology 2005;102:1014-1022.

Index

Note: Page numbers followed by f indicate figures.

A

Accessory nerve, 13, 14f, 15f
Achilles tendon, 197f
Adhesive capsulitis, 23, 227-228
Adrenaline
  in ankle block, 209
  safety and utility of, 226
Anesthesia
  general, for thoracic paravertebral block, 219
  local. *See* Local anesthetics.
Ankle, anatomy of, 195-199, 197f-200f
Ankle block, 203-210
  anatomic considerations in, 205
  anesthesia for, 209-210
  failure of, 205, 232
  indications for, 205
  technique for, 205-209, 206f-209f
Anterior lumbar plexus blocks
  femoral nerve
    continuous, 143-152
    single-injection, 141-143, 141f-143f
  lateral cutaneous nerve of thigh, 157-159, 158f, 159f
  obturator nerve, 153-157
Anterior tibialis tendon, 197f
Arm slings, 30
Arthroscopy, knee, 223
Axilla, innervation of, 87-95, 90f-98f
Axillary artery
  anatomy of, 97f
  in axillary block, 101, 101f
Axillary block, 99-105
  continuous, 102-105
    anesthesia for, 105
    catheter removal in, 105
    indications for, 102-103
    technique of, 103-105, 103f
  failure of, 231-232
  single-injection, 101-102
    anatomic considerations in, 101
    anesthesia for, 101-102
    indications for, 101
    technique of, 101, 101f, 102f
    ultrasound-assisted, 101, 102f
Axillary nerve, anatomy of, 3f, 95, 97f

B

Bleeding
  compartment syndrome and, 230
  psoas compartment hematoma and, 163
Botulinum toxin, for thoracic outlet syndrome, 230
Brachial plexopathy, 226-227, 229
  decompressive surgery for, 223, 228-229
  differential diagnosis of, 23, 227
  gender differences in, 227
  pathogenesis of, 227
  signs and symptoms of, 23, 226-227
Brachial plexus
  dermatomes of, 43f
  distal. *See also* Brachial plexus cords.
    anatomy of, 3f, 65-66, 67f-73f
  divisions of, 3f
  neurotomes of, 15, 16f, 41, 42f
  osteotomes of, 44f
  proximal, anatomy of, 3-17, 3f, 6f, 59f
  terminal branches of, 3f
Brachial plexus cords, 65-73
  lateral, 3f, 65, 66, 67f, 68f, 72f, 73f
  medial, 3f, 66, 69f-71f
  posterior, 3f, 66, 72f, 73f
Brachial plexus root block. *See* Cervical paravertebral block.
Brachial plexus roots, 13-14
Brachial plexus trunks, 13-14
  inferior, 3f, 13-14
  middle, 3f, 13-14
  superior, 3f, 8, 13-14
Bupivacaine
  for ankle block, 209-210
  for femoral nerve block, 143
  for interscalene block
    continuous, 36-37, 37f
    single-injection, 28-29
  for lateral cutaneous nerve of thigh block, 158
  for supraclavicular block, 60
  for thoracic paravertebral block, 219
Buprenorphine
  for axillary block, 102
  for femoral nerve block
    continuous, 152
    single-injection, 143
  for infraclavicular block, 81
  for interscalene blocks, 28-29
  for popliteal sciatic nerve block, 191

C

Calcaneal nerve, 198f
Carpal tunnel, median nerve injury and, 225
Casts, compartment syndrome and, 230-231
Catheter, tip-protrusion marking on, 34, 34f, 50f
Catheter leakage, from skin bridge, 84

Catheter tunneling
with skin bridge, 148, 149f-151f
catheter leakage and, 84
without skin bridge, 148, 151-154f
Cervical paravertebral block
anatomic considerations in, 15-19, 17f-20f
anesthesia for, 52
catheter removal in, 52
dermatomes for, 43f
duration of, 233
failure of, 231
indications for, 41, 228, 231, 233
neurotomes for, 15, 16f, 41, 42f
osteotomes for, 44f
superficial cervical plexus sparing in, 15
surface anatomy for, 17-19, 18f-20f
technique for, 15, 17, 20f, 41-52, 45f-51f
trapezius–levator scapulae window in, 15-17, 17f
ultrasound-assisted, 50, 51f
Cervicosympathetic chain, Horner's syndrome and, 17
Common peroneal nerve, 164f
anatomy of, 173, 174f, 176-181, 179f, 180f
traction injuries of, 226
Common peroneal nerve block, indications for, 226
Compartment syndrome, 230-231
Coracoid process, 65, 65f, 66f

D

Deep peroneal nerve, 197, 197f, 198f, 200f
Deltoid muscle, 65, 66f
Dexamethasone
for axillary block, 102
for femoral nerve block, 143
for infraclavicular block, 81
Diabetes mellitus, ankle block in, 205
Distal brachial plexus, anatomy of, 65-66, 67f-73f. *See also* Brachial plexus cords.
Dorsal pedis artery, 200f
Dorsal scapular nerve, 3f, 8, 12f
Dorsal venous arch, 200f
Double crush injury, 228

E

Elbow
blocks around, 119-124
indications for, 121
median nerve, 122-123, 122f
musculocutaneous, 121-122, 121f
radial nerve, 122, 122f
rescue, 119
ulnar nerve, 123-124, 123f
innervation of, 107-117
Epinephrine
in ankle block, 209
safety and utility of, 226
Extensor hallucis longus tendon, 197f
External jugular vein, 6f

F

Femoral artery, 128f
Femoral branch of genitofemoral nerve, 164f
Femoral nerve
anatomy of, 127-133, 128f, 129f, 132f, 156f, 164f
quadriceps vs. sartorius contraction and, 133
Femoral nerve block
continuous, 143-152
anatomic considerations in, 143-144
anesthesia for, 143, 144f, 151-152
catheter placement in, 144, 145f
catheter removal in, 150-151, 154f, 155f
catheter tunneling in, 148, 149f-154f
failure of, 232
indications for, 143, 232
Raj test in, 149-150
technique for, 145-148, 145f-148f
with popliteal sciatic nerve block, 191
single-injection, 141-143, 141f-143f
anatomic considerations in, 141
anesthesia for, 143
indications for, 141
technique for, 141-143, 141f-143f
ultrasound-assisted, 141, 142f
with sciatic nerve block, 141
Fractures, compartment syndrome and, 230-231
Frozen shoulder, 23, 227-228

G

General anesthesia, for thoracic paravertebral block, 219
Genitofemoral nerve
femoral branch of, 164f
genital branch of, 164f
Great saphenous vein, 200f

H

Hematoma, in psoas compartment, 163
Hemorrhage. *See* Bleeding.
Hereditary neuropathy with liability to pressure palsies, 229
High-yield blocks, 233
Hilton's law, 155, 223-224
Horner's syndrome, 17
Hypertrophic spondylosis, 229

I

Iliohypogastric nerve, 164f
Ilioinguinal nerve, 164f
Inferior brachial plexus trunk, 3f, 13-14
Infraclavicular block
continuous, 81-85
anesthesia for, 84
catheter removal in, 85
duration of, 233
failure of, 231
indications for, 81-82, 231, 233
technique of, 82-84, 82f-84f
single-injection, 77-81
anesthesia for, 81
duration of, 233
indications for, 77, 233
neurotomes for, 77
technique of, 77-81, 77f-81f
ultrasound-assisted, 78, 79f

Interscalene block, 22-37
continuous, 30-37
anesthesia for, 36-37
catheter removal in, 37
dermatomes for, 30
failure of, 231
indications for, 30, 228, 231
neurotomes for, 30
osteotomes for, 30
technique for, 30-36, 31f-37f, 225
single-injection, 23-29
anesthesia for, 28-29
dermatomes for, 23, 25f
failure of, 231
indications for, 23, 231
intraforaminal needle placement in, 225
neurotomes for, 23, 26f
osteotomes for, 23, 24f
Raj test in, 28
technique for, 23-28, 27f-29f, 225
ultrasound-assisted, 28, 29f
Intervertebral disk disease, 229
Intervertebral neuroforamen, catheter placement in, 224-225
Ischemia, in compartment syndrome, 230-231

K

Knee arthroscopy, 223

L

Labat's approach, 176
Lateral brachial plexus cord, 3f, 65, 67f, 68f
Lateral calcaneal nerve, 198f
Lateral cutaneous nerve of thigh, anatomy of, 127, 128f, 131f, 132f, 156f
Lateral cutaneous nerve of thigh block, 157-159, 158f, 159f
anatomic considerations in, 158
anesthesia for, 158-159
indications for, 157-158
technique for, 158, 158f, 159f
Lateral femoral cutaneous nerve, 164f
Lateral pectoral nerve, 3f
Lateral plantar nerve, 198f
Levator scapulae muscle
anatomy of, 17, 19f, 20f
nerve to, 8-13, 13f
Levator scapulae-trapezius window, in cervical paravertebral block, 15, 17f
Levobupivacaine
for interscalene block, 36-37, 37f
for lateral cutaneous nerve of thigh block, 158
for supraclavicular block, 60
Ligamentous laxity, in thoracic outlet syndrome, 230
Local anesthetics
epinephrine with, 209, 226
for ankle block, 209-210
for axillary block
continuous, 105
single-injection, 101-102
for cervical paravertebral block, 52
Local anesthetics—cont'd
for femoral nerve block
continuous, 143, 144f, 151-152
single-injection, 143
for infraclavicular block
continuous, 84
single-injection, 81
for interscalene block
continuous, 36-37
single-injection, 28-29
for lateral cutaneous nerve of thigh block, 158-159
for obturator nerve block, 156-157
for popliteal sciatic nerve block
continuous, 194
single-injection, 191
for psoas compartment block, 169-170
for subgluteal sciatic nerve block
continuous, 188-189
single-injection, 185
for supraclavicular block, 60
for thoracic paravertebral block, 219
long-acting, 233
Long thoracic nerve, 3f
Longus colli muscle, nerve to, 3f
Lower limb
compartment syndrome in, 230-231
dermatomes of, 135f
neurotomes of, 136f
osteotomes of, 134f
Lower subscapular nerve, 3f
Luer lock, in continuous interscalene block, 36, 37f
Lumbar paravertebral block. *See* Psoas compartment block.
Lumbar plexus
anterior, anatomy of, 125-133
posterior, anatomy of, 163, 164f
Lumbar plexus blocks
anterior, 139-159. *See also* Anterior lumbar plexus blocks.
failure of, 232
posterior, 163-170. *See also* Psoas compartment block.

M

Major pectoral muscle, 65, 66f
Medial brachial plexus cord, 3f, 66, 69f-71f
Medial calcaneal nerve, 198f
Medial cutaneous nerve, 3f
Medial pectoral nerve, 3f
Medial plantar nerve, 198f
Median nerve, 3f
anatomy of
at elbow, 109-112, 110f, 113f-115f
in axilla, 89-91, 92f, 93f
in distal brachial plexus, 65, 66, 67f
in upper arm, 115, 117f
ischemic injury of, 225
sensory neurotomes of, 89, 92f
Median nerve block
at elbow, 122-123, 122f
at wrist, 225
Median nerve entrapment, 229

Meniscectomy, 223
Mepivacaine, for supraclavicular block, 60
Meralgia paresthetica, 158-159
Midazolam, for thoracic paravertebral block, 219
Middle brachial plexus trunk, 3f, 13-14
Minor pectoral muscle, 65, 65f
Musculocutaneous nerve, 3f, 101
  anatomy of, 65, 67f, 95, 97f
  in axilla, 93, 96f, 97f
  sensory neurotomes of, 96f
Musculocutaneous nerve block, at elbow, 121-122, 121f

N
Needles, selection of, 224
Nerve blocks. *See* Regional anesthesia *and specific nerves.*
Nerve injury
  double crush, 228
  in compartment syndrome, 230-231
Nerve stimulators. *See specific blocks.*
Nerve to levator scapulae, 3f, 8-13, 13f
Nerve to longus colli, 3f
Nerve to sartorius
  anatomy of, 127-133, 164f
  sartorius vs. quadriceps contraction and, 133
Nerve to scalene, 3f
Nerve to subclavius, 3f
Neuropathy, pre-existing, 226-230

O
Obturator nerve, anatomy of, 127, 128f, 130f, 132f, 154-155, 156f, 164f
Obturator nerve block, 153-157
  anatomic considerations in, 154-155
  indications for, 143, 153-154
  technique for, 155-156, 156f, 157f
"Opening up the space"
  in axillary block, 103
  in femoral nerve block, 147
  in infraclavicular block, 83
  in interscalene block, 32
  in popliteal sciatic nerve block, 193
  in psoas compartment block, 167-168
  in subgluteal sciatic nerve block, 188

P
Pain management. *See* Local anesthetics.
Paravertebral blocks. *See* Cervical paravertebral block; Psoas compartment block; Thoracic paravertebral block.
Pectoral muscles, 65, 66f
Pectoral nerves, 3f
Peroneal artery, 200f
Peroneal nerve
  common, 164f
    anatomy of, 173, 174f, 176-181, 179f, 180f
    block of, 226
    traction injuries of, 226
  deep, 197, 197f, 198f, 200f
  superficial, 197, 197f, 198f, 200f
Phrenic nerve, 3, 3f, 6f, 7f, 17, 18f
Piriformis muscle, 173, 174f
Plantar nerve, 198f
Pleural injury, in supraclavicular block, 57, 225
Pneumothorax
  supraclavicular block and, 57, 225
  thoracic paravertebral block and, 213
Popliteal sciatic nerve block
  continuous, 191-194
    anatomic considerations in, 192
    anesthesia for, 194
    indications for, 191-192, 225-226
    technique for, 192-194, 192f, 193f
  single-injection, 189-191, 190f, 191f
    anatomic considerations in, 190
    anesthesia for, 191
    indications for, 189-190, 225-226
    technique of, 190, 190f, 191f
Posterior brachial plexus approach. *See* Cervical paravertebral block.
Posterior brachial plexus cord, 3f, 66, 72f, 73f
Posterior femoral cutaneous nerve, 164f
Posterior lumbar plexus block. *See* Psoas compartment block.
Posterior tibial artery, 200f
Posterior tibial nerve, 197-199, 197f, 199f, 200f
Proximal brachial plexus
  surface anatomy of, 3-13, 3f-15f
  transectional anatomy of, 15-17, 17f, 18f
Psoas compartment block, 163-170
  anatomic considerations for, 163, 164f
  anesthesia for, 169-170
  indications for, 163-170, 233
  technique for, 165-169, 165f-169f
Pudendal nerve, 164f
Pulses, in compartment syndrome, 230-231

Q
Quadriceps contraction, vs. sartorius contraction, 133

R
Radial nerve
  anatomy of, 3f
    at elbow, 109, 110f-112f
    in axilla, 89, 90f, 91f
  in axillary block, 101
  sensory neurotomes of, 89-91, 90f
Radial nerve block, at elbow, 122, 122f
Raj test
  in axillary block, 101
  in femoral nerve block
    continuous, 149-150
    single-injection, 143
  in interscalene block, 28
  in subgluteal sciatic nerve block, 188
Regional anesthesia. *See also specific nerves.*
  alternatives to, 232-233
  anesthesia for
    general, 219
    local. *See* Local anesthetics.
  block selection for, 223-224, 233
  brachial plexopathy and, 226-227

Regional anesthesia. *See also specific nerves.*—cont'd
compartment syndrome and, 230-231
complications of, 223-234
contraindications, 232-233
duration of, 233
equipment in, 224
existing neuropathy and, 226-230
failed/incomplete blocks in, 231-232
for subacromial decompression, 228-229
frozen shoulder and, 227-228
hereditary neuropathy with liability to pressure palsies and, 229
high-yield blocks in, 233
indications for, 223
overblocking in, 232-233
pitfalls in, 223-234
sites to avoid in, 224-226
technique selection for, 224
thoracic outlet syndrome and, 229-230
vs. systemic analgesics, 232
Remifentanil
for subacromial decompression, 229
for thoracic paravertebral block, 219
Reperfusion, compartment syndrome and, 230
Rescue blocks, at elbow, 119
Ropivacaine
for axillary block
continuous, 105
single-injection, 101-102
for cervical paravertebral block, 52
for femoral nerve block
continuous, 152
single-injection, 143
for infraclavicular block
continuous, 84
single-injection, 81
for interscalene block
continuous, 36-37, 37f
single-injection, 28-29
for lateral cutaneous nerve of thigh block, 158
for popliteal sciatic nerve block
continuous, 194
single-injection, 191
for psoas compartment block, 169-170
for subgluteal sciatic nerve block
continuous, 188-189
single-injection, 185
for supraclavicular block, 60
for thoracic paravertebral block, 219

S

Sacral plexus, anatomy of, 171-181, 173f-180f
Sacral plexus block. *See also* Sciatic nerve block.
indications for, 223
Saphenous nerve, 127, 129f, 132f, 164f, 197, 197f, 198f, 200f
Sartorius muscle
contractions of, vs. quadriceps contraction, 133
nerve to, 127-133, 127f, 133f
Scalene muscle(s)
in thoracic outlet syndrome, 229-230
nerve to, 3f
Scapular nerves, 3f, 8, 12f
Sciatic nerve, 164f
popliteal, anatomy of, 176-181, 177f-180f
subgluteal, anatomy of, 173-176, 174f-176f
Sciatic nerve block, 183-194
failure of, 232
popliteal
continuous, 186-188, 191-194
indications for, 143, 225-226
single-injection, 189-191, 190f, 191f
subgluteal
continuous, 186-188
indications for, 143, 225-226
single-injection, 185-186, 185f, 186f
surface landmarks for, 176, 176f
transgluteal, 225-226
with femoral nerve block, 141
Shoulder
frozen, 23, 227-228
innervation of, 3-17, 3f-7f, 9f-18f
Skin bridge, 148, 149f-151f
catheter leakage from, 84
Slings, 30
Small saphenous vein, 200f
Spinal accessory nerve, 3f
Spinal cord injury, 224
Spondylosis, hypertrophic, 229
Sternocleidomastoid muscle, 6f
Subacromial impingement, 226-227. *See also* Brachial plexopathy.
decompression for, 223, 228-229
indications for, 23, 228
diagnosis of, 228
Subacromial injection test, 228
Subclavian artery, 65, 65f
Subclavian vein, 65, 65f
Subclavius muscle, nerve to, 3f
Subcostal nerve, 164f
Subgluteal sciatic nerve block, 225
continuous, 186-188
anatomic considerations in, 186-187
indications for, 186
technique of, 187-188, 188f, 189f
indications for, 225-226
single-injection, 185-186, 185f, 186f
Subscapular nerves, 3f
Sulcus ulnaris block, 225
Superficial cervical plexus block, 15
Superficial peroneal nerve, 197, 197f, 198f, 200f
Superior brachial plexus trunk, 3f, 8, 13-14
Supraclavicular block, 57-60
anatomic considerations in, 57, 58f, 59f
anesthesia for, 60
indications for, 57, 225
pneumothorax and, 57, 225
technique for, 57-60, 59f, 60f
ultrasound-assisted, 60, 61f

Suprascapular nerve, 3f, 8, 11f
Sural nerve, 197, 197f, 198f, 200f
Systemic analgesics, vs. regional anesthesia, 232

T

Tendons, of ankle, 197f
Thoracic outlet syndrome, 229-230
Thoracic paravertebral block, 211-219
  anatomic considerations in, 215, 216f
  anesthesia for, 219
  complications of, 213
  indications for, 213
  multiple-level injections in, 214-215
  pneumothorax and, 213
  technique of, 215-219, 217f, 218f
  test dosing in, 219
Thoracic paravertebral space, anatomy of, 215, 216f
Tibial nerve, 164f
  anatomy of, 173, 174f, 176, 177f, 178f
  posterior, anatomy of, 197-199, 197f, 199f
Tip-protrusion mark, 34, 34f, 50f
Tourniquet sites, nerve block placement and, 190
Transgluteal sciatic nerve block, 225-226
Trapezius muscle, 17, 19f, 20f
Trapezius–levator scapulae window, in cervical paravertebral block, 15, 17f
Tunneled catheter. *See* Catheter tunneling.
Tuohy needle, 224

U

Ulnar nerve, 3f
  anatomy of
    at elbow, 110f, 112, 116f, 117f
    in axilla, 91, 94f, 95f
    in distal brachial plexus, 66, 70f
  sensory neurotomes of, 94f
Ulnar nerve block, at elbow, 123-124, 123f
Ulnar nerve entrapment, 229
Ultrasonography
  in axillary block, 101, 102f
  in cervical paravertebral block, 50, 51f
  in femoral nerve block, 141, 142f
  in infraclavicular block, 78, 79f
  in interscalene block, 28, 29f
  in obturator block, 157
  in supraclavicular block, 60, 61f
Upper limb
  compartment syndrome in, 230-231
  dermatomes of, 4f
  neurotomes of, 9f
  osteomes of, 5f
Upper subscapular nerve, 3f

V

Vertebral artery, 15-17, 17f
Vertebral vein, 15-17, 17f

W

Winnie's point, 8, 23, 29f
Women
  brachial plexopathy in, 227
  frozen shoulder in, 228-229
  thoracic outlet syndrome in, 230
Wrist, median nerve block in, 225